ENCYCLOPAEDIA
OF
INDIAN MEDICINE

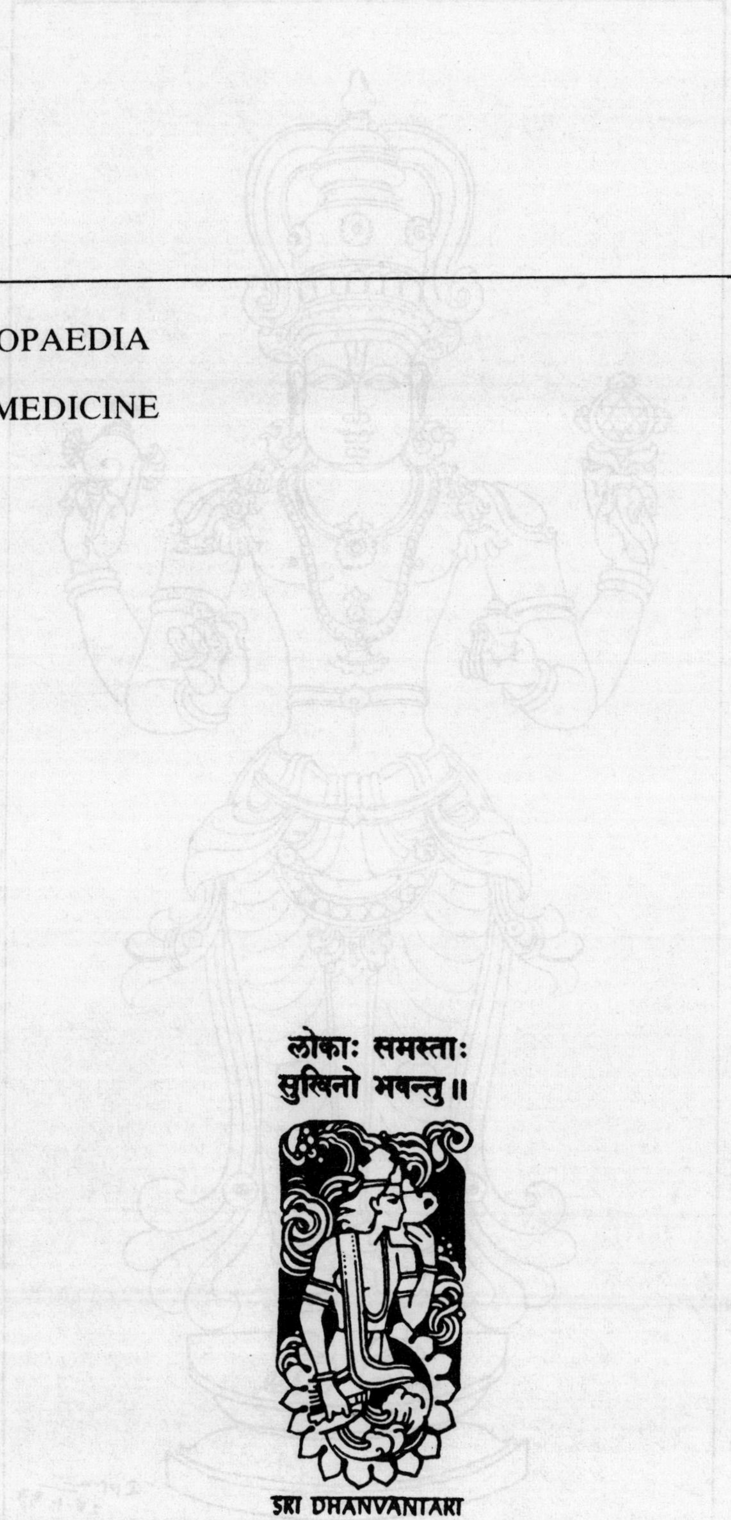

लोकाः समस्ताः
सुखिनो भवन्तु ॥

SRI DHANVANTARI

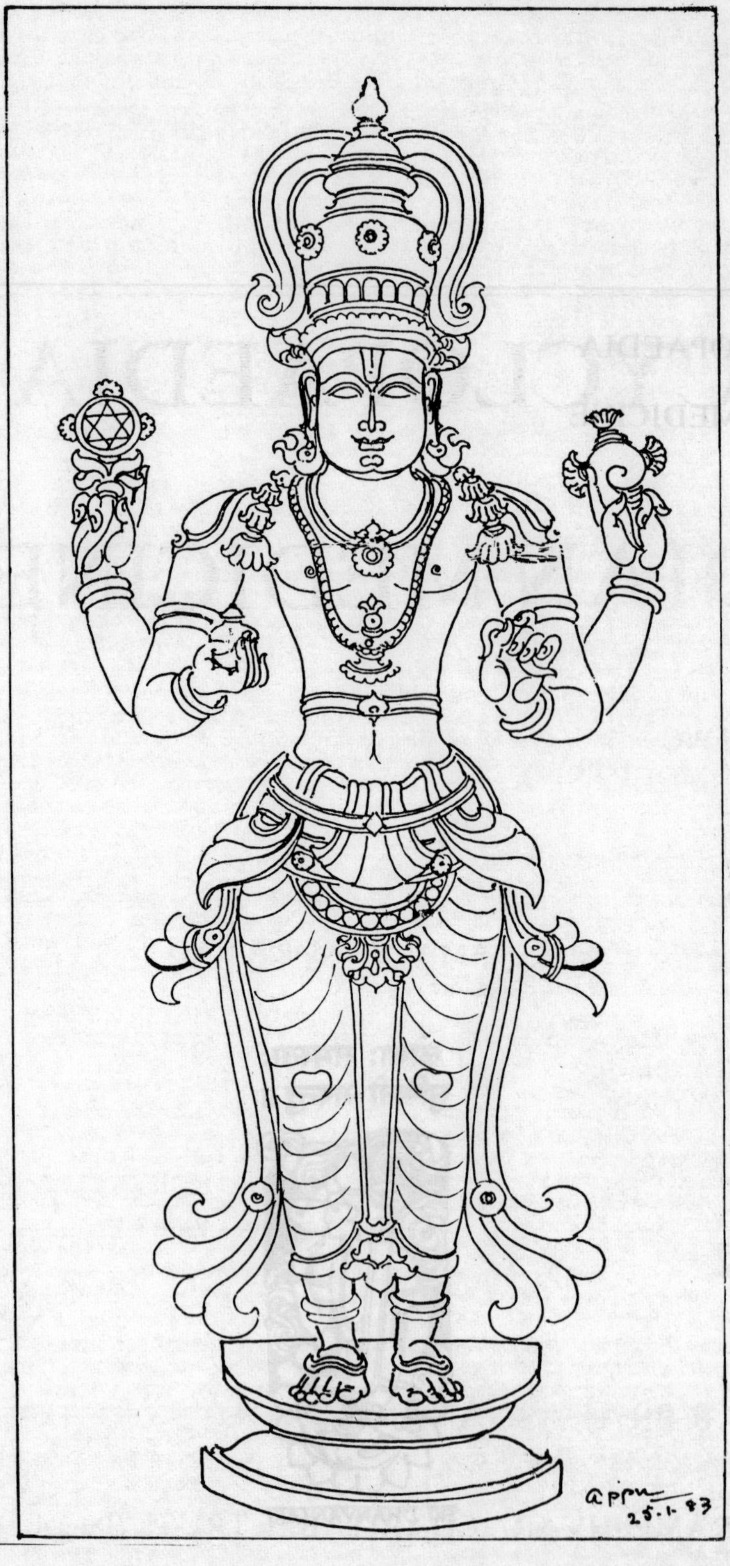
appu
25.1.83

ENCYCLOPAEDIA OF INDIAN MEDICINE

VOLUME TWO
BASIC CONCEPTS

Editor
Vidyalankara PROF. S. K. RAMACHANDRA RAO
President, Ayurveda Academy, Bangalore

WITH ASSISTANCE OF
Dr. S.R. SUDARSHAN

POPULAR PRAKASHAN BOMBAY

On behalf of
Dr. V. PARAMESHVARA CHARITABLE TRUST, Bangalore

ENCYCLOPAEDIA
OF
INDIAN MEDICINE PROJECT

VOLUME TWO

Sponsored by
Dr. V. P. Parameshvara Charitable Trust
Bangalore

Chairman
Dr. V. Parameshvara
M.B.B.S.,F.R.C.P. (London), F.A.C.C.,F.C.C.P.,F.I.C.A.,
F.I.S.E.,F.A.I.I.D.,M.S.A.,F.I.A.M.S.,F.I.C.N.

Editor
Vidyalankara Prof. S. K. Ramachandra Rao
President, Ayurveda Academy, Bangalore

First published 1985
First Reprint 1998
Second Reprint 2005

ISBN : 81-7154-256-5

(3303)

Printed in India by :
Taj Press
Noida (U.P.)

Published by RAMDAS BHATKAL for
Popular Prakashan Pvt. Ltd.
35-C Pandit Madan Mohan Malaviya Marg,
Tardeo, Mumbai-400 034

PREFACE

Indian religions are well known in the world. The philosophical systems that emerged on the Indian soil have also engaged the attention of scholars all over the world. India's achievements in the field of science and technology have also been recognised. However, the fact that India developed a system of medicine, thousands of years ago, has not received wide coverage in the world. And that the system thus developed is still prevalent among the masses of India is likewise not generally known, even to historians of medicine.

There are manifold reasons for this general ignorance of Indian medicine among historians of medicine, medical practitioners outside the country and intelligentsia interested in the problems of health and disease. One is, absence of authoritative and well documented publications in English by Indians, dealing with this branch of medicine. The European indologists who have taken an interest in Indian medicine and have written on the subject do not seem to carry much credibility, because they are alien to the traditional details which are indispensable to the understanding of the spirit, outlook and value of Indian medicine. The literature available on this topic written in the traditional style of Indian languages have proved to be enigmatic to the modern reader. A great need is, therefore, felt for an authentic publication which communicates to the modern mind the traditional wisdom of India concerning medical practice.

The Encyclopaedia of Indian Medicine in six volumes has been planned to fulfil this need. The first volume provides the historical perspective as well as acquaintance with the medical literature in India. The volume has been prepared by Vidyalankara Prof. S.K. Ramachandra Rao, who hails from a family of traditional physicians and is the President of the Ayurveda Academy, Bangalore. Besides being a Sanskrit scholar and well versed in Ayurveda, he has also been a scientific worker, having headed the department of Clinical Psychology at the National Institute of Mental Health and Neurosciences, Bangalore (with which he is still associated as consultant to the Ayurvedic Research Unit).

The second volume deals with the concepts that characterize the Indian system of medicine. The aspects of health, hygiene, health care, medicare, treatment and prevention are covered in this volume.

The volume will be followed in due course by other volumes dealing with basic ideas, methods of clinical investigation, therapeutic procedures, pharmaceutical practices and materia medica of Indian medicine. It is hoped that a comprehensive and factual knowledge of Indian medicine will be available to the world when the series is completed.

Bangalore
June 23, 1987

V. PARAMESHVARA
Chairman

INTRODUCTION

Indigenous medical wisdom in India known as Ayurveda goes back to a hoary past. Even in the early strands of the Vedic corpus belonging to a period several centuries prior to the Christian era, we find references not only to medical practice but to elaborate medical theories. Medical wisdom in India was systematized at a slightly later period, and a remarkably rich medical literature has grown up since those days. Medical practice based on this systematization has continued to our own day, despite the growing popularity of Western medical practice.

Indian medical wisdom has unfortunately been confined to India; and the West is largely ignorant of it. Even in India, the traditional medical practice seems to be losing contact with the system as it was crystallized over two thousand years ago. This is so because much of the early and core medical literature, which is in Sanskrit, is still in manuscripts, hidden away in libraries and private collections; only a few major texts like Charaka's *saṁhita,* Suśruta's *Saṁhita* and Vāgbhaṭa's *Sangraha* and *Hṛdaya* have been printed and translated into English. The influence of the philosophical systems, especially of Sāṁkhya and Nyāya-Vaiśeshika, on medical thought in India has not been sufficiently appreciated. The generation of practising physicians who are also scholarly has almost disappeared. Thus the authentic tradition of Indian medical thought has not yet been presented to the modern mind. The medical world at large is almost entirely ignorant of the relevance or the value of Ayurveda.

The present series of volumes constituting *The Encyclopaedia of Indian Medicine* is an attempt to present in a manner that would appeal to the modern mind the theoretical and practical issues as was formulated in Ayurveda several centuries ago. In so doing, we have relied entirely on original texts, which constitute the nucleus of Ayurveda, and on the commentarial literature thereupon, and have attempted to reconstruct the authentic perspective of Ayurveda The following volumes have been planned and are under preparation:

Volume I Historical Prespective
Volume II Conceptual Framework
Volume III Clinical Examination and Diagnostic Methods
Volume IV Diseases: Drugs and their Preparations
Volume V Materia Medica (in two parts)
Volume VI Folk Medicine

These volumes of the *Encyclopaedia of Indian Medicine* have been planned to appear in two phases, each complete in itself; the first phase comprising of three volumes viz. Volume I: Historical Perspective; Volume II: Conceptual Framework; Volume III: Clinical Examination and Diagnostic Methods and the second phase comprising of volumes dealing with diseases, drugs and their preparations, materia and medica and folk medicine. The first phase is now completed and three volumes that are now being issued represent a comprehensive and self-contained account of the general and fundamental aspects of Ayurveda covering all the theoretical involvements of Ayurvedic practice. Work on the second phase is in progress.

Ayurveda being a system first and practical discipline next, there is here an elaborate conceptual framework, involving numerous well-connected ideas concerning health and disease. Unlike other systems of medicine (barring the Chinese), Ayurveda leans heavily on philosophical and metaphysical orientations of the Darsanas, principally Samkhya, Nyaya and Vaiseshika and considerably on Yoga. The well-being of the individual is treated not only as a medical issue, but as a total affair involving the body, the mind and the spirit. Further, the idea of medical care emphasises equally the preventive and curative aspects. There is thus in Ayurveda an extensive and eminently practical literature concerning health and hygiene. This volume deals with all significant and basic concepts regarding health, hygiene, therapy, treatment methods and medical care. Philosophical formulations as can be gleaned from the definitive texts are also included here.

It has been kept in mind by those who are involved in this Project that the purpose of any encyclopaedia is not only to provide information but to relate it. The entries are designed to introduce the reader to the basic principles guiding Indian medicine in the context of the country's geography, history and culture. Care has been taken to present the details objectively, and in accordance with the traditional framework. We have refrained from taking sides in the controversy regarding the relative merits of the different systems of medicine.

While the present Encyclopaedia is ultimately based on the original texts, commentaries and annotations in Sanskrit, a large number of works on Ayurveda written and published in English and in some of the Indian languages (Hindi, Kannada, Telugu and Tamil) have been consulted, as also many elderly specialists in this system of medicine. We are indebted to all these authors and scholars. But the formulations of the concepts and their applications have uniformly been made in accordance with the original textual tradition disregarding later versions, evaluations and amendments.

The enlightened interest of the eminent cardiologist of Bangalore, Dr. V. Parameshvara has originated this project, and has been sustaining it. Being himself a physician trained in the best traditions of modern medicine, he is interested in the world getting acquainted with the contributions of traditional medicine in India so that there could be greater benefit to mankind.

I am grateful to my son Dr. S.R. Sudarshan, who has helped me in the preparation of this volume, and to my student Prof. M. Sridhara Murthy for preparing the typescript for the press.

Bangalore S.K. RAMACHANDRA RAO
Editor

CONTENTS

ABBREVIATIONS & MAJOR REFERENCES

AD	Aruṇadatta (Sarvānga-sundara)
AHR	Ashtāṅga-hrdaya (Vāgbhata)
AR	Āyurveda-rasāyana (Hemādri)
AS	Ashtānga-samgraha (Vāgbhata)
ASM	The Ayurvedic System of Medicine (Nagendranath Sen Gupta)
BP	Bhāva-prakāśa (Bhāva-miśra)
BPN	Bhāva-prakāśa-nighantu
BR	Bhaishajya-ratnāvalī
BS	Bhela-samhitā (Bhela)
BYT	Brhadyoga-tarangiṇī
CHKP	Chakrapāni-datta on CS
CS	Charaka-sámhitā
DMA	Digestion and Metabolism in Ayurveda (Dwarakanath)
DN	Dhanvantari-nighaṇṭu
DGV	Dravya-guna-vijñāna (P.V. Ṣarma) in 4 parts
FAM	Fundamentals of Ayurveda Medicine (Bhagawan Dash)
GN	Gada-nigraha
GNS	Gaṇa-nath Sen
HIM	History of Indian Medicine (Girindranath Mukhopadhyaya) in 3 vol.
IA	Introduction to Ayurveda (Chandrashekhar G. Thakur)
KS	Kāśyapa-samhitā
MN	Mādhava-nidāna (Mādhava-Ḳara)
MPN	Madana-pāla-nighantu
MV	Madana-vinoda
NIS	Nibandha-samgraha (Ḍalhana on SS)
PRM	Paryāya-ratna-mālā
PS	Pratyaksha-śārīram (Gananath Sen)
RJN	Rasa-jala-nidhi (Bhudev Mukhopadhyaya)
RN	Rāja-nighantu
RRS	Rasa-ratna-samucchaya (Nityanātha)
RN	Rāja-vallabha Nighantu (Nārāyana-dāsa-kavirāja)
RV	Rgveda
RVS	Rasa-vaiśeshika-ṣūtra (Nāgārjuna)
SAS	Śārngadhara-samhitā
SDN	Sodhala-nighantu
SDS	Śiva-dāsa-sena
SK	Sāmkhya-kārikā (Īśvara-Krishna)

SKD	Śabda-kalpa-druma
SM	Siddha-mantra
SN	Śāligrāma-nighaṇṭu
SS	Suśruta-samhitā
SSSS	Śusruta-samhitā : A Scientific synopsis (P. Ray et al)
SSM	Śabda-stoma-mahānidhi
STH	Sthāna
SU.	sūtra
SY	Siddha-yoga (Vṛnda)
VJ	Vaidya-jīvana (Lolamba-rāja)
VRM	Vaidyaka-ratna-mālā
VSS	Vaidyaka-śabda-sindhu
VYK	Vyākhyā-kaumudī
VYMK	Vyākhyā-madhu-kosha
YR	Yoga-ratnākara
YV	Yajur-veda.

ENCYCLOPAEDIA OF INDIAN MEDICINE

The Conceptual Context of Indian Medicine

The Conceptual Context of Indian Medicine

(1)

Although Indian medicine emerged from folk practices, it developed, unlike in other countries except Egypt and China, within a well-defined philosophical framework. It is, therefore, that Indian medicine has remained a consistent system of thought, besides being an integrated approach to the problems of health and disease. Further, it did not develop a philosophy in course of time as drugs came into use and cures were effected, but, on the contrary, drugs were administered with a resulting cure on the basis of a philosophy that was crystallized at its earliest stage of development. It was theory that determined the practice in Indian medicine; and not the other way round.

Indian medicine did not however adopt any particular philosophical system as a mere intellectual exercise. Its alignment with the already stylized system of thought (like the Sāṁkhya and the Nyāya-vaiśeshika) was motivated by the practical considerations involved in man's happiness here and now. The conceptual context that was provided for Indian medicine was thus pragmatic and materialistic. It had little use for purely metaphysical, ethical or religious issues.

The affiliation of Indian medicine to the two philosophical systems, Sāṁkhya and Nyāya-vaiśeshika is marked. It is not difficult to see what prompted this preference. Both the systems were essentially rational in approach. They sought to understand man, not as a special creation of God, but as a detail in the natural world, as a product of evolution and as sharing with all other living beings the mechanism of life as well as the quality of consciousness. Both systems emphasized the value of the evidence of the senses and of human reasoning.

The basic assumptions of Indian medicine are the theory of the material constitution of human nature (the theory of pañchabhūta), and the explanation of human behaviour in its normalcy as well as in its disturbance on the basis of the tripartite categorization of influences (the tridosha doctrine). The former was borrowed from the Nyāya-Vaiśeshika system, while the latter was taken from the Sāṁkhya. It is important to recognize that the details of the two systems were not contrary to each other, although they varied. In fact, the details were complementary to each other. The Nyāya-Vaiśeshika system may be said to have contributed the basic physics and chemistry, while the Sāṁkhya system provided biology and physiology. Indian medicine achieved an effective integration of these contributions. An illustration of this can be seen in the explanation of diseases both as contained in the cause (sat-kārya-vāda of Sāṁkhya) and as an original production of symptoms and effects (ārambha-vāda of Nyāya-Vaiśeshika).

Indian medicine thus represents a level of systematization that was higher and more meaningful than either the Nyāya-Vaiśeshika or the Sāṁkhya. The conceptual coordinates of this systematization as found in the seminal works of CHARAKA, SUŚRUTA and VAGBHAṬA are obviously derived from these two systems, but they are free from narrow metaphysical constraints within which the systems worked as mere intellectual disciplines.

(2)

It is hard to identify the period when thought in this country began to be systematized. The Vedas do not betray this tendency; the Upanishads (early ones) do, though faintly. But the Upanishads represent doctrines taught principally by the conformists, and conclusions arrived at in conferences following the vedic tradition. There were, however, non-comformists and protestants even during the earliest of periods, even among the vedic philosophers themselves.

There were also thinkers and leaders who were altogether outside the vedic fold, and who belonged probably to a pre-vedic tradition. These were collectively designated as 'vrātyas', which for us today is an expression of uncertain meaning. But included in the collection were magicians, medicine-men, physicians, mystics, materialists, mendicants, wandering 'madmen', fire-eaters, poison-swallowers, libidinous pleasure-seekers as well as austere ascetics.

The word 'vrātya' comprehends a multiplicity of folk traditions and regional cults that resisted absorption into the vedic fold, or were more or less unaffected by the vedic impact. Some of these practices were monstrous and primitive, violent and erotic, and others were sophisticated and refined, evolved and austere. The great tradition known as the Tantra, with its almost infinite ramifications all over the country, is a survival of this Vrātya culture. Although it came to be associated rather closely with the vedic tradition in course of time, it was recognised widely and consistently as non-vedic, if not in fact as anti-vedic. The tāntric tradition must have been so widely spread and so deeply-rooted that the new culture could not brush it aside, much less wipe it out; the laws of coexistence prompted not only recognition but also assimilation.

It would appear that while 'vrātya' was the folk nomenclature, 'tantra' was the cult-word. Tantra connoted not only a characteristic way of thinking and knowing but signified a set of practices and exercises. The two aspects naturally supplemented each other, and together they constituted an integrated religious philosophy. There are indications that this religious philosophy, broad-based and multi-faceted, was current when the Upanishads were being composed, perhaps in a different region but within the zone of contact.

There has been much speculation as to who the vrātyas were at all. J. H. Hauer has hazarded a guess that the vrātyas were the forerunners of the latter-day yogis. Gough thought that yoga was derived from the 'ecstatic rites of savages'. S. K. Belvalkar and R. D. Ranade, who agreed with him, described his savages as 'wandering swarms of ascetics'. These were no doubt clever conjectures; although convincing evidence came much later and from other sources, they were responsible for the general belief that the origins of the Yoga system, far from being bound up with PATAÑJALI, were lost in remote antiquity, stretching anterior to the vedic period. PATAÑJALI, as is well known, was only an editor, not the founder of the system (even according to his commentators).

The Yoga that we are acquainted with today, that is to say, the Yoga that was accepted and sanctified by the vedic tradition, is clearly a late arrival, a modification of the earlier one, with a strong theistic bias. It was VYĀSABHĀṢYA on PATAÑJALI'S *Sūtras* that gave Yoga the present outlook and attitude. VĀCHASPATI, VIJÑĀNABHIKṢU, and BHOJA followed his lead and made Yoga acceptable to Vedānta. This is a development which began around the tenth century and reached its completion in the sixteenth century, that is, the period of VIJÑĀNABHIKṢU, the author of *Yogavārttika* (which fully reconciled the yoga ideology with the Vedāntic standpoint). The process took several centuries and had a background of several thousands of years, during which period there was a shift even of the major premises with a view to achieving conformity (however artificial) with the vedic tradition.

If Yoga in its early phase represented the ascetic and ecstatic practices of the vrātyas, its theoretical groundwork was supplied by the Sāṁkhya; and its practical application was to be seen in Āyurveda.

Parallel to the transformation of Yoga from primitive, atheistic and heterodox practices to the sophisticated, theistic, and orthodox system, was the development of the original materialistic Sāṁkhya of the pre-vedic tāntric tradition into the later theistic Sāṁkhya of the *Mahābhārata* and the *Bhagavad-Gītā*. IŚVARAKRSHNA'S Sāṁkhya marked a significant stage in the sytematization of this viewpoint, even as PATAÑJALI'S Yoga was in the systematization of Yoga. The Sāṁkhya that the vedic tradition found somewhat acceptable (even though unwillingly) is the work of IŚVARAKRSHNA. But the unknown author of *Kapila-sūtras* (about 1400 A.D.) and his commentators ANIRUDDHA (fifteenth century) and VIJÑĀNABHIKṢU (sixteenth century) worked out fully its compromise with Vedānta, involving a theistic orientation.

(3)

Both Sāṁkhya and Yoga have been regarded since the sixteenth century as orthodox (āstika) systems, that is to say, systems within the Vedic tradition, in contradistinction to the Lokāyata (or Chārvāka), Jainism and Buddhism which were dubbed as heterodox (nāstika) systems. But if one considers the fervour with which the *Brahma-sūtra* (about second century B.C.) and the great commentators like ŚAMKARA, RĀMĀNUJA and MADHVA attack Sāmkhya, and the suspicion with which ŚAMKARA looks upon Yoga, the acceptance of Sāṁkhya and Yoga within the orthodox-fold seems rather strained, and was with reservations. Even if the two systems were not hostile to the vedic tradition (vedaviruddha, as ŚAMKARA makes out in the case of Sāṁkhya), they were at least non-vedic in their origin and early development. They were probably rooted in the vrātya-tantra culture of the pre-vedic period.

The relation of Sāṁkhya-Yoga to the two other heterodox systems, Buddhism and Jainism, is too obvious to be ignored and too intimate to be regarded as accidental. One may not agree with Emilé Senart's contention that Buddhism is a branch of Yoga; but the Buddha is certainly a Yogi-type, and his teachings have heavily incorporated the old Yoga particulars of askesis, control, restraint, release and freedom. Early Buddhism preserved the Yogi-ideal of nirvāna. In fact, the expression Yoga is really an equivalent of samādhi (one-pointedness of consciousness) which is described as 'soullessness' (nirātmakatvaṁ), a detail which received great consideration in Buddhist philosophy. Likewise, the Sāṁkhya entered into Buddhism in a significant way; in fact, Gotama the Buddha's teacher, Ārāḍa Kālāma, was a Sāṁkhyan master.

Jainism based its theory almost entirely on the Sāṁkhya, and its practice on the Yoga. The Sāṁkhya-Yoga ideal of isolation (kaivalya) was destined to play an important role in Jaina thought. It was a variant of cessation (nirvāna) or absolute inner quiet (moksha), terms signifying alike the withdrawal of the individual spirit from all hindrances and extraneous matter. The Sāṁkhya dualism, pluralism and realism provided the groundwork for Jaina ideology; and in the Jaina thought, the goal is to be achieved by a concerted programme of askesis and self-torture–more so than in later Yoga and early Buddhism.

Medical wisdom as well as practice developed in a spectacular way within the twin contexts of Jainism and Buddhism. We not only find numerous references to medical practice in the early scriptures of these religions, but it is a fact that many of the medical writers even during the medieval ages were Buddhists or Jains.

In the historical perspective, Sāṁkhya-Yoga and Jainism-Buddhism were derived from a common nucleus that was outside the vedic tradition, at least in its early phase. But it does not mean that these ways of thinking developed entirely independent of the vedic tradition. There was, in fact, a series of successful contacts between the Upanishads and these systems. The Sāṁkhya and Yoga ideas can be discovered in the Upanishads, and the Upanishadic impact can be seen on Buddhism and Jainism. While there is some truth in the argument of Max-Müller and Garbe that the Sāṁkhya system emerged as a reaction against the monistic idealism of the Upanishads, it is possible, as Anima Sen Gupta has shown,[1] to trace the beginnings of the classical system in the Upanishads themselves. Jennings has demonstrated that Buddhist thought is heavily indebted to the Upanishads.

The Upanishads may be regarded as the most productive and highly significant period in the Vedic tradition, inasmuch as it provided the inspiration for all systems of thought in the country, orthodox or heterodox. But the systems as they got structured in course of time were significantly different from their beginnings. The beginnings of the Sāṁkhya-Yoga and Jainism-Buddhism were different from what they came to be as a result of reconstructions, reductions and systematization. The stimulus for systematization along with the direction perhaps came from the Upanishadic aspect of the Vedic tradition.

The nucleus, which, in course of time developed as Sāṁkhya-Yoga and Buddhism-Jainism, was distinguished by the exercise of human reason and an absolute reliance on human effort. Man became the focal interest; his striving was what mattered, and the goal of his striving was within the human framework. Gods were kept out and grace was dispensed with. The four great ways of thinking either rejected or minimized the involvement of supernatural principles. They were uncompromisingly realistic and pragmatic. Those who were committed to these ways concerned themselves with elimination, reduction, tranquility, withdrawal, isolation, release from distractions and hindrances.

The basic ingredients of this nucleus were, of course, the Sāṁkhya and Yoga. There is hardly any doubt that the two had a joint career from the earliest of times and even when the two were independently systematized they retained their twin-relationship. Even in a late compendium like MĀDHAVAS *Sarvadarśana-sangraha,* Yoga is described as a Sāṁkhya, 'seśvara-sāṁkhya' or 'pātañjala-sāṁkhya'. In terms of chronology, it is probably true that Sāṁkhya as a system was older than Yoga as a discipline, and that is why it is frequently asserted that Yoga was directly indebted to Sāṁkhya for its theoretical framework. But Yoga as askesis must indeed be of much greater antiquity as it was based on the most primitive urges and inclinations. And its involvement in medical practice must also be of considerable antiquity.

It is difficult to determine the exact period or circumstance of this interdependence of Sāṁkhya and Yoga. Even the *Mahābhārata* contends itself by describing them as "the immemorial twins" (sanātane dve). The Yoga ideal of isolation or emancipation as a human achievement by human effort must have promoted the exploration into human nature, the understanding of its dimensions and potentialities, and the appreciation of its limitations. It is in this context that understanding or knowledge (jñāna, gnosis) becomes essential for the work of askesis (karma). While Yoga concerned itself with the latter, Sāṁkhya sought to specialise in the former.[2] It was inevitable thus that the two systems had to function as twins, as equally valid, and as interdependent.

The expression 'tantra', applied to Sāṁkhya, Yoga and the medical texts, in fact comprehends both the aspects: knowledge (or theory) and askesis (or practice). The image of threads being mounted on the loom, resulting in uninterrupted weaving was in the background of this expression The derivative meaning of the word stands for 'extension', 'expansion', 'continuity', 'propagation' or more simply 'knowledge'. But it also signifies an esoteric undercurrent of magical rites and practices. It is no accident that an early Sāṁkhya text, now lost, was called *Shashthi-tantra;* and Śaṁkara explicitly mentions that Sāṁkhya is called 'tantra' (tantrākhyā). It is well-known that Yoga went usually by the name of 'Pāntañjala-tantra'. The tāntric involvement of the feminine aspect was indeed responsible for the 'pradhāna-vāda' (doctrine of the productive Mother Nature) of the Sāṁkhya, and the intriguingly helpless role played by the male purusha in it. Again, the preoccupation of the tantra with the human constitution, and especially the physical body, is to be seen in the Yoga. Sāṁkhya-Yoga thus continued the tāntric interest in understanding human nature and in effecting improvements in it.

The scene for consistent physical and psychological speculations in India was set when from the nucleus of amorphous tāntric perceptions, precepts and practices, Sāṁkhya and Yoga emerged as a composite theory-practice complex with little theistic preoccupation and religious involvement. It is from this foundation that Indian medicine gathered its conceptual context.

4

It is hard at this point of time to identify the presuppositions of the pre-Vedic tāntric cults. Probably, the usual involvements of magic, animism, agricultural rituals, fertility ideas, emphasis on the feminine, worship of the mother-goddess figures, and possession-intoxication complex were all there. R.P. Chanda, J. Marshall and K. N. Sastri have discovered some of these involvements in the Indus Valley finds. It is possible to read these elements in Rgvedic references to the religion prevailing among the masses of those days.

Atharva-veda is especially full of descriptive material concerning regional and tribal beliefs and practices answering to tāntric ideology. The mediaeval tāntric cults in the eastern regions of India and the Himālayan ranges probably represent continuation of the older tāntric cults. Many of the elements of tāntricism have survived to this day in the rural and tribal regions of the land. However, the tantra as systematized and as contained in classical and Buddhist tāntric texts cannot be credited with great antiquity. It bears a clear impact of vedāntic ideas. Many of the cults were so corrupt and so brimming with antinomian ideas that no serious philosophical system would care to own them. They survived merely as regional perversities.

The characteristic features of the tāntric tradition, however, is its reliance on the ultimacy of the feminine principle and on the mediacy of some abnormal state like intoxication. It is this that distinguishes this tradition from the vedic tradition with its heavily masculine orientation. The *Brahma-sūtra* upheld the 'brahma-vāda' (or the doctrine of the Spirit) in contradistinction to the Pradhana-vada (or the doctrine of Nature) of the Saṁkhyan thinkers. Nature is essentially the creative principle; it is inevitably linked with evolutionary change (parināma). We are reminded of the tāntric view that the entire cosmos evolves out of the primal sounds (mātrkā), the sounds themselves undergoing changes to become mystic formulae (mantra) and mystic diagrams (yantra). The vedāntic view as propounded by the *Brahma-sūtra* and as interpreted by ŚAṀKARA favoured the transformation-view (vivarta-vāda), and criticized the evolutionary theory of the Sāmkhya (parināma-vāda). It also emphasized the role of purusha (the male), which in Vedānta stood for Brahman, bringing about the phenomenal world by an unreal transformation. Even when the Sāṁkhyans conceded the existence of the theistic purusha (or rather purushas) it was but secondary in importance (apradhāṇa) apropos the prākṛti.

Based on the tāntric foundation, Sāṁkhya emerged as a strong protagonist of the materialistic,naturalistic and pluralistic viewpoints. The Nyāya-Vaiśeshika system also developed the same tendencies. Dominated by these aspects and not being excessively preoccupied with religious practices, Sāṁkhya developed easily into a psychological system. And the psychological orientation formed so early in the history of Indian thought was bound to leave its clear impression on subsequent ways of thinking. It is not unlikely that the later Upanishads themselves were indebted to an extent to the Sāṁkhya outlook, the crystallization of which was in all probability contemporaneous with the early Upanishadic thought. The Sāṁkhyan orientation undoubtedly inspired the early Buddhist psychology and influenced the Jaina psychological speculations.

It is difficult at this point of time to reconstruct the Sāṁkhya ideology of the Upanishadic period, more so the pre-Upanishadic Sāṁkhya thought. There is a persistent belief that the beginning of the Sāṁkhya system can be traced in the Upanishads themselves. Attempts have been made to recover the Sāṁkhya ideology in *Kaṭha* and *Śvetāśvatara-Upanishads*. But the ideology is as old as the vedas.

Sāṁkhya as a system, of course, became well-known even in orthodox circles from the days of the Kārikās of ĪŚVARAKṚSHṆA, which according to S.N. Dasgupta were composed only around 200 A.D.[4] Mention is made of two ancient texts[5], now no longer extant: *Māṭhara-bhāshya* and *Atreya-tantra* which were next in importance only to the celebrated *Shashti-tantra*, a work which also is now lost[6].

Charaka-saṁhitā contains an account of Sāṁkhya, very different from the account of Sāṁkhya in ĪŚVARAKṚSHṆA'S *Kārikā*. And CHARAKĀ continued the tradition of ATREYA-PUNARVASU, the Ātreya probably of the lost Sāṁkhya-tantra mentioned above. *Ahirbudhnya-saṁhitā*, *Mahābhārata* and *Bhagavad-gītā* contain Sāṁkhya accounts.

Several Purānas including *Bhāgavata* find occasion to mention and explain the Sāṁkhya thought. These accounts are not only not identical but contain significant variations despite the protestations of *Bhāgavata-purāṇa* (11, 22) to the contrary.

The claim of the commentators about the unbroken continuity of the Sāṁkhya tradition is hard to maintain. The *Mahābhārata* itself mentions three distinct schools of Sāṁkhya[7] one postulating twenty-four categories (tattvas) which were all material, leaving no room for the spirit; the other twenty-five, including the purusha as the conscious self; and the third twenty-six, including God as the supreme being (īśvara)

The last mentioned school is the theistic Sāṁkhya, acceptable to the Vedic tradition and advocated in the epic. The second of the schools is identified with the classical dualistic Sāṁkhya, propounded by ĪŚVARAKṚSHṆA and attacked by orthodoxy. The first school appears to have been the original stratum, materialistic and atheistic, the Sāṁkhya type ascribed to PAÑCHAŚIKHA and represented in *Charaka-Saṁhitā*.

The Sāṁkhya tradition ascribes its first formulation to the sage KAPILA who communicated the doctrines to his disciple ĀSURI, who in turn taught them to PAÑCHAŚIKHA. Not much is known about KAPILA or ĀSURI. There are *sūtras* in the classical style ascribed to KAPILA, but they are clearly of late origin. If we may judge by the *Bhāgavata-purāṇa* account of KAPILAŚ Sāṁkhya, it was theistic in orientation[8].

There is an argument that Sāṁkhya was originally theistic and that it was PAÑCHAŚIKHA who gave the atheistic slant to it[9]. The argument, however, is based on accounts occurring in avowedly theistic works like the *Mahābhārata, Bhāgavata, Ahirbudhnya-saṁhitā* and the Purānas. It appears more probable, as already noted, that the tradition was originally atheistic and continued to be so during the days of PAÑCHAŚIKHA and CHARAKA, until ĪŚVARAKṚSHṆA (200 A.D.) carved out what is known as the classical Sāṁkhya by the introduction of a quasi-theistic element[10].

It has not been sufficiently appreciated that PAÑCHAŚIKHA, who is said to have lived contemporaneously with early Buddhism, was a brilliant psychologist who gave Sāṁkhya its characteristic outlook. *Mahābhārata* (12, 219) contains an account of PAÑCHAŚIKHA'S Sāṁkhya[11]. HARIHARĀNANDA-ĀRAṆYA has edited and annotated the *Sāṁkhya-sūtras* of PAÑCHAŚIKHA[12]. One may glean from these accounts that he set the scene for psychological speculations in our country. It was but natural that the medical writer CHARAKA relied heavily on his analysis and explanations. Āyurveda as a practical discipline naturally profited much by adopting the Sāṁkhya ideology of PAÑCHAŚIKHA.

5

PAÑCHAŚIKHA and CHARAKA retained the relationship with the tantric tradition by subscribing to the primacy of body principle (deha-tattva). Unlike the Lokāyatas or the early Buddhists, they believed in the existence of soul or self (or person, purusha). And they even admitted that the soul or self could occur as the transcendental self or Purusha, uncaused and eternal, unmanifest and beyond comprehension. But more important in their system was the empirical or the phenomenal self (sometimes called Jīvātman or embodied self), in contradistinction to the transcendental Purusha (called paramātman).

The expression purusha here comprehends both these aspects (or rather states). And Purusha is not a principle of consciousness, as it is in the other systems of thought. Not that PAÑCHAŚIKHA and CHARAKA brush aside consciousness as merely an expression, or as a mere accidental occurrence; the principle plays a very important role in their system. But consciousness is an emergent phenomenon, arising out of the mind-body complex that is alive; the phenomenal self merely upholds it.

For PAÑCHAŚIKHA and CHARAKA, human constitution is of great interest and pragmatic value, for emancipation (apavarga) as well as health (ārogya). They recognize in man's constitution several elements, organized meaningfully and purposefully. The elements entering into this organization are technically known as 'categories' (tattvas). And they are counted as twenty-four; in two groups, prakṛti (nature, in the sense of causative factors) and vikāras modifications thereof, in the sense of effects). Included in the former group are eight categories: five subtle elements, 'consciousness-stuff' (buddhi), 'egoity' (ahaṁkāra) and the 'unmanifest' primordial principle (avyakta). The latter group consists of sixteen factors: five gross elements with specific characteristics, five organs of knowledge, five organs of action, and mind.

What we call man is only a conglomeration (a heap, rāśi), a gestalt, a configuration, a pattern composed of discrete but interrelated items. It is a body-mind complex. While the soul partaking of the nature of divine spirit or of the nature of an inner controller is not acceptable to this school of Sāṁkhya, they do accept the phenomenal self, which is the real experiencer. The expression 'heap-person' (rāśi-purusha), which these thinkers employ, is an interesting one. It is psychologically very suggestive and significant, as it emphasises the organizational aspect.

The phenomenal self is not pure consciousness, the reflection of which is caught up in 'the consciousness-stuff' (buddhi) as some schools of Sāṁkhya hold. The self somehow[13] gets related in a characteristic manner with the elements mentioned above, and renders them organized, integrated, enlivened, and patterned. And consciousness emerges sui generis from this organization which is described as the phenomenal self or the 'heap-person'.

Consciousness belongs to this organized heap, but is in no sense the essential nature (svarūpa) of the Self. In its transcendental aspect, there is no consciousness. Consciousness is a quality that emerges as incidental to the involvement of Self in the phenomenal mass. PAÑCHAŚIKHA holds that consciousness continues only as long as one is alive; at death it ceases. In this sense, it may be said to belong to the Self, and to be founded on the Self. It is likened to a light that radiates all round. The entire body-mind complex becomes aglow with consciousness.

The phenomenal self in this way becomes aware of the world around and feelings within, because of the involvements of sense-organs and mind. Experiences occur within this frame-work; knowledge, feeling, and action as also pleasure and pain are events that occur only here. The ancient Sāmkhyan thinkers coined a remarkably modern expression, 'field' (kshetra). The psychological complex that we call man represents essentially a field wherein the body, senses, mind, ego and the elements operate as forces; all the dimensions of experience are to be located in this field, and are explained as due to the operation of the field forces.

However, both PAÑCHAŚIKHA and CHARAKA recognize that the field, the forces of which are in an incessant flux, retains continuity and identity as long as the phenomenal self is involved in it, and that consciousness which occurs as a general 'field-quality' has a source (or core) on which it is founded, but which does not become manifest, or get committed to the field in an absolute manner. This unmanifest (avyakta) aspect of the field is its necessary background and support. This is figuratively spoken of as 'the field-knower' (kshetrajña).

But knowledge here does not involve the instrumentality of the senses and mind, or of the ego: it is mere awareness. There is an intriguing statement ascribed to PAÑCHAŚIKHA[14], wherein he refers to "the fourth principle of unconditioned awareness" which does not mutate and which is an unconcerned witness, (the other three principles being the guṇas which constitute the fabric of phenomenal existence). The commentator explains[15] that consciousness of the details of the phenomenal world (saṁvedana) is possible only because of the subliminal awareness which is inverted on itself (pratisaṁvedana). This latter is called pure-consciousness or mere (undifferentiated) 'I-feeling', different from the ego but basic to it. This inverted process of awareness itself is styled 'consciousness-stuff' (buddhi-tattva). It is dynamic, being composed of the three guṇas. But the subject of this awareness, static and beyond the influence of the modes of being or guṇas, is the unconditioned 'person' (purusha).

PANCHAŚIKHA and CHARAKA regard the ultimate truth as 'the unmanifest in the state of person' (purushāvasthamavyaktam). It is a unified category, comprehending both nature (prakṛti) and spirit or person (purusha). Nature involves the spirit in an unmanifest condition. It is, therefore, that CHARAKA groups the categories only into nature (prakṛti) and the modifications thereof (vikāras). The involvement of the unmanifest in the psychological complex is brought about by the inverted awareness (pratisaṁvedana).

(6)

Vyāsa cites an unidentified authority: "The phenomenal process on the part of the primal material is for the purpose of self-expression"[16]. It is explained that self-expression is twofold: involvement of the static and unconditioned self in the phenomenal existence (experience, bhoga), and realization that the self, in fact, is distinct from phenomenal existence (discrimination, viveka, or isolation, kaivalya). The former expression results in evolution (sarga) while the latter is spoken of as involution or dissociation of the Self from phenomena (apavarga). Both modes of self-expression involve ceaseless and continuous change from one state to another, one projected plane (āyatana) to another. This change (or mutation) is technically termed 'evolution' (pariṇāma); and the thought is of great significance in the Sāmkhya-Yoga thought. The progressive involvement in phenomenal existence comes in for discussion in the Sāṁkhya works, while Yoga is especially interested in the progressive disengagement of the self from phenomenal involvement.

The basic propositions of early Sāmkhya were really simple. The world that we experience is real; it is evolved, and is subject to incessant change. There are subjects of experience (purushas), objects of experience (artha) and instruments of experience (indriya). The subjects are numerous, each distinguished by a psychological complex called 'body' (deha). For evolution, or for experience, these subjects are not really important, they do not materially matter. What matters is nature and that is really important (pradhāna). The expression pradhāna, almost an equivalent of prakrti (nature in the sense of primal constituent or essential materiality) acquired great significance in the Sāṁkhya thought, so much indeed that the system came to be known as 'pradhānavāda'.

Nature, in contradistinction with the unmanifest spirit, is productive (prasavadharmī) and this is so because of the gunas that constitute it. Gunas are objective and ultimate constituent elements of experience; they are the modes of being. They are infinite in number, but are for the sake of understanding grouped into three types according to perceptibility (sattva), mutability or activity (rajas), and inertness (tamas). The guna theory in Sāmkhya has always been important. In the classical Sāmkhya and theistic Sāṁkhya, it developed into an elaborate doctrine. Guna is frequently substituted for the expression prakṛti[17]. The real dualism is between the guna (becoming) and purusha (being).

Even PAÑCHAŚIKHA, the early teacher, spoke of gunas as active constituents (kartārah) as opposed to the inactive purusha[18]. Gunas are doers in the sense of productive agents; they are the factors that are responsible for evolution as well as involution. These agents cooperate, interact and act together; they also strive for differential survival and specific dominance. The Sāṁkhya theory regards the phenomenal world as a tangled scene of the primal constituents, each one of them struggling for expression and ascendancy, and the other two struggling for the suppression of such expression and ascendancy.

These constituents patterned in one manner become responsible for the material world of physical objects and events; patterned in another manner, they result in the mental world of perceptions, feelings, thoughts and desires. These are two different lines of development, but the stuff of development is the same; and the source is a common one. Physics and psychology thus have a common origin; and the fundamental laws are the same, although the lines of development are understandably different.

It is interesting that the Sāṁkhya thinkers strike a modern note when they postulate that all evolution starts from the disturbance of an original state of equilibrium (sāmyāvasthā), wherein the primal constituents (guna) are all perfectly balanced. But then somehow[19] there is disturbance, and consequently the struggle for ascendancy is instituted among the primal constituents. Like the Lokāyatas, the Sāṁkhyans, in keeping with the tāntric tradition, hold to natural laws (svabhāva) as responsible for evolution. They do not think it necessary to posit any cause beyond nature (nimittāntaranirapeksha). As a result of this disturbance, mahat takes shape; from the general ground of the unmanifest, a figure emerges from this initial spurt of activity (for that is what mahat means).

The ground-figure analogy is a perfect one: the unmanifest like the ground, is without characteristics (aliṅga) or nature, while the mahat, like a figure, is really a sign or a symbol (liṅga). The former is static and stays behind, while the latter is dynamic and moves forward. It is called 'the spread-out one' because of its universality. It is a category that is common to all persons, like the 'common human archetype', and is therefore responsible for the objective character of the world for all of us alike. Experiential reality for all is projected from this source within each one of us. In its public or world aspect it is called mahat (the 'great one'), and in its private or individual aspect it is called buddhi ('consciousness'). The former aspect is cosmic, while the latter psychological. But in reality it is but one category (buddhi-tattva).

Mahat or buddhi is the primary phenomenon or evolute. It is the very first category to appear above the threshold of manifestation. And it is made up of the primal guṇas which have been shaken up, and each of which has started struggling for ascendancy; and the sattva prevails here over the other two. This represents the first phase of evolution at the cosmic as well as the individual levels. It is, for this reason, described as the 'seed of the phenomenal extension' (prapañchabīja). It is determinate, with ascribable qualities and identifiable function.

PAÑCHĀDHIKARAṆA, a Sāṁkhya teacher who came after PAÑCHAŚIKHA but before the formation of classical Sāṁkhya, held that out of the womb of the unmanifest pradhāna emerges a category which is altogether indeterminate and without any specificity whatsoever, prior to the formation of mahat[20]. Shall we call this the urge for expression coming closely on the heels of disturbance, or is it a homeostatic impulse, projecting the entire series of evolution so that the creation (sarga) will ultimately bring about the elimination of the disturbing factor (apavarga)? In a sense, Sāṁkhya considers evolution and elimination as complementary to each other.

It is important to remember that the emergence of phenomena is not only a cosmic affair. More significantly, it is an individual affair. The Sāmkhya thought recognizes a sort of psychophenomenology (pratyayasarga) which is a descriptive analysis of subjective processes, eight primary mental dispositions and their derivative dispositions, all answering to a four-dimensional psychic model, the dimensions being misperceptions (viparyaya), inadequacies (aśakti), satisfactions (tushṭi), and achievements (siddhi).[21]

The mahat is obviously exceedingly subtle: it is not extended in space, and cannot be perceived by the senses or by the mind. It is 'great' in the sense of being the recipient of knowledge of all things. It has no limitations as regards comprehension; and, in fact, it is fundamental to knowledge of whatever kind. PAÑCHAŚIKHA and CHARAKA take it in the sense of 'mere I-ness' (asmītimātra). It is the subjective counterpart of the objective 'mere isness' (tan-mātra) of things.[22] Functionally, this is the linking factor between the objective particulars and the self (purusha), which are otherwise totally isolated. According to VĀCHASPATI'S interpretation, it is so transparent and so dominantly sāttvic that the reflection of the self is caught in it, and when this is done, the process acquires the quality of consciousness.

The changes that occur in the buddhi are necessarily, though erroneously, referred to the self, and they are construed as the Self's own experiences. In reality, however, the self is neither the agent of action nor its locus. The apparent identification of the self with the 'consciousness-stuff' is responsible for all phenomenal existence. The Sāṁkhya speaks of the emergence of 'phenomenal self' (pratibiṁba-purusha), which is in the nature of an image of the self caught in the 'consciousness-stuff'. It is a reflex image that forms the core of individual existence, and becomes involved in all subsequent experiences, subjective and objective.

The buddhi being the link between the Self and nature, partakes of the attributes of both. It 'knows' as well as 'works'. It is mere awareness; and is also an inclination for phenomenal involvement. There is in it an activity-orientation, although it is primarily sāttvic in constitution. It is interesting that in this system of thought the 'life-force' (prāṇa) is looked upon as an aspect of this principle. If buddhi emphasizes the consciousness aspect of the mahat category, prāṇa symbolizes its power as activity. VIJÑANABHIKSHU, a later authority, regards the five-fold vital currents (vāyu) as merely different functions of the mahat in an extended sense.

Arising from the 'consciousness-stuff' (buddhi) and projected from it is egoity (ahaṁkāra), the dynamic principle of specific individuation. This projection is said to be necessitated by a stress condition (disturbance) within the 'consciousness-stuff'. The 'mere I-ness' of it has within itself a preparedness (or set) in favour of more determinate, that is to say, better structured, figure, namely, the egoity.

The function of this egoity which is characterized by awareness of phenomenal involvement is to produce a self-regarding sentiment or what is known as self-assertion (abhimāna) or self-love. If buddhi is predominantly sāttvic, egoity is rājasic. It consists of activities of continual adjustment to the changing situational involvements. It would be wrong to regard egoity as purely a subjective affair. The subject-object distinction of the experiential world is necessary for the functioning of the buddhi. This involves phenomenological structuring, which is an achievement of egoity. The 'mere I-ness' in the prior state is undifferentiated subjectivity, while in egoity the objectivity extension is provided for it so that there comes about a well-defined sense of individuality, an ego-sense in the context of the objective world of events and experiences.

This egoity is functionally an urge for self-preservation, not only for survival of individuality but for its continuous growth in relation to the changing situational involvements. Egoity in Sāṁkhya is not looked upon as a substance but as a process (vṛtti), a ceaseless process as long as life continues in the body.

(7)

Contrary to the modern viewpoint that ego is a growth incidental to maturation, the Sāṁkhya theorists hold that egoity is an equipment even at birth, and it is because of this dynamic principle that individuation takes place and is completed. Individuation is the acquirement of characteristics (liṅga) when associated with the body. CHARAKA includes the body composed of five elements (air, ether, water, fire, earth) in the category of eight-fold nature (prakṛti) alongside 'consciousness-stuff' and egoity. This is, according to him, the fundamental psychophysical equipment.

The senses and the mind, however, belong to a different category: they are instruments of knowledge and of action. Each sense-organ is a product of the five elements; it is a physical structure with specific physiological functions. It achieves its fulfilment only when the mind works along with it; otherwise, knowledge or action is impossible. The senses thus constitute further differentiation within the individualized 'field' (kshetra) for purposes of communication and self-expression. VĀCHASPATI prefers to consider the senses and mind as evolved from the sāttvic aspect of egoity, incidental to individuation;

VIJÑĀNABHIKSU, on the other hand, takes only mind as an evolute of the sāttvic aspect of egoity, the senses being evolutes of the other two (rajas and tamas). They, however, agree with the general Sāṁkhya position that mind and the senses work together, and that both senses and mind are evolutes from egoity. Purposeful structuring of the individualized 'field' is the import of this position.

The three internal organs, 'consciousness-stuff' (buddhi), egoity (ahaṁkāra) and the mind (manas) together constitute a continuum, a psychological field that is both subjective and individualized. They are three aspects (or phases) of one internal instrument (antahkaraṇa), and represent a movement towards greater specificity and particularity, better structuring, and more efficient transaction with the world, or in other words, greater phenomenological involvement.

It is significant that the Sāṁkhya school regards the five-fold 'life-force' (prāṇa) that preserves and upholds the psychophysical constitution as signifying the joint operation of these three phases or aspects of the internal instrument. The biomotor force, it follows, is essentially psychological energy. The three aspects of this energy are said to contain within themselves the power to open and close the 'field' (kshetra). The analogy of the birds in the cage by their conjoint flight lifting up the cage and carrying it away has been given by the commentators.

'Consciousness-stuff', egoity and mind constitute the human personality (samyogi-purusha); and functionally they engender the human involvement in the phenomenal world. The Sāṁkhya theorists as well as the Yoga teachers regard this inclination for phenomenal involvement as pain-provoking (klishṭa), as an impairment or disturbance of the original state of equipoise (in the pre-mahat state), as a perversion leading to errors in knowledge and action.

Five such disturbances (kleśa) have been listed: lack or absence of the apprehension of the original nature of consciousness (avidyā), ego-dominance (asmitā), attachments (rāga), aversions (dvesha), and love of life (abhiniveśa). The first among these (avidyā) is, of course, the foundation for the rest: the utter isolate character of the self and its essential non-involvement with the psychophysical constitution or with the phenomenally presented world is lost sight of in the progressive process of individuation. The tamas initially predominates over the sāttva, and rājas takes the field utilizing sattva and tamas for continued differentiation and onward movement.

What in reality is mere conglomeration (rāśi) of categories comes to be projected as an integrated field of experience and action, with the ego as the core. Approach tendencies and withdrawal urges constitute the twin processes of involvement and disengagement, of construction and destruction, of love and hate, of building-up and breaking-down. As a result of this dual involvement, there is a certain clinging to life, an urge to preserve oneself against odds, to preserve in the involvement, and to dread isolation. This is an excellent statement of the basic dimension of man's personality. This is also a statement of his problems arising out of aspiration, anxiety, frustration, but unavoidable involvement in the worldly processes.

The thorough-going analysis of human constitution distinguished the Sāṁkhya system. There was also an attempt within the Sāṁkhya fold to formulate a method whereby the pain-provoking conditions could be eliminated. The well-known methodology in Yoga and Āyurveda deals with the statement concerning the nature of painful condition (heyaṁ), the diagnostic formulation of the causative factors thereof and the attendant conditions (heyahetuh), the statement concerning the possible elimination of the painful condition (hānam), and the prescription of a curative procedure, whereby the elimination is achieved (hānopāyah). This methodology is to be ascribed to the early Sāmkhyan thinkers like Pañchasikha.

Contact (saṁyoga) between the self and the phenomenal appearances, between being and becoming, between existence and occurrences is the real source of the transactional world, of our involvement in it and of our continued participation in its perseverance. Elimination of this contact, and the consequent isolation (kaivalya) of the Self are held out as the goal of human life. This is what is called detachment, unburdening, release, liberation, freedom (moksha).

The systematic and progressive undoing of the evolutionary process (that is to say, the work of the senses, mind and egoity) so as to regress into the original state of 'mere I-ness' (asmītimātra), undifferentiated, unconditioned, unqualified and non-particular, is the method prescribed. Evolution is an onward process of progressive differentiation and proliferation, greater and more complex structuring, multiplication of co-ordinates and dimensions, and projection of more planes of experience. It is a spreading out and hence called prapañcha. The method that the Sāṁkhya indicated (and the Yoga developed) is an involution, a backward process of gradual attenuation, closing in, and concentrating the consciousness into an undifferentiated mass (samādhi). The world then becomes a mere 'is' (asti), and the individual a bare 'am' (asmi).

NOTES AND REFERENCES

1. Anima Sen Gupta, *The Evolution of the Sāṁkhya School of Thought*. Lucknow, The Pioneer Press, 1959, p.11 f.
2. ***Bhagavad-gītā***, 3,3.
   लोकेऽस्मिन् द्विविधा निष्ठा पुरा प्रोक्ता मयाऽनघ ।
   ज्ञानयोगेन् सांख्यानां कर्मयोगेन योगिनाम्।।
3. Śaṁkara, ***Brahma-sūtra-Bhāshya***, 2,1,1
   स्मृतिश्च तन्त्राख्या परमर्षिप्रणीता शिष्यपरिगृहीता, etc.
4. S. N. Dasgupta, *History of Indian Philosophy*, Vol. I, Cambridge, The Syndics of the Cambridge University, 1957, p. 212.
5. By Guṇaratna (14th cent.) in his comm. on Haribhadra's *Shaḍdarśana-Samucchaya*.
6. An account of this work attributed to Kapila occurs in *Ahirbudhnya-Saṁhitā* ('Tattva-samāsa' section). But we cannot be sure if this was the same as the ancient *Shashti-tantra*.
7. ***Mahābhārata*, 12, 318, 72.**
   षड्विंशं पञ्चविंशं च चतुर्विंशं च पश्यति ।
8. S. N. Dasgupta, *op. cit.*, Vol. iv, p. 36. Also Anima Sen Gupta, *op. cit.*, p. 102.
9. Cf. Johnston E. H. *Early Sāṁkhya*, London, Prize Publ. Fund, 1937, **pp** 8-9; also Keit**h** A. B., *The Sāṁkhya System*, 2nd ed., Calcutta YMCA Publ. House, 1949, pp. 47-49.
10. A. K. Majumdar argues that classical Sāṁkhya was theistic.See his *Sāṁkhya Conception of Personality*, Calcutta University Press, 1930 But orthodoxy does not concede this claim.
11. **Summarized in S. N. Dasgupta, *op. cit.*, Vol. I, pp. 216f.**
12. **Apart from Charaka's account being an elaboration of Pañchaśikha's Sāṁkhya, Vyāsa's** *Sāṁkhya-pravachana-bhāshya* has preserved **twelve statements ascribed to Pañchaśikha and these have been collected and annotated by Hariharānanda Araṇya. *The Sāṁkhya Sūtras of Pañchaśikha and other Ancient Sages*, Calcutta, Motilal Banarasidass, 1934.**
13. By will, aversion, ignorance and action.
14. In Vyāsa's *Sāṁkhya-pravachana-bhāshya*, 2, 18.
    अकर्तरि च पुरुषे.....चतुर्थ साक्षिणि)
15. Hariharānanda-Āraṇya, *op.cit.*, p. 97.
    (सापि अस्मीतिरूपा आत्मबुद्धिः येन
    प्रतिसंविदिता भवति स पुरुषः)
16. In *Sāmkhya-pravachana-bhāshya*,2,23.
    प्रधानस्यात्मख्यापनार्थप्रव
17. As for instance, in the expression
    गुणपुरुषसंयोगात्सर्गः
18. Cited in Vyāsa's *Sāṁkhya-pravachana-bhāshya*, 3, 18
    अयं तु खलु त्रिषु गुणेषु कर्तृषु अकर्तरि च पुरुषे।

    It is to be noted however, that for Charaka the three gunas are merely three different mental states.
19. There is no extraneous reason for this disturbance (निमित्तान्तर-निरपेक्ष); the explanation is that the disturbance is natural (*svabhāva*). Contact with *purusha* is sometimes given as the reason, such contact resulting in *avidyā*.
20. Pañchādhikaraṇa's view is described in *Prapañchasāra-tantra-vyākhyāna*, 1st paṭala, verse 94. His name figures prominently in the list of Sāṁkhya teachers given in *Yuktidīpikā-kārikā*, 71.
21. *Sāṁkhya-kārikā*, 44-52.
22. cf. Pañchaśikha's aphorism quoted in Vyāsa's *Sāṁkhya-pravachana-bhāshya*, 1, 36.
    तमणुमात्रमात्मानमनुविद्याऽस्मीत्येव तावत् सम्प्रजानीते ।
    But Charaka does not mention the 'tanmātras'.

A

Basic Concepts (alphabetically arranged)

A

Abhimāna: Meaning 'thought of oneself', self-conception or self-regard (abhi + mān), it is said to be the integrative function of one of the internal structures of human personality, namely, ego (ahamkāra) [*See* SĀMKHYA]. In common usage, it signifies pride, arrogance, high opinion of oneself; but in philosophical parlance it refers to the erroneous notion that the physical and physiological complex of man (body, sense-organs, mind, and so on) is itself the experiencing self. In the medical context, however, it is used in the sense of 'body-awareness' (bodha), giving rise to anxiety in case of an illness. [*See also* SĀMKHYA].

Abhyanga: Included as a detail in personal hygiene, daily or periodical anointing and rubbing of body with fragrant (sometimes medicated) vegetable oils is prescribed not only for regional benefits but also for toning up the whole system. Anointing the head with oil prevents baldness and greying of hair, facilitates thick growth of soft hair, removes headache, improves eyesight, and facilitates sleep. Anointing the body removes any bad smell, fatigue, heaviness of limbs, body-pain and skin troubles; it also increases appetite and helps digestion. Putting drops of oil into the ear prevents earaches and deafness; it also helps keep the throat clear. Rubbing the feet with oil keeps the soles soft, and removes dryness, numbness, sciatic pain and cracks in the feet; it reduces heat in the body due to disturbances of the doshas and removes burning sensations and exhaustion; it improves eyesight.

Rubbing in the form of massages (udvartana) relieves the aggravation of kapha, helps reduce fat, and invigorates the limbs of the body; the skin becomes soft, lustrous and firm. Rubbing the body with oil should be followed by a bath with hot or tepid water. [*See* BATH].

Action: Action (karma) is inclination (pravrtti) which is threefold : verbal (vāk), mental (manah) and bodily (śarīra). An excessive inclination of these is known as 'abnormal utilization' (atiyoga), while a total absence of all inclinations is 'non-utilization' (ayoga). 'Wrong-utilization' (mithyā-yoga) does not belong to either of these groups but is still abnormal and it is illustrated by such behaviour as falsehood, slander, harsh speech, frivolous talk (verbal); fear, anxiety, anger, greed, vanity, envy and so on (mental); and suppression of the natural urges or forcing them, faltering, slipping (bodily). (*CS*, sūtra, 11, 39-40).

Unwholesome effects of action are caused by three factors: improper sensory objects (artha, namely contact of the sensory organs with their objects in a morbid manner, 'asātmyendriyārthasamyoga'); improper desires (kāma viz. errors of judgement, 'prajñāparādha'); and improper time (kāla, viz. improper transformation 'parināma') (*CS*, ibid. 43; and śarīra, 1,113-139; 2,40).

Ādhi: Name for discomfort, in particular mental discomforts (ā + dhyai, 'care', 'worry', 'anxiety'); it is mostly used in association with vyādhi, (disease), especially bodily. [*See* DISEASE].

Ādi-Bala-Pravṛtta: Diseases that have a hereditary origin, viz. having their origin at the time of the union of the semen and ovum of the parents (like severe skin diseases, kushṭha, and stones in the bladder, arśa). They are of two types : "coming from the mother's side" (mātrja) and "coming from the father's side" (pitṛja) (*SS*, sūtra, 24). [*See also* DISEASES].

Agada-Tantra : Strictly meaning 'drug' or 'medicine' (a-gada, freedom from affliction, disease-less-ness), the expression 'agada' is specifically used in the sense of treatment of poisonous or toxic conditions. Regarded as one of the eight divisions of Āyurveda, Agada-tantra (toxicology) deals with the effects on the human body of organic and inorganic poisons (visha), especially of the poisons arising from reptiles, insects, rodents and so on, and also with the management and cure of these conditions. [*See* TOXICOLOGY].

Age: Age (vayah) is defined as the bodily condition which is a function of time-units (*CS,* vimāna, 8,122). Human life is broadly divided into three age-groups: (1) childhood (bālyavayah), where the bodily constituents are as yet immature, tender, incapable of bodily strain, and comprising in turn of three phases: (a) 'milk-ingesting' (dugdhāśi), the first year, (b) 'milk-solids ingesting' (dugdhānnāśi), the second year, and (c) 'solid-ingesting' (anna-bhuk) thereafter; (2) middle age (madhyavayah) when the bodily constituents have matured and all the faculties are efficient, from sixteen years to seventy years, and comprising of three phases: adolescence (tāruṇya) from sixteen years to eighteen; early youth (yuvāna), from eighteen to twenty-five years; middle youth (madhya) from twenty-five to fifty years; and late youth (vṛddha), till seventy years; and (3) old age (vārdhakya) over seventy years till about a hundred years, which is the normal human life-span.

In the first age-group (childhood), the body-constituents are gradually perfected, strength is acquired, sense-functions are matured; during this period, kapha predominates. In the second (adult), the individual functions as a mature individual, fully participating in all the normal functions of human life. The body and mind are at the peak of their efficiency. The dosha pitta will be most active here. In the third (old age), the individual gradually loses his bodily strength, sensory efficiency and mental vigour, his body-constituents begin to disintegrate; the vāyu dosha predominates in this phase (*CS,* vimāna, 8,122,also CHKP).

The male is said to be an adult at his twenty-fifth year, and the female in her sixteenth year. It is then that the body constituents attain their fullest development (*SS,* sūtra, 35,13). [*See* DEVELOPMENTAL STAGES].

Agni: The concept of fire (agni) has its roots in early Vedic literature, as one of the three primal divinities : fire (agni) on earth, air (vāyu) or Indra in the mid-region, and sun (sūrya) in the upper regions (Nirukta, 4,1,11 and 7,5, 1-2). The praise of this divinity which is a principle of nature, occurs in the *Ṛgvedic* corpus in as many as two hundred hymns (for example, 1,59,5; 1,68,2; 3,3,10; 6,6,2; 6,9,7; 7,6,1 and so on). Fire is said to exist as the 'inner controller' (antaryāmi) in water (as apām napāt), in the forest trees (as dāvāgni or wild fire), in moving organisms (animals, birds and humans) as the 'digestive fire' (jāṭharāgni) (cf. *RV,* 1,70,4 and 3,22,2). It manifests itself as the Sun (āditya) in the upper region, lightning (vaidyutāgni) in the mid-region, and as submarine fire (bāḍavāgni) in the ocean (namely the nether-regions) (*RV,* 1,95,3). The identification of fire with the sun is also to be found in *Ṛgveda* (for example, 1,59,2; 1,143,2; 3,27,12; 10,88,6 and so on). The presence of the fire principle in the human body (vaiśvānara), which is responsible for digestion and metabolism is also an ancient doctrine (*CHU,* 5,11,2, Māṇḍu, 3, and Bg 15,14). Devarāja-yajva, an authority on the Vedic lore, derives the expression Vaiśvānara (bodily or digestive fire) from viśvanarā (meaning life, 'prāṇa') : "the digestive fire is the offspring of life" (Nighaṇṭu-tīkā).

The etymological meaning of 'agni' is "that which moves up" ('agni gatau', aṅgati ūrddhvaṁ gacchati) but the word is usually employed in the sense of heat and light (pāka and ushna). The entire universe is regarded as composed of two fundamental principles (powers): agni (responsible for heat and light), and soma (responsible for nourishment and growth) ('agnī-shomīyatvāt jagatah', *SS,* sūtra,4). In early medical literature, three kinds of 'fire' are distinguished : physical fire produced from fuel, and used for cooking and so on (bhaumāgni), the celestial fire produced from water and blazing across the sky (divyāgni) and the 'stomachic fire' in the body for digesting food (jātharāgni). (Cf. Sandeha-bhañjana on Vijayarakshita on *MN*). The 'stomachic fire' is not fire in the common sense of the term, but it is designated as fire because it is responsible for the heat generated in the body and it discharges the function of 'cooking' (namely, digesting food) as pāchaka-pitta (cf. CHKP on CS, sūtra, 12,11).

Further, the idea of agni in Indian medicine is indebted greatly to the Nyāya-Vaiśēshika outlook on heat (tejas) and cooking (pāka). There are in the world different kinds of 'cooking', responsible for changes, growth, decay, transformations and activities. These are due to the manifold influence of tejas (or agni) which occurs in two aspects: (1) permanent (nitya) as ultimate, extremely minute partless units of matter (paramānu), beyond the range of sensory apprehension; and (2) transient (anitya) aggregates of the former as phenomenal effects (kāryas). The source of this tejas is the solar heat, which "cooks all the three worlds" ('saurasya tejasah trailokya-pāka-hetoh').

The tejas, in this system of thought, has characteristics such as enabling things to have form, colour, visibility (rūpa) enabling things to be touched (sparśa) and thus producing the sensation of heat (ushṇa), enabling things to be enumerated (sankhyā), to have dimensions (parimāna), to be separable (prthaktva), to combine (sāmyoga), to separate (vibhāga), to be prior and posterior (parāparatva), to flow (dravatva) and to have speed in motion (vega) (cf. Vyomavatī on PRAŚASTA-PĀDA'S *Padārtha-samgraha,* and UDAYANA on *Kiraṇāvalī*).

Derived from the concept of tejas is the idea of 'cooking' (pāka), which is an essential function of tejas. The Nyāya-Vaiśēshika school of thought recognizes two kinds of cooking : conversions that occur in the nature of things as a result of the combination and recombination of the ultimate elements (pīlu-pāka, a term that roughly denotes chemical changes) and involving a change in the very nature of the thing (piṭhara-pāka, a term that may roughly mean physical changes).

The cooking process means changes that occur in different manners: combustion or burning (dahana), production of heat (tapana), transformation (parināmana), mutation (parāvrtti). All these changes presuppose the presence of 'fire' within ('antahpraveśah kṛśānoh), which provides the necessary direction and impulsion (nodana) for the changes to occur (cf. JAYANTA-BHATTA'S *Nyāya-mañjarī*). This is also styled as the 'internal fire' (antar-agni), where the expression 'fire' is used metaphorically. Indian medicine utlilzed the twin-concepts of tejas (heat) and pāka (cooking) found in the Nyāya-Vaiśēshika system of thought to explain digestion and metabolism in the human body.

Another factor involved in digestion is closely associated with agni, namely, the structure known as grahanī (*CS,* chikitsā, 15, 56-57; *SS*, śārīra, 4,18-19 and uttara, 40,169-170, *AHr*, śārīra, 3,50-53). It is so called because it receives and retains (grahanāt) food that is ingested for digestion. It is located in between the stomach (āmāśaya including small intestine) and the large intestine (pakvāśaya), in a part of the cavity (koshtha) which is the seat of the pitta-dhara-kalā [*See* KALĀ]. The main function of the part known as grahaṇī is to support pāchaka-pitta which is essential for digestion [*See* PITTA].

"The four kinds of food (eaten, drunk, swallowed and licked), descending from the āmāśaya is retained in the pakvāśaya, and in due course digested, being dried by the heat of the pitta". (*SS,* ibid.) Grahaṇī helps in separating the nutrient portions of the food (sāra) from the undigested portions (kiṭṭa). It retains the food that is not yet digested (apakva) and sends down the digested portion (pakva) to the large intestine (pakvāśaya) on either side (pārśvatah) (according to CHKP. via the left side, 'vāma-pārśvatah'). In case of a weak digestive fire, it releases only undigested food (āma)". (*CS,* ibid.).

The structure grahaṇī is supported by agni. In fact, agni is said to be located in the grahaṇī (*AHṛ,* śārīra, 3.50-53). Any impairment of agni disturbs the integrity of the grahaṇī, and any defect in the grahaṇī makes an unfavourable impact upon the agni. All diseases, especially of the abdominal region (udara), are ascribed in Indian medicine to the defects in this agni, which interferes with digestion and increases the waste products in the body (cf. *CS,* chikitsā, 1,19 and *AHṛ,* nidāna, 12,1).

There has been some discussion about the identification of grahaṇī in terms of modern anatomical and physiological knowledge. However, it is often identified with the small intestine (adho-āmāśaya), which extends from the terminal end of the stomach (ūrdhvāmāśaya) to the cecum (unḍuka), from where maladhara-kalā begins. The stomach extends from the cardiac sphincter and the fundus to the pyloric sphincter, and small intestine (adho-āmāśaya) from the pyloric antrum to the ileo-cecum. (cf. S. C. Dhyāni, in DVARAKANATH, *DMA,* pp. 37-38).

In the human body there are said to be thirteen kinds of fires or agnis: five elemental fires (bhūtāgni), comprising of physical and chemical changes that occur in the five primary forms of matter (namely, earth, water, fire, air and ākāśa) that go to compose the human body [*See* PANCHABHŪTA]; seven constituent fires (dhātvagni), comprising of the metabolic changes that occur in the seven primary constituents of the human body (namely chyle, blood, muscle, fat-tissue, bone, bone-marrow and semen) [*See* DHĀTU]; and the 'stomachic fire' (jātharāgni) which is the chief principle responsible for the digestion of food, assimilation by the organs and elimination of waste. [*See* JĀṬHARAGNI].

The elemental fires (bhūtāgni) bring about the transformation of the external and heterogeneous elements (mahābhūtas) in the surrounding of the individual into internal and homogeneous factors of the body so that the physical constitution remains a dynamic, efficient and stable organism (bhūtāgnipāka). The constituent fires (dhātvagni), located in the primary constituents of the body (tissues) bring about the assimilation of the nutrient substances (sāra) received from the 'elements' after being subjected to the fires therein (bhūtāgni-pāka), and their transformation into the necessary ingredients (tissue elements) which are homologous to the constituents. During this process, each of the constituents gives out characteristic by-products and waste-products [*See* DHĀTU and MALA].

The principal agni, however, is the one which is found in the stomach (jāṭharāgni), and is also called internal fire (antaragni), digestive fire (pāchakāgni), bodily fire (dehāgni or kāyāgni), and cavity-fire (koshṭhāgni). It is actually located between the stomach (āmāśaya) and the large intestines (pakvāśaya). It is identified with the digestive pitta (pāchaka-pitta) [*See* PITTA and DOSHA] which not only directly participates in the digestion of food, but assists actively in the function (cf. *SS,* sūtra, 21,9 and *CS,* sūtra, 12,11) of the other pittas [*See* PITTA] present elsewhere in the body. This agni is important inasmuch as it is the root of the others (the elemental and the constituent fires). It is the cause for the maintenance of heat within the system (without which the living mechanism breaks down), and is also the source of energy synthesis (which maintains health, encourages growth and mobilizes strength).

CS recommends that this agni is to be maintained by a regular and adequate supply of fuel in the form of food. The food coming from the external world is broken up, absorbed and assimilated by this 'fire'. Helping the 'fire' in this function are the samāna-vāyu (which conveys the ingested food near the 'fire' and also inflames it), moisture in the system which breaks up the components of food, and kledaka kapha, which softens the food by its viscidity. Time is another factor, for the process of digestion is actually a function of time. The above factors are to be properly combined so that the final result of digestion (namely the nourishment of the body constituents) is secured [*See* DIGESTION].

"Even as the sun stays in the heavens and by his rays dries up (or absorbs the essence of) the earth and plants, even so the fire located in the navel region of the human beings digests by its own heat the food that is eaten." (*Rasa-pradīpa*). The fire is likened to a tiny lamp enclosed in a glass case; it is covered only by a membrane ('jaraya-mātra-pracchanna'), and is located in the centre of the solar orb (saura-mandala), which in turn is located in the centre of the lunar orb (soma mandala), which is located slightly to the left of the navel' (*BP*).

Four varieties of this fire are recognized, the varieties being determined by the prevalence of the three doshas : when kapha is predominant, the fire is called slow (mandāgni); when pitta predominates, it is called intense (tīkshnāgni); when vāta predominates, it is erratic (vishamāgni); and when the three doshas are balanced, it is balanced fire (samāgni). The last one is regarded as the best, for it gives happiness and health, which result from good digestion (*MN*, 'agnimāndya-nidāna') (cf. also *SS*, 35, 30ff).

(1) The slow-fire or mandāgni in the stomach means that even normal food cannot be properly digested, and the metabolic processes are impeded owing to the influence of excess of kapha. It causes heaviness in the abdominal region and in the head, cough, or other disturbances like dyspnoea, emesis and weakness of the body. Diseases that belong to the kapha type are usually due to the slow fire (hypo-metabolism).

(2) Intense fire or tikshnāgni or atyagni is when the stomachic fire is easily and excessively excited. Under the influence of aggravated pitta, one digests large quantities of food, even if taken frequently. The digestive process is quickly over too. There is a disease called bhasmaka, which is due to exceedingly intense fire, when whatever is eaten is reduced to ash and the constituent tissues are also burnt (VIJAYA-RAKSHITA on *MN*, 6). This condition leads to a parched throat, thirst, dry lips, dry palate, heat, fainting spells, and burning sensations. This condition is comparable to the concept of hyper-metabolism (*CS*, chikitsā, 15, 217-220).

(3) Erratic fire or vishamāgni is when the stomachic fire is fanned by an excess of vāta. At times, food is properly digested and at other times, it is not digested at all; sometimes digestion is slow, and at other times normal. It produces diseases like distension of the abdomen, colicky pain, diarrhoea, ascites, heaviness of the body, dysentery, a gurgling sound in the intestines (antra-kūjana), loose motions and so on.

(4) Balanced fire or samāgni is the normal and proper functioning of the stomachic fire. It ensures complete digestion of the ingested food, without hurry or delay, and without any disturbance.

The physician understands the condition of the fire in the body of the patient by considering the ability of the individual to digest food (*jaraṇa-śakti*). This is one of the main diagnostic aids in Indian medicine. Likewise, the condition of the fire in terms of production of body heat (ushma) is termed strength (bala) which is understood by considering the ability ot the patient to perform physical exercise (*vyāyāma-śakti*) (*CS,* vimāna, 4,8). [*See also* JATHARĀGNI, DIGESTION, PITTA, GRAHAṆI, and AGNI].

Ahaṁkāra : Ahamkāra is literally that which makes for the awareness of 'I' ('ahaṁ iti jñānam kriyate anena'), but generally signifies ego or 'self'-concept, the function of which is abhimāna (or conceit) [*See* ABHIMĀNA]. In the Sāmkhya school, three varieties of ahamkāra are distinguished: (1) sāttvika (or vaikārika), from which the sense-organs and mind are evolved, (2) tāmasika (or bhūtādi) from which the five primary pristine and subtle forms of matter (tanmātras) originate; and (3) rājasika (or taijasa), which cooperates with the above two (*SK*). There is another view that mind evolves from the sāttvika variety of ahaṁkāra, while the ten organs (five of cognition and five of action) evolve from the rājasika variety. The foundation for the ego is the ātman (*Bhāshā-pariccheda*). [*See* SĀṀKHYA, MIND, SENSE-ORGANS, ĀTMAN].

Āhāra: Whatever food is eaten or drunk is called āhāra, but its properties are specified as production of immediate satisfaction (sadyas-tṛpti), generation of bodily strength (bala) and maintenance of the physical con stitution (deha-dhārana) (*SS,* sūtra, 1,27).

Food is classified into two types : 'wholesome' (hita) contributing towards health, and 'unwholesome' (ahita), responsible for illness. The former establishes the bodily constituents in a state of natural balance (prakrtau), and corrects the errant constituents; the latter creates imbalance by excessively exciting one or more of the bodily constituents. Therefore, care must be taken to eat proper food, in a proper measure, so as to continue to be in good health and to prevent disturbances of body and mind (*CS,* sūtra, 5, 13). [*See* HEALTH, HYGIENE, SEASONAL CONDUCT].

Articles of food are classified in several ways. One of them is in terms of the manner of ingestion : eatables (aśita), beverages (pīta), linctus (līḍha),masticable (khādita). (*CS,* sūtra, 28, 3). Another is with regard to the preparations: corns, pulses, meat, vegetables, fruits, greens, wines, water, milk and preparations of milk, products of sugarcane, delicacies (krtānna, literally 'prepared food'), and side-dishes (āhārayogin) (*CS,* ibid., 5-7). Still another classification refers to the personality types that relish certain kinds of food : sāttvika, rājasika and tāmasika (*Bhagavadgītā*, 17, 8-10). Taste (rasa) is an important consideration in the selection of food, and hence the classification of food in terms of the six tastes [*See* TASTE].

Food is 'broken up' by water when ingested, and is thus prepared for digestion. Food that is assimilated in the body is transformed into the body constituents, Chyle and so on in order, and thus becomes responsible for vitality (ōjas). [*See* BODY CONSTITUENTS, DIGESTION, VITALITY]. During the process of digestion and metabolism, the nutritive portions of food (sāra-bhāga or prasāda) are separated from the waste products (kiṭṭa-bhāga). The primary transformation of food that provides the nutritive element to the body is called 'the essence of food' (anna-rasa, or rasa). The waste product is eliminated (*See* MALĀ) (*SaS,* 1,6,6). [*See also* FOOD].

Aitihya : Traditional knowledge, (contained in works like the Vedic texts which are ascribed to divine origin and works of enlightened sages prompted by compassion for the suffering humanity) which has the characteristic of instructions from a competent and well-meaning authority (āptopadeśa) (*CS,* vimāna, 8,41) [*See* EXAMINATION, PRAMĀNA, ŚABDA

Alkali : Alkalis (from Arabic *al-qualiy*, 'qualay'; 'to roast in a pan') or caustics have been in use in Indian medicine since very early times (*CS*,1,27, and *SS*, 1, 11 also *Bower's Mss*, and so on). The Sanskrit name for them (kshāra) is derived from its capacity to quickly eliminate impurities ('ksharati malam yo śīghram'), and especially from its action in removing diseased portions of skin, muscles, and so on ('kshāraṇāt, dushṭa-tvaṅg-māmsādi-chalanāt') (cautery).

Many kinds of alkali have been known, but most frequently used are:(1) potassium carbonate prepared from ashes of barley-ears (yava-kshāra); (2) refined natron (svarji, sarjikā), sodium nitrate; (3) salt-petre (ūshara-kshāra); (4) sal-ammoniac (navasāra) which is classed also under uparasas, for it has some mercurial properties; and (5) borax (ṭankaṇa). Among them, three (natron, salt-petre and borax) are obtained from the earth, while the first (potassium carbonate) and also other alkalis are extracted from the ashes of the parts of trees and plants such as palāśa (*Butea frondosa*), aśvattha (*ficus religiosa*), kuṭaja (*Hollarrhena antidysenterica*), vibhītaka (*Terminalia belerica*), snuhi (*Euphorbia nerifolia*), arka (*Calotropis gigantea*), apāmārga (*Achyranthes aspera*), chitraka (*Plumbago zeylanica*), punarnavā (*Boerhoavia diffusa*), ārdraka (*Zinziber officinale*), mūlaka (*Raphanus sativus*), tamarind, beans, sesasum seeds and ears of barley.

General properties of alkalis include being light, warm, acrid, moistening. They are all digestives; and they increase appetite, reduce kapha, destroy intestinal worms, cleanse, heal wounds, and open the boils. But they cause inflammation and increase the tendency to haemorrhage (raktapitta). They are indicated in conditions of tumour in the belly, piles, chronic diarrhoea, diabetes, stones in the kidney and colic. The carbonate of potash (yavakshāra) is pungent, soft and light; it helps discharge of urine; it is also a laxative. It is recommended for intestinal obstruction (ānāha), anaemia, asthma, enlargement of the spleen and heart diseases, besides the conditions mentioned above. It is said to be "like unto fire" (vahni-sama); and it destroys semen. Its internal administration is said to dissolve urinary calculi. Refined natron (sarji-kshāra, crude carbonate of soda, washing soda) is very similar in action to the carbonate of potash, equally "like unto fire", pungent, hot and acrid; it impairs semen. It is recommended in conditions of asthma, intestinal obstruction, enlargement of liver and spleen, piles, flatulence and boils.

Salt-petre (ūśara-kshāra, bhauma-kshāra) is light, soft, moistening, digestive, and capable of easily spreading throughout the system. It increases appetite, pacifies vāta, and removes belching winds (udgāra); but aggravates pitta, and impairs strength. It is useful in constipation, colic, intestinal obstruction, intestinal worms, and tumours in the belly.

Borax (*tankaṇa*) occurs in two kinds, the pure white crystal (sita), and the dirty white lump (piṇḍa). The former, which is the better of the two, is pungent, hot, rough, acrid; it is a digestive and laxative; it pacifies kapha, vāta, and is useful in wasting diseases and conditions of poisoning. The latter, which shares many of the properties of the former, pacifies kapha but aggravates pitta and vāta. It increases the digestive power; and it is useful in conditions such as cough, asthma, dysmenorrhoea and inorganic poison.

Alkali is classified into two groups : solid (kaṭhiṇa) and liquid (tarala). The solid alkali is meant for external application (pratisārya) and is used as an ingredient in medicines (prayojya). The liquid alkali is given for drinking along with rice-gruel, wine, curds, buttermilk, decoction or warm water in several disease conditions. To obtain liquid alkali, the solution of ashes mixed with water is heated till the solution becomes red, clear, acrid and sticky. However when it is further heated, the solution solidifies (*RJN*). External application is indicated in conditions like ringworm, leucoderma, leprosy, ulcer, chloasma, warts, external tumour, inflammation of the gums, fistula, and sinus. Internal administration is recommended in conditions of diabetes, stones, internal tumour, piles, fever, biliousness, giddiness, poisons, spells of fainting, cataract, and in several diseases of children and the aged (*RJN*).

Alkali, when it is properly prepared, must be white in colour, smooth and soapy to touch, neither too strong nor too weak, not spread beyond the area on which it is applied, and should act speedily and successfully (*SS*). [*See* PREPARATIONS.]

Āmāśaya : Literally this means 'receptacle for undigested food'. This refers to the organ of digestion located between the navel region (nābhi) and the breasts (stana) (*BP*); namely, the stomach, a part of the gastro-intestinal tract (mahā-srotas). It has two sections : upper (ūrdhva) and lower (adho), consisting of the stomach and the small intestine (kshudrāntra or pachyamāna-āśaya). [*See* ANTRA, ĀŚAYA, DIGESTION]

Āmaya : Disease in general. But the structure of the word signifies the diseases which originate in disturbances of digestion ('āma-samuttha', āma meaning 'uncooked' or 'undigested'): indigestion, constipation, dyspepsia. The background thought is that most of the diseases have their source in attaching stress (root 'ming' meaning stress, violence, injury, hiṁsāyām) to the place or process of digestion. [*See* DISEASE]

Aniyata-vipāka-vāda : The view that during digestion and assimilation of food, the tastes are transformed on the principle of 'the stronger one suppressing the weaker'. The taste that is powerful naturally tends to inhibit the taste that is mild and the resultant (post-digestive) transformation is determined by the taste that is powerful. It is difficult to ascertain which of the tastes would become powerful and when ('kadāchit kasyachit saṁbhavāt'). The power of the taste is known only when it becomes dominant. ('balavattvam vyaktatvena') (cf. *SS*, 1,40). [*See* VIPĀKA, DIGESTION.]

Antra : Meaning 'connecting organs of the body' (antyate saṁbaddhyate), it refers generally to the parts known as entrails, intestines, or bowels, located in the middle portion of the human body (which, in turn, consists of the four extremities, (that is, the hands and legs, head, and trunk or middle portion) (cf. *SS*, śārīra, 5,2). They, together with the bladder (vasti) and anus (guda), are formed out of the essence of blood and kapha, heated by pitta and associated with vāta (*SS*, śārīra, 4,26). In an adult male, the total length of these parts are said to be fourteen cubits (cubit is three vyāmas and a half), while in the female, twelve cubits (*SS*, ibid., 8).

The large intestine (pakvāśaya) is known as *sthūlāntra*, and the small intestine (pachyamānāśaya) *kshudrāntra*. They are situated in the lower portions of the region of the stomach (āmāśaya), and include the organ known as grahaṇī, where the digestive 'fire' is located. [*See* GRAHAṆĪ].

Among the diseases of antra are 'rumblings in the bowels' (antra-kūjana), inflation of bowels or indigestion (antraṁdhami), inguinal hernia or rupture (antra-vṛddhi), and worms in the intestines (antrāda) (*SS*, nidāna, 1, etc.)

Anumāna : Inferential knowledge, dependent upon rational thinking (yukti). Examples given are deducing the action of 'stomachic fire' from the individual's capacity to digest food, presence of the individual's strength from the efforts he can put forth, and the presence of the sense-organs from apprehensions. (*CS*, vimāna, 8,40). [*See* PRAMĀNA]

Anupāna : A fluid vehicle prescribed to be used while taking medicine, or a drink prescribed to be had soon after medicine is taken (post-prandial drink). The purpose is to facilitate the absorption or assimilation of the drug in the system, or to increase the efficacy of the drug. "Even as oil dropped on water spreads quickly, the medicine spreads in the body as a result of the prescribed vehicle" (*SaS*, 2, 6, 4 and 5). It also checks the undesirable side-effects of the drug.

The vehicle is prescribed according to the constitution of the patient, the condition of the dosha in his body, and nature of the drug to be administered. In conditions where vāta is aggravated, the vehicle must be unctuous and hot; in pitta, unctuous, sweet and cold; and in kapha, coarse, severe, and hot.

The main vehicles are water (cold or warm), honey, ghee, butter, sugar, jaggery, buttermilk and milk. Sometimes, a medicinal preparation (like fresh or inspissated juice, decoction, cold or hot infusion) itself may serve as a vehicle for other medicines prescribed. Drugs are also occasionally employed as vehicles of other drugs.

Such liquid vehicles are indispensable when drugs are given in the form of powders, pills, boluses, thickened extracts, and pasty masses. The measure of the vehicle varies according to the dosha which is being sought to be corrected : if vāta, three palas (a pala is roughly four tolas in weight); if pitta, two palas; and if kapha one pala.

Examples of vehicles indicated in different ailments are: warm water in indigestion; butter-milk in dysentery; ghee in intestinal colic; honey in chronic fever, bronchial asthma and typhoid; water mixed with honey in obesity; old ghee in insanity; buffalo's milk in insomnia; water in which hot gold is dipped in abnormal thirst; honey in vomiting; cow's urine in rheumatism; juice of ash-gourd in stranguary; and meat-juice in emaciation. Herbs used as vehicles include āmalakī (*Emblica officinalis*) in obstinate urinary disorders (diabetes, etc.), pippalī (*Piper longum*) in splenic disorders, amṛta (*Tinospora cordifolia*) or vasikā (*Adhatoda vasica*) in diseases caused by the vitiation of blood, hiṅgu (*Ferula foetida*) in colic, bhārgi (*Clerodendrum serratum)* in asthma, guggulu (*Commiphora mukul*) in wounds and boils, lodhra bark (*Symplocos crataegoides*) in menorrhagia and other gynaecological disorders and viḍaṅga (*Embelia ribes*) in parasitic infection. Mineral products are also used as vehicles, although seldom, like mineral pitch (śilājatu) in tuberculosis and iron-rust (maṇḍūra) in anemia (*VJ*).

Included in the category of anupāna, although not exactly answering to the description, are prescriptions like sleep in diseases due to indigestion, and activities conducive to cheer up people in diseases involving fright (cf. *VJ*). The drink used for post-prandial purposes must generally have properties contrary (viparīta) to the properties of food that the patient takes, but not be deleterious to his body-constituents. In diseases due to vāta-aggravation, the post-prandial drink must be unctuous and hot. (*CS*, sūtra, 27, 319-324). The usefulness of the drink is determined both by the nature of the drink itself and the nature of the food that goes before it (*Chkp* on the above).

Generally, the post-prandial drink refreshes the patient (tarpayati), bestows a pleasurable feeling (prīṇayati), contributes energy (ūrjayati), nourishes (bṛṁhayati), and affords satisfaction (paryāpti); it also helps digestion by breaking the food down, softening it, and aiding assimilation (*CS*, ibid. 325).

Apāna : The aspect of the bodily wind (prāṇa) that goes out through the lower portion of the body, that is anus (guda). It pushes the ingested food down, and helps in the elimination of urine, faeces, and semen. [*See* MALA *and* VĀTA].

Arishta (Rishta) : Literal meaning is 'that which strikes, hurts or kills' (rish himsāyām̐), the expression signifies unfavourable symptoms, symptoms that forebode certain death (niyata-marana-khyāpaka-liṅgam, *MN*). The knowledge of this is regarded as helpful to a physician in order to ascertain the possibility of cure with regard to a case in hand. Without understanding the unfavourable symptoms, one will be unable to judge when a disease has become incurable; and by seeking to cure an incurable disease, the physician is likely to lose his practice, reputation, friends and goodwill among the people (*CS,* sūtra, 10, and *Chkp* on it). The physician should also be able to distinguish between secondary diseases (upadrava) and moribund conditions (rishṭa) (cf. also *AHr,* 2, 171, 5). It is because of the importance of the unfavourable symptoms to the physician that *Charaka-Samhita* takes up this matter (Indriya-sthāna) even before the topic of treatment (Chikitsā-sthanā) is dealt with (*Chkp* introduction to chapter 5).

Even as a flower is the sure indication of the fruit that will eventually come into being (*CS,* 5, 2, 3), as the smoke suggests the invariable presence of fire, and the thick cloud the possibility of rain (*AHr,* 2, 5, 1), unfavourable symptoms indicate that death is round the corner. When the unfavourable symptoms have gathered, death cannot be avoided; and there can be no death without unfavourable symptoms (*CS,* 5, 2, 5). *Chakrapāni* discusses in this context the problem of timely and untimely death (kāla-mrtyu and akāla-mrtyu). He cites a view that unfavourable symptoms occur only in cases of natural and timely death (that is, death in old age); and that even the best of treatment done then would be in vain. According to this view, the unfavourable symptoms that occur in other cases could be remedied, and death could be prevented. *Chakrāpani*, however, argues that unfavourable symptoms precede timely as well as untimely death; and they may flash forth in a moment's time (*CS,* NS ed. p. 357).

The physician should look for clues that are unfavourable before he begins his treatment. Of these, some are not dependent upon the patient (purusham̐ anāśritāni); for example, messengers, informants, and other conditions that are external to the patient. The physician must in this case bring to bear his skill, intelligence, past experience, and learning to make adequate inferences (yukti) regarding the patient's condition. Other clues are dependent upon the patient himself (purusha-samśrāyani), like disturbances or changes (vikrti) in complexion, speech, odour, movements and so on that have occurred in the constitution of the patient (prakrti) with due regard to his social class, economic status, age, and individual differences as well as the time of the year and place where the patient is residing. (*CS* 5, 1, 4-7). This classification also underlines the distinction between internal (ābhyantara) and external (bāhya) factors that suggest the moribund condition of the patient (*NiS* and *Chkp*).

Among the internal factors, a further subdivision is made between the changes (vikāra) in the normal nature of the body (śarīra-prakrti-viparyaya), and changes in the normal conduct or behaviour (śīla) (*SS*). Sometimes, simultaneous changes in body as well as conduct can be observed.

Another classification rests on the symptoms that are irreversible (sthāyī) and reversible (asthāyī). The former are indications of certain death, while the latter are brought about by the abundance of disturbances in the doshas and would be eliminated when they are made to subside (*AHr* 2, 5, 3). This corresponds to the classification of unfavourable symptoms into invariable (niyata) and variable (aniyata); and among the conditions that can reverse the moribund condition are included rasāyana-preparations, austerities (tapas), and repetition of sacred formulae (japa) (*SS,* sūtra 28).

Symptoms foreboding death are said to arise from one or more of three sources : (1) wrong treatment of the disease (vishamopachāra), that is, the treatment that goes contrary to the constitution of the patient; (2) past actions (pūrva-karma), or actions done in previous births; and (3) natural process of decay in all beings (svabhāva). Corresponding to this tripartite division, we have other conditions (*NiS*): dependent upon the patient himself (vyakti-vyapāśraya), dependent upon supernatural factors (daiva-vyapāśraya) and the very nature of things (svābhāvika).

The medical ethics insist that the physician should not divulge, even when pressed, the unfavourableness of symptoms, or the approaching of death, to the patient or to his relatives (*AHṛ* 2, 6, 129). He must refrain from causing anxiety or sorrow for the persons concerned (*CS*, 5, 12, 63). Nor should he, when convinced that death is certain and close at hand, launch on any treatment, taking care however not to reveal to the relatives the hopelessness of the case (*CS*, 5, 12, 62-64). Indeed, he should tell them that the symptoms are favourable, although they appear altogether unfavourable (ibid. 65). The idea is that the patient must be allowed to die peacefully, without interfering with the natural processes of disintegration.

The medical texts contain elaborate enumerations of unfavourable symptoms with regard to the physical appearance of the patient, his sensory functions, his behaviour (bodily, mental and speech) and bodily conditions (*CS*, chap. 5, *SS*, 1, 31-34). There are also accounts of unfavourable symptoms which are specific to different diseases (*AHṛ*, 2, 6-128).

In these accounts, excellent medical gleanings get mixed up with common folk beliefs (like omens, portents). But there is an attempt to construct a systematic outlook on the problem of the moribund condition, as for instance, in the Indriya-sthāna chapter of *CS*. [*See* DEATH, DISEASE, MEDICAL ETHICS].

Arka : Distilled or concentrated aromatic waters (aquae, arka) are used both in Āyurveda and Yunāni, especially because they can be preserved for longer periods of time than the infusions. They contain volatile constituents of drugs in the medium of water; they are also described as weak and simple solutions of volatile oils.

They are prepared by pounding the drugs, soaking them in water for a night-and-day (that is, 24 hours) and then distilling the whole (drugs as well as water) in a sealed distill (arka-yantra) until the black fumes begin to escape through the exhaust. Care should be taken to prevent the vapours from escaping, and to obtain uniform concentration of drug essences in the several distillate takings. Different kinds of fire (slow-fire, smoky-fire, steady-fire, medium-fire, coarse-fire and so on) are employed. While preserving, it is important to see that the volatile oils do not get lost owing to loose lids. While administering, an equal quantity of water is added.

Arka is also the name of a medicinal plant (*Calatropis gigantea*). [*See* PREPARATIONS].

Ārogya: Literally meaning diseaselessness, it means health, lightness of body (lāghava), efficiency of limbs (pāṭava) (*RN*), and that which brings about happiness (sukhāvaha) (*SaS*, 1); it is indicated by happiness which arises from an equilibrium of the body constituents (*CS*, sutra, 9, 4). Health is extolled as necessary for the achievement of all the four objectives of life, namely virtue, wealth, pleasures and salvation. [*See* HEALTH].

Āsava-Arishṭa: Considered in early literature as synonymous, the two expressions refer to medicated spirituous liquors, prepared by allowing the drug, juices, or decoctions mixed with sugars (honey, jaggery, treacle) in earthern jars to remain for a long time for vinous fermentation (sandhāna). Later, a distinction was made between āsava, which is the fermented fluid got out of the fresh juices of plants, and arishta, which is the fermented product when decoctions are used. The former is prepared without making use of fire, while the latter is prepared with boiled decoctions (*SaS*, II, 2). The usual proportions of the ingredients are : medicinal substances (in powder or decoction) 1¼ seers; water 32 seers (a little more than 29 kilograms); treacle 12½ seers; (a little more than 11 kilograms); honey 6¼ seers. (a little more than 5 kilograms).

When the whole is laid aside for fermentation, the alcoholic content in the liquors may be upto 12 per cent by volume. The drinks are usually sweet to taste, aromatic and slightly acid. They function like mild wines; but along with the property of liquor, there also remains the property of the drugs or the extracts used. They are easily digested, and are hot (ushṇa) in effect. They are stimulants, stomachics, tonics, alteratives, and febrifuges.

There are several varieties of such alcoholic medicaments: wines (sīdhu), which are fermented products of raw (śīta-rasa-sīdhu); or boiled juices of drugs (pakva-rasa-sīdhu); liquors (surā), which are products of fermented 'boiled food' (paripakvānna-sandhāna-samutpanna); the frothy scum floating on the surface or the clear take of the above (prasanna or surā-manda); the heavier portion of the same (kādambarī); the thick sediment at the bottom (jagala); and a thicker under-layer (medaka); liquor fermented from dates and palmyra fruits (vāruṇī), tubers and fruits (plantain, grapes and so on) mixed with salts and oils allowed to ferment (sūkta), sweetish fluids (like sugar-cane juice) fermented in the pot, buried in a heap of grains (chukra), grains of yava soaked in water and fermented (tushāmbu), the same grains dehusked and boiled, and fermented in water (sauvīra), cereals boiled in water and fermented (kañjikā), tubers like carrot and sesamum seeds, mixed with a fluid and allowed to ferment (sandakī), and so on.

These are prescribed in several pathological conditions, for example, kañjikā in loss of appetite and indigestion; tushāṁbu in digestive troubles, weak heart, anaemia and intestinal worms; sandakī in disorders of vāta. [*See* PREPARATIONS].

Āśaya: The word 'āśaya' (from śerate, 'to rest on') means seat or receptacle. It refers to the cavities or viscera in the body, where the doshas, body constituents (dhātus), and by-products (mala) are contained (avasthāna-pradeśa, *NiS* or *SS*, sārira, 4,5).

There are seven āśayas in men and eight in women. Common to both men and women are: (1) receptacle of the bodily wind or vāta (vātāśaya), the middle and end portions of the large intestine (pakvāśaya); (2) receptacle of pitta (pittāśaya), namely, liver (yakrt) and the part known as grahanī (*See* GRAHANI); (3) receptacle of kapha (kaphāśaya, sleshmāśaya), that is, the lungs (pupphusā); (4) receptacle of the blood (raktāśaya), the heart (hṛdaya); (5) the stomach and the small intestine (āmāśaya); (6) the end portion of the small intestine and the beginning of the large intestine (pakvāśaya) including caecum (unduka); and (7) the receptacle of urine (mutrāśaya), that is, the urinary bladder (vasti) and the kidneys (vṛkkau) (*SS*, ibid., 5, 7).

The receptacle which is additional in women is the uterus (garbhāśaya) and is connected with the breasts (*SS*, ibid. 8). [*See* BODY (HUMAN).]

Ashes: Known as bhasma, they are medicinal preparations, where herbs or minerals are pulverized or, more often, calcined by fire. [*See* BHASMA].

Asthi: Translated as bone or as bone-tissue, this is counted as the fifth among the seven body constituents. Derived from fat (medas) and generative of bone-marrow (majjā), it discharges the important functions of supporting the body and nourishing bone-marrow. The subtle form of fat (medas), 'cooked' in its own 'fire' (medāgni) and frozen by the action of the wind in the body becomes bone, 'the core of the whole system' (sāram sarva-vigrahe). Fat is said to form a compact mass of earth, fire and wind elements by its own heat; and this mass is known as bone, in which the earth element predominates although wind is present in the pores. Bone, during the course of being 'cooked' in its own 'fire' (asthy-agni), remains as bone in its concrete and structural aspect, but transforms itself as bone-marrow in its subtle aspect. [*See* DHĀTU, DHĀTVAGNI].

Asthi is the hardest structure of the human body, and because of it the body stands firm and straight. 'Even as the tree stands firm because of the hardwood that runs through within it, the body stands firm because of the hard-bones (asthi-sāraih)' (*SS*, śārīra, 21). When the fleshy parts are fastened securely to the bones by means of big veins (sirā) and muscular bands (snāyu), the organs are well protected and do not slip away (ibid, 23). Even when the skin and flesh loosen themselves, crumble and decay, bone will not; it is the most enduring portion of the body-constituents.

Bone is heavy, rough, stable and gross in its characteristics. Teeth are derived from bone as secondary constituents (upadhātu); nails and hair are waste-products from bone.

That bones are numerous and varied in nature and function has been recognized from Vedic times. The accounts included in the Vedic texts enumerate as many as 360 bones, the number retained in *CS, AS* and *AHṛ*. But *SS,* which is more reliable, for it is based on dissection and surgical considerations, counts only 300 bones. Of them, 120 are in the extremities (lower 60, upper 60), 117 in the trunk (pelvic cavity 5, sides 72, back 30, chest 8, collar-bone 2), and 63 above the clavicles (neck 9, wind-pipe 4, jaws 2, teeth 32, nose 3, palate 1, ears 2, temples 2 and cheeks 2, 6 in the cranium).

Bones in the body are of five main types : (1) kapāla (flat), in the knee-joints, shoulders, hips, cheeks, palate, temples and cranium; (2) ruchaka (lustrous), for example, the teeth; (3) taruna (cartilaginous) in the nose, ears, throat, and eye-sockets; (4) valaya (curved or irregular) in the wrist, ankles, sides, back, chest and abdominal regions; and (5) nālaka (long and tubular), the remaining bones (avaśishṭāni) (*SS,* śārīra, 5, 21).

Bones are further divided into (a) movable (chala, diarthrosis), such as those in the four extremities, waist and jaws, and (b) immovable (sthira, synarthrosis), the rest of the bones (although some of them have slight movement). There are also 210 joints (sandhi, articulation) of bones, 68 in the extremities, 59 in the trunk, and 83 in the neck and in the region above it. Joints are classified according to their forms (hinged, ball-and-socket, raft, seam-like, crow-beak, circular, conch-shell-involution and so on) and locations (finger-joints, knee-joints, elbows, shoulder-joints, hip, anus, neck, spinal column, and so on) (ibid., 22-28).

Among the diseases pertaining mainly to bones are hypertrophy of bones (adhyasthi) and of teeth; tearing pain in bones and in teeth, colicky pain in bones and teeth, pathological conditions of hair and nails. [*See* also DHĀTU]

Ātaṅka : Disease, ailment. More specifically anguish, born out of the realization that one, being diseased, is no longer capable of normal living (with regard to food, conduct, enjoyment); it brings into bold relief the fact that ill-health makes life miserable (taki kṛcchra-jīvane). [*See* DISEASE]

Ātman: In the philosophical context of Āyurveda, soul (ātman) has been accepted as distinct from the psychophysical complex known as the body and as responsible for the feeling of 'I' (egoity), actions, experiencing the fruits of actions, passage from one body to another, and memory in the individual (*CS*, śārīra, 1,52). It is different from the purusha, who is a conglomeration (rāśi) of twenty-four material categories of existence, and who is produced by the actions prompted by ignorance, intentions and aversions (*See* PURUSHA).

But the soul that is relevant to the medicinal framework is an empirical one, namely, as an agent of cognition (jñah) when associated with the five faculties of sensation (indriya), mind (manas) and individual but undifferentiated consciousness (buddhi) (*CS*, ibid., 54). The soul that is devoid of the association with these factors is of no interest to the Āyurvedic physician; it simply does not exist ('na hy eko vartate', *CS*, ibid., 58). Although it is conceded that the soul by its nature is free from modifications (nirvikārah, devoid of pathogenicity), and eternal, he becomes the cause of consciousness (chaitanye kāraṇaṁ) when associated with the mind, specific properties of the primary forms of matter and the sense-faculties (*SS*, sūtra, 1, 56).

Consciousness is a quality that the material aggregates altogether lack. Aggregates are collectively called corpus or field ,'kshetra', namely, all that is excluded from the unmanifest, 'avyakta' and this is the significance of soul as the principle of consciousness (chetañavān) that lights up this corpus (hence, kshetrajña); and is therefore, the cause of all action (*CS*, ibid., 65 and 76).

The empirical soul (bhūtātmā) is unitary, but altogether beyond comprehension by the instruments of cognition. It is all-pervasive, but individualized owing to association with the sense-organs which in turn are associated with phenomenal objects. It is a witness (drashtā, *SS*, sūtra, 1,56; and sākshī, *CS*, śārīra, 1,83) of all actions and modes of being.

According to *Charaka-Saṁhitā* (śārīra, 3,8-10) the foetus is derived from the soul, and gets the designation 'jīva' (individualized soul). It is owing to this that the individual takes birth in a particular womb (yoni), has specific life-span (ayus), is aware of himself (ātma-jñāna), has a mind (*manas*) and sense-organs (indriyāni), inhales and exhales (prānāpānau), can motivate and sustain the sensory-functions (prerana and dhāranā, *Chkp* 'indriyēnā eva'), acquires a definite form (ākrti-viśesha) and complexion (varna-viśesha), experiences pleasure and pain (sukha-duhkhe),has desires and aversions (icchā-dveshau), consciousness (chetanā), perseverence (dhṛti), intellect (buddhi), memory (smṛti), ego (ahaṁkāra) and can exert himself (prayatna) (*CS*, ibid. 10).

"Along with the body (śarīra) and mind (sattva), the soul (ātmā) constitutes the tripod of life (tridaṇḍa), sustaining the phenomenal world. This indeed is the sentient purusha, the subject-matter of medicine" (*CS*, sūtra, 1,46-47). This soul is located in the heart (hrdaya), along with the chyle (raśa), the three doshas, intellect (buddhi) and mind (sattva). (*CS*, sūtra, 30,4, 'hrdi samsrtam,' cf. also *CS*. chikitsā, 24, 35). [*See* PURUSHA, SĀMKHYA]

Atyagni: Meaning excess of fire, it refers to the abnormal condition of digestion, when the digestive fire (jātharāgni) is excited by the prevailing influence of pitta. Even large quantities of food ingested frequently, are quickly digested. The condition is also called tīkshṇāgni (severe fire) or bhasmaka (reducing food to ashes). Digestion in this case is followed by conditions like parched throat, lips, palate, along with heat and burning sensations. [*See* AGNI, JĀTHARAGNI, DIGESTION, PITTA]

Aupamya: Knowledge derived from the observed similarity between things (analogical reasoning) like the rigidity of the muscles (in the disease called dandaka) and the rigidity like that of a stick (danda), the bow-like posture of the body (in the disease called dhanus-sthaṁbha) and the shape of a bow (dhanus), and the efficiency of a good physician and the efficiency of a clever archer (*CS*, vimāna, 8,42). [*See also* PRAMĀNA]

Aushadhi: Derived from oshadhi ('medicinal herb') the word is generally employed for all drugs, especially of vegetable origin. According to *Charaka-Samhitā* (sūtra, 26,12), there is no substance in the world which does not have some medicinal use but one must consider the method of use (yukti, *Chkp.* upāya) and the purpose (artha, *Chkp.* prayojana) or the disease-condition before employing any substance as a drug; careful selection of the substance is therefore indicated. Some substances need to be treated before they can be wholesome for the body; otherwise their effect would be undesirable. Certain combinations of substances are generally unsuitable for the body in normal health but they can be pressed to an advantage in some disease conditions. Even poisons have a therapeutic value, provided one knows how and when to use them. Generally, the considerations for the selection of a substance as a drug include the nature of the substance, the nature of the disease, time of the year, place where the patient resides, his habits of food and conduct and so on (*Chkp* on the above).

Drugs are effective owing to several factors. Some drugs become effective in certain conditions by their very nature (like dantī, *Baliospermum montanum,* as a purgative, and precious stones as anti-toxic); some by their specific properties (like drugs of bitter taste and coldness in fever); some by both of the above factors (like cow's milk boiled with a gold ring in it acts as an aphrodisiac). [*See* MEDICINE]

Avalehya : Meaning extract or electuary, it is a medicinal preparation meant to be licked or lapped up by the tongue (from *lih,* 'to lick'). It acquires the consistency of a thick paste, suitable for licking, after the strained decoction (kvātha) is boiled down; sugar or jaggery is added to it. It is also called leha or prāśa. [*See* CONFECTIONS]

Avastha-Pāka : Also called 'pra-pāka' (preliminary digestion), the term signifies the digestive process in the gastro-intestinal tracts in three successive stages (avasthā) (*CS* 6,15,9-11). *Chkp* describes this as the sequence of 'subtle digestion' (anu-pākakrama). The three stages are : (1) 'sweet' cooking (madhura), when the frothy kapha (gelatinous mucus) emerges, also called the undigested stage (āma-avasthā); (2) transformation into sour taste (amla-bhāva or acidulation), which is subsequent to the above (paraṁ). As the food is pushed downwards from the āma-region (stomach) owing to the action of the biomotor force or vāyu, the pellucid non-solid pitta (accha-pitta, *Chkp* gives aghane as the synonym of accha) arises. The stage is described as 'partly digested' (vidagdha or pakvāpakva); and the region is known as pachyamāna-āśaya (duodenum), which is native to pitta; and (3) the final transformation into pungent taste (katu), when the partly digested food is pushed into the pakva-āśaya (small intestine) where the faecal matter is formed as a byproduct of complete digestion, (paripindita-pakva, *Chkp* 'mala-rūpatayā pakva'), dried up by the 'digestive fire'. The uprising of vāta takes place at this stage.

The three doshas emerge in accordance with the prevailing tastes of the food as it is digested in the three regions of the digestive tract : kapha in the first region when sweet taste prevails, pitta in the second region when sour taste prevails; and vāta in the third region, when pungent taste prevails. The region of the sweet taste is said to be in the area above the heart; the kapha that arises here provides strength to the body. The region between the heart and the navel is the area of the sour taste; pitta arises here. Below the navel region, which is the region of pungent taste, is where the vāta is generally (prāyah) generated; (cf. *Chkp* on *CS* 6,15,11; cf. also *AHṛ,* 2,3,55-58). It is the region in which digestion takes place that determines the taste and the dosha.

Fold is completely digested here, and got ready for vipāka (also called nishṭhā-pāka). [*See* VIPĀKA] Chakrāpani argues that kapha and pitta are aroused and increased in the digestive stage (avasthā-pāka), whereas in the post-digestive stage of assimilation (nishthā-pāka) the production of the doshas is in the form of faecal matter (mala-rūpatayā) (on *CS*, NS., p.513). [*See* DIGESTION]

Āyus : The literal meaning is duration of life; but as the subject-matter of Indian medicine (Āyurveda), it means 'life' or 'the quality of life' : beneficial (hitaṁ), not beneficial (ahitaṁ), happy (sukhaṁ) and unhappy (duhkhaṁ). (*CS* sūtra, 1,41). The aim of Āyurveda is to make known this quality of life, and the conditions which contribute to a beneficial and happy life. The physician's skill consists in transforming the unhappy quality of life to a happy one, that is, free from diseases which torment the body and mind. The happy quality of life is that which helps one to accomplish the three objectives of life, namely, virtue, wealth and enjoyment; unhappiness in life is what interferes with this.

Life (jīvita) is the organization (saṁyoga) of body (śarīra) and soul (jīva). The span of time that is distinguished by the continuation of this organization is the duration of life (āyu) (*BP*), which in the present day (asmin kāle) is for human beings optimally a hundred years. The *Charaka-Saṁhitā* (sūtra, 1,42) defines life as the organization of body (śarīra), organs of sense (indriya), mind (sattva), and self (ātmā) as the operative principle of conscious organization (jñāna-pratisandhātā). The body is material, being composed of five primary forms of matter (bhūta); and so are the sense organs. Although the structure of the body includes the sense-organs, they are mentioned separately in the above definition because of their transactional importance (*Chkp* on *CS*, ibid., 42) for the self; sense organs are the instruments of action and experience. Mind makes action and experience possible. The organization of these factors is governed by an unseen force (adṛshṭa-niyantrita, *Chkp,* ibid).

The organization of body, mind and self is likened to a tripod (tri-danda), and the entirety of the behaviour of living beings rests on this (*CS*, ibid, 46). Each of the three constituent factors is indispensable for life and for all actions in life.

The *Charaka-Saṁhitā* enumerates several synonyms for life or vital power, each emphasizing an aspect of this organization : (1) 'upholder' (dhāri), for the organization supports the body and does not allow it to disintegrate and decay while it lasts; (2) 'life' (jīvitam), for it renders the body alive by bringing into being the 'life-breath' (prāna); (3) 'constant mover' (nitya-ga), for it constantly moves out of the body, which is transient (*Chkp*); or 'constant companion' for it is invariably present in all the various functions of body and mind, and in development (chaya) or decay (apachaya); and (4) 'uninterrupted continuity' (anubandha), amidst a succession of bodies during the course of transmigration.

Life is said to rest on three factors even as a house on pillars: food, sleep and restraint in sexual activity (*CS*, sūtra, 11,35; also *AHr*, sūtra, 7,52). When endowed with health, strength and vitality, then bodily vigour, complexion, building up of the body, elimination of waste and so on are accomplished. Disturbances in the body are caused by deficient, excessive or improper indulgence of these three.

The physician is required to examine carefully the 'vital power' (life) of the patient before he commences his treatment, for only if the vital power is adequately present, treatment is likely to be successful (*BP*, I,5,1). Patients in this context are classified as 'long-lived' (dīrghāyu) or 'spent lives' (gatāyu). The patient whose senses function in a reasonably efficient manner, who has adequate warmth in the body, who is not troubled by excessive thirst or by perspiration, nor by any thick phlegm in the throat or by high temperature, whose tongue is soft, who breathes only through his nostrils, who sleeps well in the night, and whose body has a bright complexion belongs to the former group; and he can profit by treatment.

The patient who hears sounds when no one else hears them, or does not hear sounds that others can hear, who takes hot things for cold and cold things for hot, shivers with cold while the body has a high temperature, cannot feel the touch or pressure, cannot smell properly, sees bright light in darkness or dull light during day-time, who sees visions in the sky and whose body loses its normal lustre belongs to the latter group; treatment is not likely to save his life in this case (*BP*, ibid.).

The life-span of an individual is determined by two factors working together: 'fate' (daiva, past actions) at the moment of conception and 'effort' in later life (purushakāra, present actions). A strong 'fate' invariably overcomes 'effort', but a weak 'fate' can be overcome by effort (*CS*, vimāna, 3, 28-33). Therefore, the life-span is not always predetermined, and one should not despair or be reckless. It is possible to prolong one's life by his 'effort' on proper lines, or cut short his life by negligence and bravado, unless 'fate' is very strong (*CS*, ibid., 36). [*See* ARISHTA, ĀYURVEDA, BODY]

B

Bath : A daily bath in the morning is recommended in the Āyurvedic manuals as hygienically sound, and the Smṛti texts insist that a bath is obligatory before any ritual. Among the virtues of a daily bath that are listed in the texts are : it gives strength, increases appetite, invigorates the digestive process, nourishes the body, gives a long life, increases the vitality (ojas), improves the semen and cheers the mind. It also cleans the body, clears the skin of dirt and itches, reduces morbid heat in the body, removes drowsiness and fatigue, eliminates thirst and inflammation, diminishes the effect of toxins (visha), helps reduce fat, and improves eyesight.

A bath generally means bath over the head. And cold water is to be preferred, except in winter and spring when tepid (koshṇa) water may be used. When one is fatigued by manual labour or tired after a journey, hot water is advantageous; but habitual bathing in hot water is bad for the eyes. A bath in tepid water is beneficial to all three doshas and pacifies all the seven body constituents (dhātus). A bath in very hot water is positively harmful: as it aggravates pitta and impairs health. A bath in cold water is especially recommended in conditions such as biliousness, burning sensations, giddiness, fainting spells, toxic states, blood impurities, haemoptysis,swelling of body, putrefaction of food in the stomach (without digestion), dryness of mouth and throat, and hangover after excessive drinking of alcoholic beverages. A bath in cold water, which must be had only in the morning, corrects the disturbances of vāta and kapha.

However, an oil bath or bath (over the head) of any sort is not indicated in fever, aggravation of kapha, dysentery, indigestion, constipation, chronic diarrhoea, loss of consciousness, consumption, asthma, diseases of the head, eyes, ears and nose. [*See also* HYGIENE, DAILY-ROUTINE].

A bath in hot water after rubbing the whole body (and especially the head) with oil (produced from sesamum or other vegetable seeds) is known as abhyaṅga. Applied first to the head, oil has a beneficial influence on the whole system, spreading to all parts through the internal channels (srota) (*Chkp*). It tends to soothe the skin, the cutaneous pores, veins and arteries. "Even as water poured at the roots would help sprouts to grow on the tree, oil applied on the head and on the body would help grow the body constituents" (*SS*). [*See* ABHYAṄGA].

Among the benefits of regular abhyanga are : it prevents aging, equalizes the body constituents (dhātu), pacifies vāta, cures intractable headaches, invigorates the sense-organs, improves eye-sight, physical strength and mental cheer, makes the skin bright, soft and free from dirt, removes fatigue, facilitates sleep, acts like a hair-tonic (preventing hair from falling or greying, and making the hair-roots firm), and refreshes the individual (*Mpn*).

Oil is recommended to be applied especially on the head, with the above advantages. Oil drops also may be introduced into the ears, to remove torticollis, lock-jaw, deafness, and the aggravated vāta. Oil may also be rubbed into the feet to prevent roughness, dryness, numbness, strain and cracking of feet; it will remove sciatica and constriction of vessels and ligaments of the feet and legs; it will also improve eye-sight.

However, abhyaṅga is contra-indicated in conditions of recent fever or indigestion (which are aggravated and become obstinate due to abhyanga). Those who vomit (or are made to vomit, as a curative procedure) and those who have taken purgatives (virikta) and douches (nirūḍha) should avoid abhyanga, as it will lead to a loss of the digestive power (*RJN*).

Abhyaṅga in the sense of rubbing oil over the body is recommended as beneficial after physical exercise. It is said not only to enhance the good effects of exercise but also to prevent aggravation of the doshas. According to *SS* (chikitsā, 24, 13-23), application of oil to different parts of the body (face, head, ears, and so on) invigorates the local areas (preventing wrinkles on the face, causing growth of thick, soft and luxuriant hair, preventing ear-ache), and also benefits the entire system, because the oil applied on the surface of the body is soon absorbed by the capillaries which are present all over the surface of the body and conveyed to the general system (*SSSS*).

Bhaishajya : Meaning the activity pertaining to medicines and curative procedures (bhaishaja, from bhishag, 'physician', 'healer'), the expression signifies all healing methods, including rituals and incantations, which are conducive to health (*CS*, sūtra, 1,134). Its synonyms are bheshaja, agada, aushadha and āyurdravya (*VRM*). [*See* MEDICINE].

Bhaishajya-Kalpanā : [*See* PHARMACY]

Bhasma: These are medicinal preparations once extensively used in Indian medicine and even now widely employed in the Siddha system of medicine. [*See* SIDDHA SYSTEM] They are alkaline ashes (calx prepared by a process of calcination) derived from organic as well as inorganic substances. Vegetable drugs containing alkali ingredients are powdered coarsely, or cut into tiny bits and burnt until they are reduced to ashes. Such organic bhasmas are useful inasmuch as they are (unlike the crude organic drugs) available at all times, preserved for great lengths of time, ready-made; and they are as effective as the other preparations like liquid extracts and decoctions.

In greater use, however, are the mineral and metallic bhasmas, which involve physico-chemical action in order to activate inorganic substances. They are either activated principles (sattva) or organic chemical compounds (salts). Various medicinal herbs are allowed to act on metals and other inorganic substances, so as to transfer the herbal properties to the latter, and also to render innocuous the metallic poisons. Such preparations are regarded as easily absorbable in the human system and productive of a maximum effect in a minimum dosage. They also include interaction of two or more inorganic substances (like tin, vaṅga, and orpiment, haritāla), which is said to be more powerful in action. These preparations are less easily assimilated in the system, and may at times generate toxic symptoms.

Usually, bhasmas represent oxides of metals intended for internal use. Crude metals (such as gold, silver, copper and so on) are initially purified (by employing vegetable oils, fresh juices of plants, or decoctions of dry drugs) so that they become fit to be used medicinally. They are then made into small circular cakes, and dried before being roasted in a kiln-like structure (puṭa), oxidized and finally reduced into an extremely fine powder. A pinch of these reduced particles when gently put in water will float on the surface. If this test (vāritaraṇa) is satisfied, the bhasma is in a state to be easily assimilated in the general system and influences metabolism. There is another test, when the pinch of reduced particles is pressed between fingers, the pinch will be imprinted by the lines of the fingers, and the lines of the fingers will be filled with these particles (rekhā-pūrṇatā).

The reduction of the mineral or metallic substances into a completely calcinated and powdery form may sometimes require repetitions of calcination.

Well-known bhasmas include those of copper (tāmra), mica (abhraka), gold (svarṇa), iron (kānta), purified iron filings (loha), dross iron (maṇḍūra), lead (nāga), tin (vaṅga), corals (pravāḷa), conch-shells (śaṅkha), copper pyrites (svarṇa-mākshika) and yellow orpiment (tālaka). Animal products are also used for calcination (for example, deer's antlers in śṛnga-bhasma). [*See* PREPARATIONS, SINDURA]

Bhāvanā: Maceration of powders (vegetable or mineral) in various fluids (such as expressed juice, decoction and so on) of a quantity sufficient to moisten and cover the powders entirely : the mixture is then dried in the shade (cf. *SaS,* II,6,6). The whole process takes a day-and-night (namely, twenty-four hours) to be completed. It is usual for the process to be repeated several times (two to seven) and in several fluids, so that the mass that results has in it the active principles of all the drugs and the fluids.

Bhishak: Literally 'one who frightens away the disease' ('bibheti rogo yasmāt'). The word signifies a physician or healer, who prevents the occurrence of diseases, cures the diseases when they occur and thus accomplishes all objectives (*CS,* sūtra, 1, 135). His function is to maintain the health of people and restore their health when disturbed (*CS*, ibid.; 134).

The physician must be learned in the classical texts of medicine, and must undergo practical training under competent masters. One who is both learned and trained will be successful as a physician. If he is merely learned, he will be frightened when a patient approaches him, even as a coward would be on the battle-field; if, on the other hand, he is merely trained, he would be rash and will not be respected. Like a bird, flying with both wings, the physician must be both learned and trained. Drugs given by an ignorant or untrained physician may be indeed efficacious, but the patient must avoid such a physician, as those drugs when used by such a physician may turn harmful (*SS*, sūtra, 4, 47-51).

Medicine, which is the main cause of cure, needs to be properly selected and administered; and this is done by the physician. Hence the importance of consulting a physician.

The physician occupies the leading position in the four-fold props of medical practice [*See* PROPS OF MEDICAL PRACTICE] (*CS*, sūtra, 9,10). He must interest himself in the ideological framework (śāstra), in understanding the import thereof (artha-vijñāna), in the practical application of that knowledge (pravṛtti), and in actual practice of the medical profession (karma-darśana). This is how he can become a 'saviour of lives' (prāṇābhisara). He must be familiar with diagnostics, aetiology, therapy and prevention of diseases, for these constitute the four aspects of treatment (*CS*). The physician must constantly refresh his intellect for the sake of effective treatment. His knowledge must include textual acquaintance (vidyā), rational approach (vitarka), special knowledge with insight (vijñāna), good memory (smṛti), devotion to the profession (tatparatā) and continuous effort (kriyā). Such a physician is never unsuccessful; and he is the one who bestows happiness on living beings (*CS*, ibid., 18-23).

'Being master of only one branch of learning' (namely, medicine) no one is able to ascertain the real import of learning. Therefore, the physician must be acquainted with several disciplines and see which are interconnected with his own chosen branch of study and practice. He must also reflect on them and endeavour to apply them in his practice. The physicians who neglect to be well and widely informed and who are indifferent to the practice are in truth thieves and robbers' (*SS*, sūtra, 4,7-8). [*See* PHYSICIAN]

Bhrūna: [*See* FOETAL DEVELOPMENT]

Bhūta-Vidyā: One of the eight branches of Āyurveda, devoted to the treatment of diseases which are mainly mental. The classical description is 'the pacification of demons, ghosts, elves, nymphs, ancestral spirits, reptile spirits, planetary deities, and so on' (*SS*, sūtra, 1). But the symptoms are all psychological, and often the treatments prescribed are also rational. The physician is asked to examine the state of knowledge (jñana) of the patient, his behaviour (cheshṭā), speech (vāk), bodily strength (bala), courage (paurusha) and other details (*AHr*, uttara, 4). Eighteen kinds of diseases in this category are recognized, and the lunar period in which each of them gets aggravated is also mentioned (*AHr*, ibid., and *Vaidyasangraha*, 4).

Blood: Literally 'coloured', 'reddened' (from rañj), the word rakta signifies blood, one of the seven body constituents (dhātu). [*See* DHĀTU] It is formed from chyle (rasa), which in turn is derived from the assimilated food in the body when rañjaka-pitta [*See* PITTA, DOSHA] acts upon it. The blood's chief function is to nourish the other body-constituents (muscle, adipose tissue, bone, bone-marrow and semen), as it is circulated in the body by the heart [*See* HEART] in specific channels [*See* SROTAS]. Blood is responsible for the bodily strength and the glow of complexion. It brings into being muscle as a body-constituent. The amount of blood in the body is sufficient to fill open and hollowed hands placed side by side (añjali) eight times. [*See* DHĀTU, RAKTA]

Body (Human): Called 'śarīra' (from śīryate, 'easily broken down' or śriyate, 'supports') The body is the foundation for consciousness (chetanādhishthāna), the abode of experiences for the self (ātman) and a conglomeration of the five primary forms of matter and their modifications (*CS,* śarīra, 6). The background for the Āyurvedic concept of body is to be found in the Sāṁkhya system [*See* SĀṀKHYA], where the conglomeration of the eight forms of prakṛti (the five primary forms of matter, namely, earth, water, fire, air and ākāśa; the unmanifest ego and consciousness) and the sixteen modifications thereof (vikāra, five organs of sense, five organs of action, five objects of sense-perception and mind) provide the material cause (upādāna-kāraṇa) for the body. Together with purusha (the principle of consciousness), which occurs as the self (ātman), thus vitalizing by its presence the otherwise inert conglomeration of the eight-fold prakṛti and sixteen vikāras, and providing the subjective framework to it, we have twenty-five categories (tattva), the working model of which is the human body that is alive and conscious. The self functions as the unifying cause (samavāyi-kāraṇa) for this complex of categories known as the body.

The commingling of the semen (śukra) and ovum (śoṇita) in the mother's womb is regarded as the efficient cause (nimitta-kāraṇa) for the human body. It is in the womb that the eight-fold prakṛti and the sixteen modifications are 'possessed', 'ridden', or made interdependent (saṁmūrcchitam, *SS,* śarīra, 5,3) by the self. In fact, what is called foetus is the enlivened mass of prakṛti and its modifications. The presence of the self in the womb is responsible for the developmental process that is inherent in the foetus. The self, is thus intimately involved in the developmental experiences and assures the survival of the mass of prakṛti and its modifications known as jīva-ātmā, whose energy (to enliven the body, to endow awareness on it, and to generate behaviour, volition and cognition) is represented by the vital currents (prāṇa). The coexistence of the vital currents and the physical complex of prakṛti and its modifications is the necessary and sufficient condition for the body to discharge its normal functions. The individual body, thus, is known as shaḍ-dhātuka ('made up of six constituents', namely, the five primary forms of matter, the mahābhūtas, and the self as the sixth).

The five primary forms of matter help the foetus grow : ākāśa provides space and scope for changes and growth; 'air' helps the structuring of the physical mass into parts, organs and limbs, constituents (dhātu) and by-products (mala); 'fire' helps metabolism and mutation of the tissues; 'water' moistens and cools the mass, and eliminates the heat and violence involved in metabolism and mutation; and 'earth' stabilizes the organization and provides firmness and form to the mass (*SS,* ibid).

When the foetus, in this manner, develops all its organs and limbs (that is, hands, feet, tongue, nose and so on), constituents and byproducts, it is called the 'human body' (śārīra). The human body has six main parts (aṅga): four extremities (śākhās, upper two arms, and lower two legs), the middle portion or trunk (madhya), and the head (śirah) (*SS,* ibid.). The different members of the body or limbs are called 'pratyaṅgas', like the head, the belly, the back, the navel, the forehead, the nose, the chin, the bladder, the throat, the nostrils, the shoulders, the heart, the liver and spleen, the kidney and so on.

There are also networks of nerves, arteries, veins or ducts (śirā, dhamanī), channels of circulation (srotas), bones and their joints (asthi), visceral cavities (koshṭha), muscles and ligaments (peśi, snāyu, kūrcha), tendons (kaṇḍara) and sutures (sevanī). The three bodily doshas (vāta, pitta, kapha) and the seven body constituents (dhātu, chyle, blood, tissue-fat, muscle, bone, bone-marrow and semen) are also included in the enumeration of the members of the body.

The limbs and organs are enumerated and described with reference to their locations, structures and functions in the Āyurvedic texts, especially in Suśruta-Saṁhitā (śarīra, 4-7). Generally, the list of organs is given as below (*VSS*) : the basic structures for sensory apprehension (adhishṭhāna), 5; the actual sense-organs (buddhīndriya) 5 (ears, eyes and so on); the organs of action (karmendriya) 5 (hands, feet and so on); the heart as the seat of consciousness (hṛdaya) 1; the seats of the vital currents (prāṇa, head, throat, heart, umbilicus, anus, bladder, vitality, semen, blood and flesh) 10; the visceral cavities (koshṭha, umbilicus, heart, lungs, liver, spleen, kidneys, urinary bladder, pelvic colon, stomach, colon, rectum, anus, small intestine, large intestine and omentum) 15; members like navel, thighs and so on (pratyaṅgāni, like calves, muscles of thighs, buttocks, testicles, phallus, groins, hips, pelvis, abdomen, breasts, muscles of arms, chin, lips, gums, palate, tongue, cheeks, ear-orifices, eye-orbits, and so on), 56; the tendons and ligaments (snāyu) 900; the veins, arteries, etc (sirā) 700; the ducts etc. (dhamanī) 200; muscles (peśī) 500; the vital spots, (marmasthāna) 107; bones (asthi) 300 (according to *SS,* 360, according to *CS*); bone-joints or articulations (sandhi) 200.

The body constituents (dhātus)and other essential substances in the normal individual occur in specific quantities (measured in terms of añjali or 'cupped hands, joined' of the individual himself); chyle (assimilated food), 9 añjali; blood, 8 añjali; faecal matter, 7 añjali; kapha, 6 añjali; pitta, 5 añjali; urine, 4 añjali; unctuous portion of muscle or muscle fat (vasā), 3 añjali; fat or adipose-tissue (medas), 2 añjali; bone-marrow (majjā), 1 añjali; fat inside the skull (mastishka), semen (śukra) and phlegmatic vitality (ślaishmika-ojas) each ½ añjali; (*CS,*śarīra, 7,15).

These parts of the body are dominated by one or more of the five primary forms of matter: gross, stable, heavy, hard and rough parts (like bones, teeth, nails, skin, tendons, and smell and olfaction) by earth; liquid, mobile, slow, unctuous, soft parts (like chyle, blood, muscle-fat, urine, sweat, kapha and pitta, tastes and gustation) by water; warm, colourful and lustrous substances (like pitta, body-colours) and vision by fire; bodily processes (like breathing in, breathing out, opening and closing of eyes, contraction, expansion, locomotion, retention), touch and tactile faculty by air; and sounds, open spaces within the body, speech, subtle tubular vessels and auditory organs by ākāśa (*CS,* ibid, 16).

While the major organs and limbs of the body could be identified and enumerated, minute and subtle units (paramāṇu) are actually innumerable and beyond sensory apprehension. They combine and separate, in order to actualize the bodily processes as a result of vāta uniting with the nature of the impact of past actions (karma-svabhāva) (*CS,* ibid., 17).

In general, the human body is regarded as composed of six main parts (aṅga): the four extremities (arms and legs), trunk (the middle portion and the head), called respectively śākhā, madhya and śiras (*SS,* śarīra,5, 3). There are also specific limbs (pratyaṅga): head, back, navel, forehead, nose, chin, bladder and throat (one of each); ears, eyes, nostrils, eyebrows, temples, shoulders, cheeks, armpits, breasts, testes, sides, buttocks, arms, thighs, knee-joints and so on (two of each); fingers and toes (ten of each); internal channels (srotas) (nine in number) (distinguished from the above which are visible from outside) such as eyes, ears, mouth, nostrils, anus and urethra (in males and in females, milk-ducts 2 and channels to carry off the menstrual fluid in addition to the above) all of which are outward-oriented. (*SS,* ibid., 4).

There are also skin (with seven layers) kalās, the seven body-constituents (dhātus), waste-products (mala) like urine, faeces and sweat, the three doshas (vāta, pitta and kapha), spleen, liver, lungs, colon, caecum heart, cavities (viscera), intestines and kidneys (*SS,* ibid. 6). [*See*, ĀTMA, BLOOD, BONE, DHAMANĪ, MARMA, ORGANS OF SENSE, PAÑCHABHŪTA THEORY, RASA, PEŚĪ, SĀṀKHYA, SIRĀ, SNĀYU].

Body-Constituents: [*See* DHĀTU]

Bone : Known as asthi (from as, 'to spread out'), it is one of the seven body-constituents (dhātu), derived from adipose-tissue (medas) when it is cooked in its own 'fire' and purified by 'wind'. It serves as the main prop (sāra) for the body, even as the sap is for the tree. It is heavy, rough, gross and stable. Therefore, it supports the entire body, and in particular the musculature.

The *Charaka-Saṁhitā* (śārīra, 7) and *Ashtānga-hrdaya* (śārīra, 3) enumerate 360 bones in the body, while *Suśruta-Saṁhitā* (śarīra, 5) counts only 300.They are located in the six main parts of the body: arms, legs, trunk and head. The enumeration of bones according to the *Charaka-Saṁhitā* takes this form:

Teeth 32, roots of teeth 32, nails 20, hands and feet 20, fingers and toes 60, heels 2, lower parts of palms 2, hand-joints 4, foot-ankles 4, elbows 4, lower parts of thighs 4, knees 2, knee-bends 2, upper parts of thighs 2, arms and shoulders 2, lower parts of the temples 2, palate 2, hips 2, pubic-bone 1, upper coccyx 1, lower coccyx 1, back 35, neck 15, clavicle 2, chin 1, lower jaw-bones 2, forehead 2, eyes 2, cheeks 2, nasal bones 3, ribs and spine 72, temples 2, head 4 and breast 17. [*See* ASTHI].

Bone-joint : Called sandhis, they are the joints of the bones. As the hard core inside the trunk supports the tree, so the bones, which are the pith (sāra) of the organism, support the body; and muscles attached to the bones firmly by means of veins (sirā) and ligaments (snāyu) keep the bones in their positions. The discrete bones discharge their functions as a result of the joints that are provided (*SS*, śarīra, 5,22).

Joints in the human body are 210 in number: 68 in the extremities (śākhā, arms and legs), 59 in the trunk (koshṭha), and 83 in the region above the clavicle (grīvaṁ pratyūrdhva). Joints are of two types: (1) movable (cheshṭāvantah, diarthrosis), namely those situated at the four extremities (hands and legs), in the waist and jaws; and (2) immovable (sthira, synarthrosis), and all the other joints of the body. (*SS*, ibid., 23).

Joints are classified into eight kinds according to their form: (1) kora (hinged or lap-shaped), like those in the fingers, wrists, ankles, elbows and knee-joints; (2) ud(l)ūkhala (ball and socket), like those in the axilla (shoulder-joint), jaw and hip; (3) sāmudga (back of the palm), like those in the region of anus, vagina, shoulders and hips; (4) pratara (raft or irregular), like those in the neck and the spinal column; (5) tunnasevanī (seam-like or dove-tailed), like those found in the pelvis and forehead; (6) vāyasatuṇḍa (crow's beak), like those on either side of the cheek-bones; (7) maṇḍala (circular), like those encircling the nāḍī of the heart, throat, eyes and bladder (kloman); and (8) śaṅkhāvarta (involutions of conch-shell), like those found in the ears and nostrils. [*See* BODY and BONE].

Brain : Acquaintance with the brain (mastishka) as an organ of cognition within the head (śiras) is as old as the *Atharva-veda* (for example, *AV*, 10, 2, 6, 8 and 26). The head was regarded as the most important of all the organs, for the vital centres as well as all the sensory functions are dependent upon it (*CS*, sūtra, 17,12). It (mūrdhā) was considered as one of the three centres of life in human beings [the other two being heart, (hrdaya) and bladder, (basti)] (*CS*, siddhi, 9,9).

Its importance was derived from the fact

that it was associated with the mind (manas), which was the regulating organ for the senses (*BS,* 6,8,2). According to this authority (Bhela), mind was located between the top of the head (śiras) and the palate (tālu) (ibid.). He distinguished manas from chitta, the latter being located in the heart [*See* MIND].

Besides the expression mastishka for the brain (as the seat of the mind and senses, according to *BS*), the *Charaka-Samhita* also uses the expression 'mastuluṅga' (meaning brain-matter) (*CS,* siddhi, 9,101). The two expressions, however, connote the same object, that is, the brain which is of the nature of an unctuous mass (*CS,* śarīra, 7,15 *Chkp* 'śirogata-sneha', the sneha of the cranium) and which weighs half an añjali (cf. *CS,* ibid. 'mastishkasya ardhāñjalih').

The *Suśrutā-Saṁhita* (chikitsā, 3, 47) takes mastuluṅga in the sense of brain, for it prescribes packing the wound by applying honey and ghee for seven days, when the skull (kapāla) has been fractured, without, however, injuring the brain (mastulungād vinā), but he omits to describe it as a fat-tissue (medas) when dealing with the 'medodhara-kalā' (*See* KALĀ) (*SS,* śarīra, 4, 12), as *Ashtāṅga-Saṁgraha,* for instance, does: "the sanguinous fat is called 'brain' in the head, concealed by the skull" ('tad eva śirasi kapāla-pratichannam mastishkākhyam mastulungākhyam cha', śarīra, 5, 37). [*See* MIND].

Buddhi: Literally 'that by which one knows or is aware' ('buddhyate anayā'), buddhi (from budh) is one of the inner instruments of cognition (antaḥ-karaṇa), by which one ascertains the specific characteristics of an object. It is distinguished from manas (mind) which is grouped under the sense-organs (indriya), by its determinate cognition.

Among the functions of buddhi are (1) perceptual knowledge (pratipatti), sleep which is suspension of desires and aversions (ishtānishtavipatti), deliberation and decision (vyavasāya), attention (samādhitā), and doubt (samśaya) (*Mahābhārata,* 'moksha-dharma'); or (2) perceptual knowledge (pramāna), erroneous cognition (viparyaya), imagination (vikalpa), sleep and memory (PATAÑJALI'S *Yoga-sūtra,* 1); or (3) intent application (śuśrūshā), verbal apprehension (śravana), cognition (grahana), retention (dhāranā), conjecture (ūhā), ratiocination (apoha), determination of import (artha-vijñāna) and abstract thinking (tattva-jñāna) (HEMACHANDRA. *Abhidhāna-chintāmani*). In Nyāya philosophy, buddhi which is pervasive in nature (vibhu) is of two types: objective experiences (anubhūti, namely, derived from sensory perception, inference, analogy and testimony) and memories (smrti) (*Bhāshā-pariccheda*).

Factors that interfere with the normal functioning of buddhi are sorrow, anger, avarice, passion, delusion, jealousy, envy, conceit, doubt, despondency and disgust (*Kālikā-purāna,* 18).

The heart is regarded as the seat of buddhi (chetanā) as well as of vitality (ojas) (*SaS,* 1,5,49; also *SS,* śarīra, 4, 30). When tamas overpowers the heart, sleep results (*SS,* ibid.). In the course of the foetal development, manas (which endows facility for sense-functions, which is responsible for desires and aversions, pleasure, pain and effort, (*Chakrapani* on *CS,* sūtra, 1, 49) appears at the fifth month, and buddhi in the sixth (*SS,* śarīra, 3, 35-36). [*See* MIND, SĀMKHYA].

C

Calx : [*See* BHASMA]

Channels : Called srotas, there are nine duct-like structures opening outward : two ears, two eyes, a mouth, two nostrils, the anus, and the urethra. Women have three more channels, opening outward: two breasts (for the outflow of milk to nourish the baby) and a duct to carry off menstrual blood (rakta-vaha).

The *Charaka-Saṁhita* (vimāna, 5, 9) mentions that sirā (vein), dhamanī (artery), nādī (nerve-channel), mārga (pathway), śarīra-cchidra (empty spaces in the body), sthāna (seat), āśaya (cavity) and so on are all synonyms to indicate spaces within the body for the body constituents to move about (dhātv-avakāśa). [*See* HUMAN BODY, SROTAS].

Chatushpāda : The expression signifies four essential ingredients of successful medical practice: the physician (bhishak), the drugs (dravyāni), the attendant or nurse (upasthātā) and the patient (rogī) (*CS,* sūtra, 9, 3). The meaningful and effective cooperation of these four aspects of therapeutics is likely to restore the equilibrium of the doshas that is lost in disease (*CS,* ibid. 5).

The physician must be learned in the medical texts, well trained in practice, dextrous and clean (in habits and mind). The drugs must be sufficient in quantity, suitable to the purpose, manifold in preparation, and rich in potency. The attendant must be well-versed in the art of nursing, dextrous, affectionate and clean (in habits and mind). The patient must be mindful, willing to follow the physician's instruction, confident of getting cured, and capable of communicating effectively with his physician (*CS,* ibid. 6-9). [*See* FOUR PROPS OF MEDICAL PRACTICE]

Chetana : Derived from the root chit ('saṁjñāne', 'to know') the word signifies consciousness that is individualized (viz. buddhi or mahat of the Sāṁkhya system): the means whereby one becomes aware of oneself and the things around ('chetayate anayā').

Life is described as a tripod (tridanda), the three props of which are the mind (sattva), the soul (ātman) and the body-complex (śarīra) (*CS,* sūtra, 1,46). The integration of the three units is the individual, the person (purusha), who is the principle consciousness (chetanā) and who is also the subject-matter of the science of medicine (adhikarana) (*CS,* ibid., 47). The entire world, in fact, consists of the five primary forms of matter (that is, the earth, water, fire and ākāśa, represented by the human body including the organs of cognition and action), the individual soul (ātman, including consciousness, buddhi and ego, ahaṁkāra, *Chkp* on *CS,* ibid., 47), the mind (manas), time, and space. The complex of physical factors becomes endowed with consciousness, when equipped with sense-faculties (five of cognition, five of action, and mind as the inner and common faculty); devoid of this equipment, it lacks consciousness (achetanam) (*CS,* ibid., 48).

The *Charaka-Saṁhitā* (sūtra, 1,35) speaks of 'the organized person' (rāśi-purusha) involving a multiplicity of units (twenty-four of them, *See* PURUSHA). The important unit in this organization, however is avyakta (or the unmanifest prakrti, including the purusha), which in fact integrates the constituents (melaka) and engenders experiences (bhoga-sampādaka) (*Chkp* on above). In the psycho-physical organization that is the individual, the five primary forms of matter comprehend all the units barring avyakta, and consciousness alone stands out as the sixth (*CS,* ibid., 16), that is, it is tantamount to avyakta. All the other units are inert, and, therefore, can serve only as 'tools' (karana) or instruments for the principle of consciousness (*CS,* ibid., 54); they are fields (kshetra) for this unmanifest principle to operate (jña) (*CS,* ibid., 65). This cognizing principle (kshetra-jña) is not universal and omnipresent in the medical context, but continuous and constant in individual life (*SS,* śarīra, 1,17).

The principal seat of consciousness is the heart (hrdayam, *SS,* śarīra, 4, 30 and 33) ; when this organ is overpowered by tamas (*See* TAMAS), sleep results, consciousness of oneself as well as of the world outside is suspended (*See* SLEEP). The initial involvement of consciousness in individual life occurs in the sixth foetal month (acc. to *SS,* śarīra, 3, 36; but acc. to *AHr,* śarīra, 1, in the fifth month). [*See* PURUSHA, MIND, BUDDHI, FOETAL DEVELOPMENT, SĀMKHYA].

Chikitsā: [*See* MEDICINE].

Chūrna : The word, derived from charv, 'to pound or powder', signifies the fine powder of a drug or the fine mixture of many drugs, which are cleaned, dried and then powdered separately. This form retains its potency for a year when well preserved. [*See* POWDER].

Chyle : [*See* RASA].

Confection : Thickened or concentrated solid or semi-solid extracts (avaleha, leha, 'to be licked', phanita, or rasa-kriyā; majūn, lavūk, javāriś, usārā in Yunani; confectio in Lat.), prepared by boiling on slow fire the already boiled decoction, expressed juice (after straining), until it becomes solidified or thick in consistency. The ingredients are dissolved, macerated, infused, or boiled in cold or hot water; the solution, infusion or decoction being evaporated. The indications of a properly prepared confection are : (1) it will not dissolve in water but will, on the other hand, sink and settle steadily when put in water; (2) it will be ductile when handled, it will be drawn out in continuous strands; (3) it will receive the impressions of coins on the fingers clearly; (4) it will not break into bits when it falls down; (5) it will be of fine colour; (6) it will emit a sweet smell; (7) it will evoke the proper taste when it comes into contact with the tongue and (8) it will become harder as it cools (*SaS,* II, 8,1-3).

If sugar is to be added, it should be four times that of the powder of the drugs; if jaggery, two times; if any fluid (water, milk, cow's urine), four times. The vehicles recommended for confection include milk, sugarcane juice, or some infusion or decoction, in accordance with the disease.

Considered under confections, khanda-pāka is a preparation where syrup is added to drugs in the form of a fine powder, stirring the whole over fire until an intimate mixture is obtained and reduced to fine consistency. [*See* PREPARATIONS].

Constitution: Constitution, comprehending both physical and mental characteristics, is an important consideration in Indian medicine. Called prakrti (a word of Sāṁkhyan origin, which means 'nature', a mosaic of the three gunas, namely, sattva, rajas and tamas), it means innate nature (svabhāva), character, temperament or disposition of a person. The word also means 'health' (ārogya), in the sense of the balance of the three doshas in the human constitution, that is, vāta, pitta and kapha (corresponding to the three gunas in nature) (*See* DOSHA). The three doshas being practically always unbalanced in any person, health becomes a matter of periodical disturbance and restoration of the practical balance of the three doshas.

In any person, one of the three doshas, two of them together or all three of them would be predominant, and accordingly constitutions are regarded as seven in kind: (1) dominated by vāta; (2) dominated by pitta; (3) dominated by kapha; (4) dominated by vāta and pitta; (5) dominated by vāta and kapha; (6) dominated by pitta and kapha; and (7) having all three doshas in equal proportions (*SS,* śarīra, 4, 61-62). The dominance of the doshas is determined at the moment of birth, and therefore constitutions are more or less unalterable.

The prevalence of the dosha or doshas at the time of the conception is explained thus. The three doshas pervade all over the body of every person, and determine his character, temperament, activities, and interests. They leave their impact on every tissue-cell. They are present in varying proportions in the sperm (śukra) of the male and in the ovum (śonita) of the female when they copulate. The condition of the doshas present in the two factors that unite (samyoga) in the uterus of the mother, as well as the condition of the doshas in the uterus itself determine the condition of the doshas in the zygote (that is, the person to be born). The prevalence of any dosha or doshas over the others (utkata) in the zygote stage is registered in the constitution of the newborn one (*SS*, ibid.). Thus the innate constitution is described as "determined and set into operation by the relative strengths of the doshas in the very first stage of development" (ādibala-pravṛtta).

Other factors that influence the formation of the original constitution of a person are also recognized: condition of the sperm or ovum, conditions prevailing in the mother's body (especially in her uterus) and mind, nature of the season in which the conception takes place, nature of the food eaten by the mother, regimen followed by her during the period of pregnancy, nature of the five primary forms of matter (mahābhūta) which go to constitute the foetus, family traits of the parents, locality in which the individual is born, time of the year when delivery takes place and the age of each of the parents.

When the foetus is perfectly healthy, the three doshas are in a state of complete balance (sama-prakṛti), with no dosha dominating over the others. Such a condition is rare. Usually, one or two of the doshas are moderately in excess over the others (miśra-prakṛti), without however jeopardizing reasonable health. Thus, possession of a particular constitution (characterized by the prevalence of one or two doshas) does not mean ill-health.

The constitution is an important consideration for the physician, as prevalence of one or other of the doshas in a person makes him prone to particular ailments. An individual, of vāta constitution usually succumbs to vātika-type of disease; diseases due to other doshas rarely bother him, and even if he gets them, they are usually cured. In the course of the treatment of any of his diseases, the physician takes care to prescribe drugs, food and conduct that do not aggravate the vāta-factor. Management of the patient is made possible by a knowledge of his constitution.

(1) A person with the vāta-constitution is recognized by the typical vāta-characteristics : ('ununctuous') dry and rough skin with cracks, emaciated body, dry and hoarse voice which is also low and broken, tendency to keep awake; ('light') light and jerky gait, inconsistent action, fondness for light and inconsistent food; ('mobile') unstable joints and eyes, jaws and tongue, head and shoulders, arms and legs, excessively active; ('abundance') prominent veins and tendons, talkativeness; ('quick') swift in actions and movements, quick to get irritated, quick in likes and dislikes, quick to understand and also to forget, and quick in the onset of morbid manifestations (fear, worry, and so on); ('cold') dislike for cold things, often getting spells of cold, shivering, stiffness; ('rough') rough and dry hair, scanty hair, coarse nails, rough teeth, face, hands and feet. He is short-tempered, timid, intolerant of merit in others, and fickle in friendship; and he is seen to bite his nails and gnash his teeth often. He talks more than he acts, and often talks nonsense, and his eyes flit from object to object. He loves music. His dreams are quick and fleeting, full of excitement. His disposition resembles that of a rabbit, mouse, dog, hawk, crow, or camel. He is generally moderate in wealth, has few

friends, and a moderate span of life (*SS*, ibid., 63-66).

Treatment of the diseases that usually afflict him necessitates oleation and fomentation, mild purgatives, diet of food articles that are hot, sweet and sour, massages, poultice, affusion, bath, use of fermented drinks and drugs (āsava), and various types of medicated enema. Methods of treatment involving surprise, fear and forgetting also help him.

(2) A person with the pitta-constitution manifests typical characteristics of pitta-dosha : ('hot') dislike of hot things, usually warm body (especially face and hands), tender and clear body, freckles on the skin, excessive hunger and thirst, premature greying of hair and onset of wrinkles, tendency towards baldness; ('sharp') sharp in tongue, show of strength, courage, good digestion, tendency to overact, quick in getting angry and quick also in cooling down; ('liquid') loose joints and soft muscles, evacuation (of urine and faeces) in large quantity, tendency to sweat much; ('fleshy smell') smell of axilla, mouth, head and body and ('pungent and sour') weakness of the sex urge and insufficiency of semen. He is endowed with moderate strength, and his span of life is also moderate. His memory is good, and intelligence is sharp. He has small eyes often reddish at the corners. His body colour tends to be yellowish, and his nails, tongue, and palms are coppery coloured. He dreams of burnished gold, red flowers, fire, lightning and violence. He is courageous, not easily shaken, and can give a fight; but he shows compassion towards those who seek his aid. His gait is unsteady and he often stumbles. His appearance and conduct remind one of serpent, owl, cat, monkey, tiger, bear or mongoose.

The management of the diseases that trouble the man with this constitution involve the use of ghee, oleation, purgation, use of diet and drugs which are sweet, bitter and astringent in taste, food articles that are cooling, frequent use of cold water, cooling garments, and cool flowers. Company of friends, and especially of women, music, residence in cool buildings open to moon-light and exposed to breeze, stroll in the garden, and soothing regimens are likely to hasten his recovery.

(3) A person with the kapha-constitution is recognized by traits typical of the kapha-dosha: ('unctuous') smooth and oily skin; ('soft') tender and clear complexion, pleasing appearance, large and bright eyes; ('firm') well-formed compact and muscular body, stability of bearing and gait, firmness in mind, endurance; ('dense') tendency towards plumpness of body and rotundity of organs; ('slow') slow in action, in eating food, and in movement; ('stable') endurance and forbearance (not easily irritated, nor impulsive in action), good memory, calculative in his reactions; ('heavy') walking with heavy steps (soles of feet planted firmly on the ground); ('cold') not inordinately hungry or thirsty, not sweating much, nor warm in body; ('clear') happy in his mood, pleasant in facial expression, delicate in complexion, gentle in speech, and very definite in his views and decisions. He is courageous and grateful, and is fond of articles of food that are sweet in taste. He is given to revering his elders and believing the religious scriptures. He tends to amass wealth, but is generous in outlook. His conduct reminds one of the behaviour of a lion, elephant, bull, eagle or swan.

Management of the diseases that afflict a person with this constitution involves hot and strong elimination therapies, intake of diet having ingredients that are ununctuous, pungent, bitter and astringent, use of fermented and medicated liquids preserved for a long time, and weight-reducing therapies, oil-massages and bath. Keeping awake during night, vigorous physical exercises like running, jumping and swimming, use of warm garments and indulgence in sex activity are likely to help the patient.

The constitutions that are marked by the prevalence of two doshas, · have characteristics typical of both doshas in equal proportion but in various combinations. [*See also* DOSHA]

Cure: Although all diseases are really one as a category, characterized by production of pain, they may be classified in different ways, according to their curability (sādhya), intensity (bala), location (āśraya, that is, body or mind), cause (nimitta) and the organ affected (āśaya) (*CS*, vimāna, 6,3). Curability of the disease is an important consideration for the physician.

Diseases are classified broadly into (1) curable (sādhya) and (2) incurable (asādhya). Curable diseases are further classified into (a) easily cured (sukha-sādhya) and (b) cured with difficulty (kṛcchra-sādhya). When the diseases are mild, symptoms are not complicated, the course of the disease is localized, the disease is of recent origin, the errant dosha is one only (the other two being normal) and the body is strong enough to undergo the treatment prescribed, then the disease is easily curable. When, however, symptoms are complicated, localization of disease is uncertain, the errant doshas are two in number, the disease has already spread, and the treatment involves surgery, cautery and so on, then the disease is curable with difficulty.

(1) The curable diseases are again classified into those that require mild treatment and for a brief period (alpa-chikitsā-sādhya), those where the treatment is moderate and the duration of treatment also is considerable (madhya-chikitsā-sādhya), and those that need drastic treatment involving a long period of time (ugra-chikitsā-sadhya).

(2) The incurable diseases are of two types: (a) those which can only be palliated, although not cured (yāpya); and (b) those which are altogether incurable and beyond measures of palliation (anupakramya). In the former, the patient would not have exhausted his life-span but disturbances of two of the three doshas would be so severe and the disease so deep-seated that it precludes any hope of permanent cure. The management of the disease within limits and for shorter or longer periods is possible by strong drugs and a strict regimen. The patient can be made to live with the disease and carry on the normal functions of life with some limitations. The latter are diseases where all the three doshas are severely disturbed, and where the course of disease has far advanced beyond recovery. All the parts of the body would have been affected by the disease, and sensory functions degenerated; there would also be symptoms of imminent death [*See* ARISHṬA *and also* DISEASES, DIAGNOSIS]

D

Daily Routine (Dina-Charyā): Indian medicine prescribes a wholesome daily routine or day-to-day conduct (dina-charyā), as not only prophylactic but conducive to the four objectives of life (virtue, wealth, enjoyment and liberation). All the medical manuals(for example *CS*, sūtra, 5, 7 and 8; *SS*, chikitsā, 24; *AS*, sūtra, 3 and *AHr* Āyushkāmīya, 2) treat this subject in considerable detail, and there is fair agreement with regard to major details. Many of the activities recommended in these texts as hygienic are also prescribed in the Smrti-texts as religious imperatives. The hygienic preoccupations covered under this head are said to have been taught by the ancient sages themselves, like ATREYA, (*AS*, 1,3,2) for preserving one's health (svāsthya) and promoting his spiritual welfare (dharma). Thus we find the details of the recommended routine widely in vogue in the country even to this day, especially among the folk belonging to the upper and middle classes, among whom spiritual welfare continues to be a major interest.

The recommended routine comprehends the day's requirements (both physical and mental) from the moment one gets up from a night's sleep till the day is finished and sleep comes. It covers all activities that man normally indulges in, instinctual, habitual, spontaneous, deliberate, life-preservative, aesthetically appealing, and professionally relevant; but the routine speaks of the conduct of common interest. The guiding principle is : 'good health must be preserved, and possible ailments must be prevented from occurring' (*CS*, sūtra, 5, 13). Health is the harmonious interaction of the bodily constituents so that the state of efficient normalcy is continued and the irritating anomalies are avoided (comm. on above).

One who would guard his health for a meaningful life (rakshārthām āyushah) should get up at 'early dawn' (brāhme muhūrte). Early dawn is the last watch of the night, immediately prior to sunrise at about 3.30 or 4 a.m. As soon as he wakes up at this time, he should carefully consider whether or not the food eaten during the previous day has been well digested (jīrnājīrṇe nirūpayan). The indication of good digestion is that he feels light. He should get up early only if he thus feels light. Having got up, he should attend to the calls of nature (śarīra-chintā), and finish his morning ablutions (śaucha-vidhi). Elimination of waste-products from the body early in the morning is regarded as extremely beneficent. But one should not force the bowels, but only eliminate what is ready to be eliminated ('pravartayet prachalitaṁ, na tu yatnād udīrayet'). One should not engage in any activity with burdened and ready bowels.

Cleansing the teeth comes in for elaborate consideration in the texts: the twigs of certain trees are recommended. Preparation of the tooth-brush is described; the number of times the teeth are to be brushed during the day (twice according to *CS*) is indicated and the manner of brushing the teeth and the diseases in which brushing of the teeth is not indicated are discussed. The tongue also is to be cleansed by a scraper (jihvā-nirlekhana) [*See* CARE OF TEETH].

Drinking cold water early in the morning, especially that which has been kept in a copper vessel during the night, is a favourite prescription (ushah-pāna) among the Indian physicians. [*See* USHAH-PĀNA].

The eyes are taken care of by applying an ointment of antimony sulphide (sauvīrāñjana) to the inner surface of the eyelids. Eyesight will thereby be keen, and colour-vision perfect (*See* CARE OF THE EYES).

Anointing the body with fragrant oil would help remove bodily odour, fatigue and stiffness of limbs; anointing the head with oil would strengthen the hair-roots, prevent headaches and facilitate sleep at night; oiling the ears would improve audition and keep the organ clean. Nasal treatment (nasya) by 'aṇu-taila' is recommended for preventing various kinds of nasal troubles, headache, and optical anomalies. It must immediately follow the application of ointment to the eye, for the two dhātus (kapha and vāta) excited by the application of the ointment would be pacified by the nasal treatment (*AHṛ*, 1, 3, 33).

Exercise (vyāyāma) is an important daily routine : it makes the body strong and light, facilitates digestion of food, and reduces fat; the limbs of the body become well-proportioned; it makes one enthusiastic and bright. But there are conditions in which exercise is not indicated. There are also dangers involved in excessive exercise [*See* EXERCISE]. Exercise must be followed by gentle body-massage (udvartana) : it eliminates excessive kapha, and reduces fat; it makes the limbs firm and strong and also renders the skin bright and firm.

Bath (snāna) is the next activity to be daily indulged in. It is a cleansing process : bodily dirt, perspiration, sensations of itching and scratching are thereby removed. It also invigorates the interior : the appetite is stimulated, vitality (ojas) and strength (bala) are increased. It eliminates fatigue and reduces heat in the body. Mind also is refreshed, by removing unwholesome thoughts and bringing in a measure of tranquility. While cold water is best for bath, it should not be so cold as to cause shivering. Alternately, warm water (not hot) is to be preferred. The head must be bathed in cold water, and warm water may be used from neck downwards. A bath with cold water should always begin with the head. One should not bathe for a few hours after food is taken. And a bath is not indicated in certain diseased conditions (like indigestion, rheumatism, flatulence and so on).

The intake of food (bhojana) is naturally an important detail in all discussions of health and hygiene. Books on Indian medicine contain invariably a wealth of information concerning the nutritional, corrective, and curative values of various articles of food taken daily. They also indicate what kinds of food are to be eaten, at what times of the day, in what bodily conditions, and in what seasons; what kinds of food are to be avoided and why. They provide particulars of the preparations of food also [*See* FOOD]. The general rule, however, is that food is to be taken moderately (mita), and that the food must be agreeable to one's taste and needs (hita).

Food is to be eaten preferably in solitude and silence; or alternately, in good and happy company, in a pleasant atmosphere, and in a tranquil state of mind, without indulging in loose talk or in heated arguments. Frequent intake of water while eating would interfere with proper digestion. Chewing betel leaves, areca-nut, camphor, and cardamom after food helps digestion and removes any bad odour from the mouth [*See* TĀMBULA]. There is a verse which suggests that buttermilk must be drunk after food is eaten, milk at the end of the day, and water in the morning.

Two meals a day are recommended as ideal, one around midday and the other early in the night (preferably in the evening before sunset). Eating inbetween (antarā-bhojana) can be harmful. Food during night must be light and easily digested. Physical or mental exercises soon after eating are to be avoided. While one should rest for a while after morning food, the night food must be followed by a leisurely walk (known as 'a hundred steps' śatapatha). Sleep during daytime (divā-svāpa) is not advisable, except in the hot season. And one should not go to sleep at night at least two hours after food is taken.

There are suggestions for good sleeping conditions and habits, like sleeping in the open but not all alone, going to bed with devout thoughts, and lying down on the left side of the body, being lightly dressed while asleep, having a pillow that is neither flat nor high, and a bed that is sufficiently wide, neither very hard nor soft, and so on [*See* SLEEP].

Evenings (sandhyā) are unsuited for food, sex-activity, sleep or study. Food eaten then would lead to disease, sex-activity indulged in would cause obstructed labour (mūdhagarbha), sleep would bring about misery and poverty, and study (svādhyāya) would cut life short. Evenings are meant for contemplation ('samyag dhyāyanti asmin iti sandhyā'). 'Sandhyā' is defined as the conjunction of day and night; it can be evening (sāyam-sandhyā) or dawn (prātah-sandhyā):

the common feature is the absence of the sun and the stars. Thus whatever is prohibited for the evening is also prohibited at dawn. Food and study are indicated for the day; sleep and sex-activity for the night.

The medical manuals also contain suggestions on a variety of topics connected with health-care, like the value of oil-bath, care of hair, use of mirror, manicure, uses of footwear, umbrella and walking-stick, wood out of which cots may be made, vessels in which the cooking utensils and plates may be made, cosmetics, flowers for decoration, jewels for decoration, and garments [*See* HYGIENE].

An important consideration in the daily routine is facilitating the natural tendencies of the body (vega). On no account must the urges like evacuation (urine, stool and semen), yawning, sneezing, thirst, hunger, flatulence, tears, sleep, panting after exercise and so on be suppressed. If the natural tendencies like these are checked, diseased conditions of the body may ensue (*CS,* sūtra, 7, 1-25). It does not, however, mean that no urge should be suppressed, and that life should be guided only by animal instincts. There are urges that eventually harm the body (like excessive sex-activity, overeating, immoderate sleep and so on and there are natural tendencies which are undesirable (like fear, worry, anger, harsh speech, violent adventure, quick impulses). These must of course be suppressed. In other words, each individual must exercise caution, and consider what tendencies should be allowed to be manifest and in what measure, and what tendencies must be suppressed, and how. The individual should take into account his age, general bodily condition, weather, season and the prevailing needs.

There is a verse which speaks of the broad outline of healthy daily routine : "One who sleeps on his left side (vāma-śāyī), eats twice only (dvi-bhuñjānah), urinates six times (shaṇmūtrī), evacuates twice (dvi-purīshakah), and indulges in sex-activity slightly (alpa-maithunah) will live for a hundred years". These are said to be the pillars of health : foods (āhāra), sleep (nidrā) and exercise (vyāyāma). Under the third category is included celibacy (brahmachārya) that is moderate sex-activity and not complete abstinence.

In general, the day must be so spent that the night's sleep will be comfortable [*See* EXERCISE, FOOD HYGIENE, PREVENTIVE MEDICINE, SUPPRESSION OF URGES, SLEEP DURING DAY].

Daiva-Vyapāśraya :One of the three major methods of treatment that goes back to a hoary past, and finds mention in *RV* as well as in *AV*. Distinguished from the other two viz. yukti-vyapāśraya (or rational medicine using drugs, other forms of treatment, and diet) and sattvāvajaya (or treatment by harnessing mental faculties and powers), this method relies heavily on divine intervention (daiva) (*CS*,sūtra, 11, 54).

In life, the divine or unseen element (daiva, CHKP adrshṭa, comprehends past actions and their dispositions; devāh, gods) and human effort (purusha-kāra) are together involved in health as well as in sickness. When the former is weak, human effort can surely counteract it; in any case, human effort is able to minimize the severity of disease caused by the daiva factors (*CS,* vimāna, 3,33). Diseases such as insanity, unmāda, epilepsy, apasmāra and childhood maladies like bālagraha, all of which cannot be ascribed to physical or mental causes are included in this category.

The treatment includes the employment of incantations (mantra), precious stones and sacred gems (maṇi), auspicious rituals (maṅgala), oblations (bali), gifts (upahāra), sacrifices (homa), penances (prāyaśchitta), fasts (upavāsa), benedictions (svastyayana), bowing before elders and divine beings (praṇipāta) and visits to sacred spots (gamana) etc., all of which are intended to counteract the force of unfavourable past actions (daiva) and to secure divine influence in order to eliminate the diseases. [*See* MEDICINE].

Death : Death is described as 'cessation of life' (prāṇa-viyoga). Life is the active organisation of the five primary forms of matter as foundation and the spirit as the conscious principle (*SS,* 1, 21; *CS,* 4, 6, 4). The Sāṁkhya thought looks upon life as the integration of purusha and prakṛti (the material nature of the universe as well as the body of living beings), the latter evolving 23 elements of the constitution. However, when this integration dissolves, the 24 elements are pulled apart, and death results. The Nyāya thought also regards death as the destruction of the union (saṁyogā-dhvaṁsa) of the soul with other substances. The dissolution of the active association in which the five primary forms of matter (constituting the physical frame) are found in life, is death. When the constituents of the body (that is, the dhātus) are slightly deranged,. disease is caused resulting in distress (kleśa). When, on the other hand, they are greatly thrown out of balance, the disease assumes incurable shape and death results(CHKP on *CS,* 4, 6, 4, NS ed.).

There are one hundred and one reasons for death in the human body; only one of them is natural (kāla-kṛta), while the other hundred are adventitious (āgantu) (*SS,* 1, 34, 6, the view of the Ātharvaṇas is cited). Natural death occurs when the life-span draws to a close prompted by the natural processes themselves (svabhāva-bala-pravṛtta). This is altogether an unavoidable event, and the physician's skill, or the drug's potency, is futile in this case.

The adventitious death is caused by the disturbances of the doshas and can be prevented by medicines (aushadhi), especially rasāyana, mystic repetitions and contemplation (japa, mantra) or by ritualistic oblations (homa) (Cf. *SS*, sūtra, 34, 7, where rasa and mantrā are suggested). It is, therefore, called 'untimely death' (akāla-mṛtyu), namely, death before the normal life-span is exhausted.

The physician is instructed to discern carefully whether the patient is long-lived (dīrghāyu), short-lived (alpāyu), or has a life-span which is neither long nor short (madhyamāyu). The maximum life-span of a human being is said to be one hundred and twenty years and five days [*See* AGE]. The idea about the length of the life-span is got by examination of the physical frame and the relative proportions of the limbs, ascertainment of constitutional peculiarites regarding the predominant dosha and knowledge about the unfavourable symptoms suggesting imminent death. (*SS,* sūtra, 35,3).

The cause of death is exhaustion of the life-span (āyu), of the merit responsible for life (puṇya) or of both (ubhaya). Even when the life-span or merit is not exhausted, death may occur as a result of improper food and conduct (*AHṛ,* 2,5,132). Another account enumerates, among the causes of death, wrong treatment and conduct (vishamopachāra), the force of past deeds (purākṛta-karma) and the transient nature of all life (anityatva) (*SS,* sūtra, 31,30). Wrong conduct leading to death (vishamopachāra), includes undertakings beyond one's physical capacity, refusal to be treated when ill, complete suppression of normal physical urges, and forceful elimination of waste. Wrong treatment presupposes the ignorance of the constitutional peculiarity of the patient and administration of drugs inimical to him. The force of past deeds expresses itself in fatal accidents. The third cause of death is natural.

Clinically, death is described as due to the internal fire (agni) being extinguished. It is this fire that endows on the body life-span, complexion, strength, zeal, health, and the vital force; it is responsible for respiration, digestion, blood-circulation, pulse, body temperature and so on. When the fire is put out, the body tends to become cold and rigid and all the vital functions stop.

Death invariably follows unfavourable premonitory symptoms (arishṭa) [*See* ARISHTA]. Among the symptoms of imminent death are listed heavy and strained breathing; loss of bodily heat; pain in the chest; restlessness; changes in the constitution without reason (for example, vāta-constitution suddenly becoming pitta-constitution, the generous man becoming miserly, or the brave one becoming timid); inability to hold the head in position, the sagging of the backbone; feeling that the body has become inordinately heavy or inert; dilated pupils; glassy appearance of the cornea; inability to feel the pulse at the wrist; the tongue becoming dry, dark, rough, heavy and insensitive; lips blackening, teeth changing colour and being laden with phlegm; the breath (incoming and outgoing) becoming very short or very long and carrying bad odour with it, inability to hear the sounds of thunder, waterfall, musical instruments, etc.; hearing those sounds when they are not there; inability to perceive the smell from the oil-lamp just after it is put out; perceiving one's own reflection in the mirror or in water in a deformed manner; wasting of body, despite nutritive food in abundance; lying on the back, being unable to turn his body to the right or left; stretching one's hands to find things that are not there; perceiving black, yellow and red pigments (in the absence of corresponding objects); cold sweat on the neck, chest and forehead while the rest of the body is warm; excessive sweat on the soles of the feet; sudden deformity of the nose; constriction of the nostrils; inability to perceive one's own image in the pupil of another; hunger after eating food in plenty; perceiving one's own clean and white clothes as dirty and red; and so on (*AHr* śarīra, 5; *Mārkanḍeya purāṇa,* Alarka-episode, 43).

When the patient's disturbances increase even when proper treatment is administered or when all the complications suddenly cease without any reason, it is the sign of imminent death (*SS,* 1,32,7 and 8). Diminution of blood-circulation in head (inability to lift or hold the head, feeling dizzy); coldness in hands, feet and respiration; constant drowsiness or total lack of sleep; frequent interruptions in breathing; thirst in excessive headache are also seen as unfavourable symptoms. Various bad omens and dreams foreboding death are also listed. [*See* ARISHTA].

Decoction : Known as kashāya (also as kvātha or niryūha), it is a medicinal preparation where one part of the selected drug or drugs (parts of plants, fresh or dried) is mixed with four, eight, or (more usually) sixteen (*BP*) parts of water, and the whole is boiled down in an open vessel (apidhānamukha-pātra) until one quarter of water remains. (*SaS,* II,1,2).

The substances that are used for decoctions are of three kinds: (1) soft (mrdu), for which water to be added is four times the drug, (2) medium (madhya), water added being eight times; and (3) hard (kaṭhina), water added being sixteen times.

When the food eaten has been digested, decoction must be administered twice. In case of aggravation of vāta, sugar, to the extent of one-fourth part of the decoction must be added; in case of aggravation of pitta, one-eighth part sugar; and in case of aggravation of kapha one-sixteenth part sugar must be added. If, however, honey is to be added, the proportions are one-sixteenth part, one-eighth part and one-fourth part respectively. [*See* PREPARATIONS].

Five varieties of decoctions are collectively known as pañcha-kashāya : (1) expressed juice (svarasa), (2) paste (kalka), (3) decoction (kvātha or śrta), (4) cold infusion (hima or śīta-kashāya), and (5) hot infusion (phāntā). Each of these is stronger than the following (or is in the descending order of strength, laghavah syur yathottaraṁ) (Cf. *CS,* 1,4; *SS,* chikitsā, 31; *SaS,* II, 1,1). [*See* EXPRESSED JUICE, PASTE, KVĀTHA, INFUSIONS].

There are other forms such as pānīya, which is a form of decoction prepared by boiling one part of drugs in 32 parts of water until the water is reduced to one-half. This is meant to slake thirst. Pramathya, is another decoction where drugs are first reduced to a pulp and then boiled in eight parts of water until the water is reduced to one-fourth (administered with honey).

Decoctions are classified into seven types, depending on their action on the system: (1) pāchana (solution reduced to one-half) helps digestion; (2) dīpana (reduced to one tenth) stimulates excretion; (3) śodhana (reduced to one-twelfth) eliminates waste products; (4) śamana (reduced to one-eighth) pacifies the severity of the disease; (5) tarpaṇa (allowed to reach boiling point) nourishes body constituents (dhātus); (6) kledana (reduced to one-fourth) causes anguish to the heart; and (7) viśoshi (reduced to one-sixth) promotes thirst (*HS,* 3,1).

It is important that the decoction must be taken away from the fire after the required strength is reached; otherwise the drug principles would evaporate. Once a decoction is taken away from the fire, it should on no account be boiled again. The decoction should not be blue or red in colour, thick or slimy to touch, or foul in odour.

Developmental Stages : Human life, the optimal span of which is 120 years and five days is broadly divided into three stages of development: (1) Juvenile stage (bālya), till 16 years, when the body grows in size, and the body constituents (dhātus), sensory abilities (indriya), and vitality (ojas) also develop; the period is further divided into three phases: (a) early infancy till about a year, when milk alone is drunk; (b) later childhood, till about two years, when milk is drunk as well as solid food is eaten; and (c) still later when solid food forms the mainstay; (2) Middle stage (madhya), till 70 years (according to *SS,* 1,35,29 and *AHṛ* 2,3,105, but till 60 years according to *AS,* 2,8) during which period the development of the body constituents is at a standstill; digestive power is at its best, intellect is at its height and activity at its peak (*AS*); the middle stage is again divided into three phases: (a) youth (yauvana) till 30 years, (b) fulfilment or full maturity of dhātus etc. (sampūrṇatā) till 40, when all the body constituents and sensory abilities are fully mature, and the individual is in possession of strength, ability, valour, memory, speech, knowledge and other qualities necessary for efficient life, and (c) waning or slow decrease of the above faculties and abilities (parihāni but according to *AS* aparihāni, 'non-waning', that is, remaining without increase or decrease); and finally (3) the stage of senescence (vṛddha) or old age beyond 70 and till death, when all the above faculties quickly decline, and the individual collapses 'like an old house in a storm'. (cf. *SS,* sūtra, 35,29).

It is also suggested that during the first stage kapha or śleshman will increase, contributing to speedy growth, tenderness of body and mind, charm and innocence. During the second stage, pitta is on the increase, thus making for good digestion, intelligence and activity. The last stage is characterised by the increase of vāta, leading to the disintegration of the physical system, weakening of the bodily tissues, loosening of the joints, coarsening of the skin, instability, tremor and diseases.

There is another account which emphasises the increase or decrease in the strength of body constituents and in the ability of sense-organs: Childhood (till 10 years), when the preparatory stage is set; adolescence (till 20), when physical and mental development is speeded up; early youth (till 30), when the physical lustre (chhavi) is at its height; late youth (till 40), when intellectual faculties (medhā), especially memory, are at their best; later youth (till 50), when the complexion (tvak) is still bright; early old age (till 60), when acuity of vision (dṛshṭi) diminishes considerably; middle old age (till 70), when the seminal powers (śukra) as well as vigour (vikrama) are weakened; late old age (till 100), when the abilities of the organs of action (that is, prehension, speech, locomotion, excretion and procreation) are diminished; and finally the ripe old age (till 120), when the awareness of the surrounding (chetas) too gets gradually dim. (cf. *SaS*, 1,20).

Development of Foetus : [*See* FOETAL DEVELOPMENT].

Dhamanī : Literally this means 'blowing pipes'. The dhamanīs (from the root dhmā 'to blow', *CS*, sūtra, 30) are usually translated as nerves, arteries, ducts or tubular vessels and are distinguished from sirās (veins) and srotas (channels) [*See* SIRĀ and SROTAS]. An earlier view has been mentioned and rejected in *SS* (śarīra, 9,3), that there is no distinction between these three (dhamanī, sirā and srotas), and that the dhamanīs are only modifications of sirās (cf. *RN*, 18 where sirā is identified with dhamanī). The view supported in *SS* is that they are all different in their sources, characteristics and functions. However, they cooperate closely with each other and are located in close proximity and are functionally interconnected and interdependent. They are all equally subtle (minute), and directed towards the same systemic function, namely, the maintenance of life. (*SS*, ibid.).

The dhamanīs (called nalikas or tubes in *BP*) are mainly involved in the transportation of chyle (rasa, assimilated food) to all the parts of the body and in 'blowing' air into the entire organization (*SaS*, 1,5,41). The nourishing substances are thus conveyed to all parts of the body by the action of vyāna-wind [*See* VYĀNA] through these hollow tubes. They are fundamentally twenty-four in number, and they originate in the region of the umbilicus (nābhi): (1) ten of them are ascending (ūrdhvagāh), (2) ten descending (adhogā), and (3) four course transversely (tiryaggāh).

(1) The ascending dhamanīs are responsible for functions like apprehension of sound, touch, taste, form and smell (through sense-organs), inspiration and expiration (through the nostrils and mouth), sighing, yawning, sneezing, laughing, speaking, crying and they are generally engaged in maintaining the integral functioning of the body ('śarīram dhārayanti', *SS*, ibid.). In their upward movement, they reach the heart (viz. the region where the heart is located) and there each of them ramifies into three branches. Thus, there are thirty branches. Of them, ten dhamanīs are concerned with the transportation of vāta, pitta, kapha, blood and chyle (two for each); eight carry the sensations of sound, form, taste and smell (two of each); and twelve with speech, articulation, sleep, keeping awake, shedding tears, carrying breastmilk in the case of women or semen in the case of men (two ducts for each function). These thirty dhamanīs maintain the integrity of the body above the navel region (namely, the abdomen, sides, back of the chest, neck, shoulders and arms).

(2) The descending dhamanīs push flatus, urine, faeces, semen, menstrual fluid downward so that they are ready for elimination. They descend to the seat of pitta, where they separate the digested portion of the food, and supply it to the dhamanīs that ascend and that traverse across so that the parts of the body covered by them are also nourished.

Thus the heart is provided with adequate chyle. They also help separate the waste products (like urine, sweat, faeces). On reaching the region between the stomach (āmāśaya) and large intestine (pakvāśaya), each of them ramifies into three branches. Thus there are thirty branches of the descending dhamanīs. Of them, ten are engaged in transporting solid food (to the bladder), urine (from the bladder), semen or menstrual flow (into their receptacles); semen or menstrual fluid (out of body), and faeces (into the lower intestine); and remaining eight in transporting perspiration (sveda) to the dhamanīs that course transversely. These thirty dhamanīs maintain the integrity of the body below the navel region (organs like intestine, waist, generative organs, bladder, anus, etc).

(3) The four dhamanīs that course transversely ramify progressively into finer and finer vessels, till their total number is impossible to count. They constitute an elaborate and intricate network that pervades, sustains, and protects the body as a system ('śarīram gavākshitaṁ vibaddham ātataṁ cha', *SS,* ibid., 11). The exterior openings of these finer vessels are attached to the pores of the skin, through which perspiration and chyle are conveyed.

The dhamanīs have pores in their sides which help to transport the chyle to all parts of the body thus nourishing them all alike. They are significant inasmuch as the conscious individual, residing in the body made up of the five primary forms of matter is provided with five kinds of sensations (sound, touch, form, taste, smell) and at the time of death, these dhamanīs break up the conglomeration of the five primary forms of matter (viz. the body) into its several ingredients ('pañchatvaṁ āyānti', *SS,* ibid., 11). [*See also* BODY *and* SIRA].

Dhātu : The word, meaning 'that which supports, holds aloft, sustains, nourishes' (dhāraṇāt), is employed in different senses : (1) metals (seven: gold, silver, copper, tin, zinc, lead, iron; eight, with the addition of mercury; nine with the addition of loadstone) [*See* METALS]; (2) mineral earths like red chalk (gairika) and red arsenic (manah-śilā); (3) the five primary forms of matter (pañcha-bhūta); (4) the three doshas, vāta, pitta and kapha [*See* DOSHA]; (5) the seven bodily constituents: blood and so on etc. [*See below*]; (6) semen and menstrual flow (śukrārtava, *SS,* 1,14); (7) the sense-organs; and (8) the roots of words. The usual usage in the context of medicine is in the sense of body constituents.

The body constituents are called dhātus for they support and nourish the body, themselves being stable and intact (śvayam sthitvā deham dadhati; śarīra-dhāraṇād dhātavaḥ, *SS,* 1,14). They provide the essential nutrition for the system as well as the structural framework for the physiological functions. They are responsible for the anatomical architecture of the body and the psychophysiological mechanism. They remain inside the body, each in a specific measure and all in a state of balance in the healthy individual. Any departure from the measure specific to each of them would result in disease and if not remedied would prove fatal.

They include permanent (sthāyī) constituents consisting of the enduring and basic tissues which support the body and provide structural unity, and the temporary (asthāyī) constituents which nourish, sustain and maintain the former group. These constituents are under the influence of the activity of the three doshas (namely vāta, kapha and pitta). Any disturbance in any one, two or all three of the doshas is manifested in the vitiating changes that are brought about in these body constituents. Hence the expression dūshya (corruptible) for the constituents. In turn, these constituents by their increase (vṛddhi) or decrease (kshaya) are responsible for deteriorating changes in the body.

It is usual to enumerate seven bodily constituents in a consecutive succession (dhātu-paramparā):

(1) chyle (rasa), including lymph or the circulating plasma which is primarily made

up of 'water', although other primary forms of matter are also present, and whose function is appeasement of the physiological structure (prīṇana);
(2) blood (rakta), which is primarily made up of the 'fire' element, and whose function is preservation of life (jīvana);
(3) flesh (māṁsa) (including muscles, peśi), which is primarily composed of the 'earth' element and whose function is 'sticking' (lepa);
(4) fat or adipose tissue (medas), which is also primarily made up of the 'earth' element and whose function is oleation (sneha);
(5) bone-tissue (asthi), which is predominantly made up of the 'earth' and 'air' elements, and whose function is to 'support' (dhāraṇā); the pores in the bone represent the ākāśa element;
(6) bone-marrow (majjā), which is predominantly composed of the 'water' element, and whose function is to 'fill' (pūraṇa); and
(7) sperm (semen) (śukra) in the male or ovum (ārtavam) in the female, which is predominantly made up of water, and whose function is reproduction (garbhotpāda).

Each of these constituents undergoes 'digestion' (pāka) under the influence of its own specific 'fire' (known as dhātvagni). The seven constituents represent different stages of transformation, the causative agent in each stage being the 'constituent-fire' [*See* AGNI]. Thus these are not merely anatomical and structural in import, but have specific physiological functions in a successive manner in the order mentioned above.

The seven constituents together are responsible for vitality (ojas), which makes the internal and external organs discharge their respective functions. This vitality pervades the entire body and is immediately responsible for the efficient conduct of the vital functions in the body. This principle is decreased or damaged by physical injuries, loss of sleep, hunger, excessive manual labour, grief, anxiety etc. Vitality is regarded as the quintessence of all the seven body constituents and as the final purpose towards which the seven factors strive [*See* VITALITY].

There is a discussion whether vitality could be regarded as the eighth constituent. Although its location is principally in the heart, it has its own characteristics (like cold, unctuous, white in colour with tinges of red and yellow, acc. to *AHṛ*), and it occurs in specific quantity ('eight drops'). It only supports the body but does not nourish it and as such it cannot be regarded as a dhātu. It is sometimes regarded as an upa-dhātu (derived constituent), produced from the seventh constituent viz. sperm (śukra) (*SaS*). The general feeling is that it is the essence of the functioning of the seven body constituents, and not a constituent in its own right (*AHṛ,AS*).

Each constituent is said to be transformed into the succeeding one, as chyle into blood, and blood into muscle, etc. Transformation, however does not mean the cessation of one while the succeeding one gets formed. Nor does it mean that the preceding and the succeeding constituents remain in different quantities, one less and the other more. The idea of transformation of one constituent into another in a succession involves the continuous existence of all the seven constituents in unaltered proportions (in normal health), and intimate interaction between them.

Each of the constituents has three transformational aspects: a concrete, structural (anatomical) aspect (sthūla), a subtle functional (physiological) aspect (sūkshma), and an aspect of secretions or 'waste products' (mala). Structurally the constituents are distinct and localized and therefore recognized as such. Functionally, they are integrated and directed towards vitality. During this dynamism, each constituent approaches the nature of the succeeding constituent. It is in this context that the concept of 'constituent fires' (dhātvagni) acquires relevance. The seven 'fires' are merely modalities of the 'body-fire' (kāyāgni). As a result of the action of these 'fires' (viz. principles behind the transformations that continually occur in the constituents), the twin processes of assimilation of the nutrient substances (sāra) and the production of 'waste products' (mala) go on ceaselessly. The former means the causation of the succeeding constituent while the latter involves a byproduct which may be eliminated from the system. [*See* MALA].

The first constituent, viz. chyle (rasa), which is formed as a result of the assimilation of food that we eat, gets 'cooked' by the 'chyle-fire' (rasāgni), and, as a result, transforms itself into three aspects: the concrete, structural part which is 'chyle' proper (rasa-dhātu); the subtle, functional part which is blood (rakta) (viz. succeeding constituent); and the eliminable waste, phelgm (kapha). Likewise blood in its turn gets 'cooked' by the 'blood-fire' (raktāgni) and gets transformed into three aspects: blood as the concrete, structural aspect, flesh (māṁsa) as the subtle functional aspect (viz. the succeeding constituent) and 'bile' (pitta) as the waste-product.

Transformation in the muscle, when cooked by 'flesh-fire' (maṁsagni), involves flesh as the concrete aspect, fat (medas) as the subtle aspect and secretions in ears, nose, eyes and penis as the waste-products. Transformation in fat, when cooked by 'fat-fire' (medāgni), involves fat as the concrete aspect, bone (asthi) as the subtle aspect and sweat as the waste-product. Transformation in bone-marrow, when cooked by 'marrow-fire '(majjāgni), involves bone-marrow as the concrete aspect, sperm (śukra) as the subtle aspect, and the butter-like exudations from the eye and the oily exudations from the skin as waste products.

Finally, transformations in the sperm, when cooked by 'sperm-fire' (sukrāgni), involves sperm as the concrete aspect, and vitality (ojas) as the subtle aspect. Vitality is not a consequent 'constituent' (dhātu), and therefore the chain of transformations stops at this stage. And there are no waste-products in 'sperm-fire cooking' (Dalhana on *SS*, 1,15).

The concrete aspect is also called the 'permanent constituent' (sthāyı); it is the supporting structure. The subtle aspect of each constituent is what reinforces and nourishes the succeeding constituent, by joining itself with the latter (except in the case of the final constituent, viz. sperm). The nourishment of the constituents is sequential, according to *CS* (chikitsā, on 'grahaṇī') : chyle nourishing blood, blood nourishing flesh, flesh nourishing fat, and so on (kshīra-dadhi-nyāya). *SS* (sūtra, 14), however, argues that it is the chyle (rasa) that actually nourishes all the other constituents, not, however, all at once but in a sequential order. The illustration of the waters of one canal irrigating the different parts of a field, some near and some distant, is given (kedārī-kulya-nyāya).

The food that we eat contains elements that nourish all the seven constituents. When it is digested by the 'body-fire' (jāṭharāgni), the substantial part thereof (sāra) ascends to the heart region and joins with the chyle (rasa), reinforcing and nourishing it. It is then transmitted to all parts of the body through the other constituents. The substantial portions of the food therefore constitute the primary nourishing factors. Chyle, the first constituent, is the source of the entire human organism. It is necessary that one should strive to preserve chyle by proper food, drink and conduct. It is this chyle that gets transformed into sperm (śukra) in males and ovum in females at the end of a month (cf. *SS,* sūtra, 14, 11-14). The period of subsidence of the substantial portions of the digested food in each constituent is said to be 3,015 kalā (roughly about five days). Thus for chyle to get transformed into sperm (or ovum) requires 19,090 kalās of time (or a month), according to *SS;* but PARĀŚARA holds that seven days are enough (cited by CHKP, *CS*, chikitsā, 15, 21).

The seven constituents have their specific functions in the body; chyle nourishes the body, enlivens the mind, and strengthens blood; blood endows bright and clear complexion, nourishes flesh and invigorates the life-process (jīvayati); flesh strengthens the body and nourishes fat-tissue; fat-tissue gives unctuous quality to the body, causes perspiration, gives steadiness to the limbs and nourishes bone-tissue; bone-tissue supports the body and nourishes bone-marrow; bone-marrow fills the bone, endows strength to the body, enhances interest in life (prīti), and nourishes sperm; and sperm gives courage to man (ovum timidity to women), enhances health, encourages love and helps in the act of reproduction (*SS,* sūtra, 15, 7).

By the increase or decrease in the quantity of each constituent, specific disorders are caused. By an excessive increase of chyle (plasma), nausea and increased flow of saliva result. Increase of blood makes the face flushed, reddens the white of the eyes and fills the veins to their fullest capacity. Increase in flesh causes rotundity of the buttocks, lips, arms, thighs and penis, and makes the body heavy. Increase in fat-tissue renders the skin oily, makes the sides and belly bulky, causes a fetid smell in the body and encourages cough and dyspnoea.

Increase in bone-tissue (excessive ossification) makes for the formation of extra-teeth and abnormal bony structures. Increase in bone-marrow results in the heaviness of eyes and of all limbs. Increase in sperm leads to excessive exudation of semen and formation of gravels in the bladder (known as śukrāśmarī) (*SS,* śutra, 15, 18).

Abnormal decrease of chyle (plasma) causes pain in the heart, tremor, palpitation, feeling of emptiness and abnormal thirst. Decrease of blood makes the skin coarse and causes craving for sour food, drink and cold things. Decrease in flesh leads to emaciation of buttocks, cheeks, arms, thighs, breasts, neck and calves of legs, the arteries become lax and flabby, the body appears dry and inert, limbs are afflicted with aches. Decrease in fat enlarges the spleen, loosens the joints and renders the skin coarse and dry. Decrease in bone-tissue results in pain in the bones and in the bone-joints, decay in teeth and weakening of gums and dryness of body. Decrease in bone-marrow also leads to sharp pain in the bones and bone-joints and degeneration in the quality of semen. Decrease in sperm results in pain in the penis and testes, incapacity for sexual congress and emission of blood-stained semen (*SS,* ibid, 10).

Besides the seven constituents, there are seven 'secondary constituents' (upa-dhātu) derived from them as by-products. Their main function is to support the body. From chyle are derived breast-milk (stanya) and menstrual blood (ārtava, rajas) both in women; from blood, tendons (kaṇḍara) and blood-vessels (sirā); from flesh, fat (vasā) and six layers of ligaments (snāyu); from bone, teeth (danta); from bone-marrow, hair on the head; and from sperm, vitality (ojas). [*See* UPA-DHĀTU].

There is a discussion about the propriety of inclusion of breast-milk as a secondary constituent. *NiS,* however, regards it as a potential constituent for the infant (on *SS,* sūtra, 14, 10). Likewise menstrual blood, which closely resembles normal blood is sometimes excluded from the group of secondary constituents. But *Chkp* argues that its characterization as a constituent is justified because it is intimately related with the normal biological functions (on *CS,* chikitsā, 15, 17).

Tendons (kandara) are responsible for different kinds of motion (extension, contraction, flexion, etc) in the body; they are sometimes regarded as not different from gross nervous tissues or ligaments (snāyu) (cf. *CS*, chikitsā 15, 17). Blood-vessels (sirā) are channels, 700 in number through which blood flows; they sustain and nourish the body (*SS*, śarīra, 7, 3). Fat (vasā) not only supports the anatomical structures but nourishes them also. When the body is starved of food, the system utilizes this fat for subsistence and for enabling the normal metabolic processes. Ligaments, which serve to render the body well-knit and strong bind the several structures (like muscles, bones, joints) so that the body is able to withstand pressure and has better endurance (*SS*, sūtra, 5, 30-34). Vitality (ojas) which is the final derivative pervades the entire physical constitution and is responsible for all vital functions. [*See also* ASTHI, MĀMSA, MEDAS, MAJJĀ, RASA, RAKTA, AND ŚUKRA].

Digestion : 'Food sustains life and so all beings seek food. Food, properly digested not only maintains the body but promotes complexion, clarity of mind, good voice, brilliance, satisfaction, nourishment, strength and memory' (*CS*, sūtra, 27, 349-50). The body itself is the outcome of food. But food that is ill-digested can be a source of all ailments (*CS*, ibid., 28, 45). Therefore, digestion is an important consideration for a physician.

Digestion of food (which comprehends metabolism) depends upon the 'fires' in the body (agni), which are thirteen in number: 'stomachic fire' (jātharāgni), five 'elemental fires' (bhūtāgni, the elements or primary forms of matter being earth, water, fire, air and ākāśa), and seven 'constituent fires' (dhātvagni, the primary constituents of the body being chyle, blood, muscle, fat-tissue, bone, marrow and semen). (*See* AGNI, JĀTHARĀGNI, PAÑCHABHŪTA THEORY, and DHĀTU]. Digestion of food (anna-pāka) thus has three distinct and successive phases : jātharāgni-pāka, bhūtāgni-pāka and dhātvagni-pāka.

Digestion proper takes place in specific regions of the gastro-intestinal tract (anna-pāka-nādī or mahā-srotas) which is about twenty cubits long and which consists of mucosal linings (covering membranes called kalās, which also secrete and absorb) and muscles (peśī), extending from the mouth (mukha) to the rectum (guda). The principal regions that are involved in the digestive process are the oral cavity (mukha), the tract from throat till the stomach (viz. anna-vaha-nādī, corresponding roughly to oesophagus), the stomach (āmāśaya), the small intestine (kshudrāntra or pachyamānāśaya) containing the duodenum (grahanī, where the digested food is retained), above the navel region, and the large intestine (pakvāśaya or sthūlāntra), which ends with the rectum (guda). (*Ātreya-samhitā,* cited in VSS). Metabolism takes place in the respective elemental ingredients in the body (bhūta) and in the seven constituents of the body (dhātu).

'Agni' which is essential for digestion and metabolism is present in the body in the form of pitta. As it is responsible for digestion, it is called 'pāchaka-pitta', 'koshthāgni' 'jātharāgni', 'audarya-tejas' or 'kāyāgni', all referring to intestinal digestion, with the end-results (vipāka) of three tastes : sweet (madhura), pungent (katu) and sour (amla). (*See* VIPĀKA). This 'agni' is located in the region between the stomach and the large intestine, above the umbilicus (nābhi) and below the liver (yakrt) (*SS*, sūtra, 21, 10). This is known as the 'seat of pitta' (pittāśaya, also called agnyāśaya). Sometimes it is identified with the structure known as grahanī (e.g. *CS*, chikitsā, 15, 56). [*See also* GRAHAṆĪ].

Digestion as activity of this 'agni' is concerned with conversion of the external and heterogeneous food into internal and homogeneous mass (pāka), breaking down of the composite and complex food into its component factors which are assimilable in the body (anu-pāka), and separation of the nutrient substances that must be assimilated from the indigestible matter that needs to be thrown out of the body (sāra-kiṭṭa-vibhajana). As soon as the food is placed in the mouth, its taste is perceived by the bodhaka-kapha present in the tongue and the pharynx, and then the food is broken down by the tejas-factor present in the salivary secretions (lālā). This is known as the preliminary phase of digestion (pra-pāka, CHKP on *CS*, chikitsā, 15, 9) [*See* PRAPĀKA]. It is followed by the ushering of the food into the stomach by the action of prāṇa-vāyu (*CS*, chikitsā, 15, 6, and *SS*, nidāna, 1, 13). The kledaka-kapha present in the stomach moistens the food (by the gastric mucous or secretions), disintegrates it and liquifies it. (*SS*, sūtra, 21, 12 and *AHṛ*, sūtra, 12, 16). Thus the food is made ready for 'intestinal digestion' (jātharāgni-pāka), the outcome of which is the conversion of the food (which has undergone prāpaka) into the tastes as end-products : sweet (madhura), sour (amla) and pungent (kaṭu). This is known as vipāka (cf. *AHr*, sūtra, 9, 20) [*See* VIPĀKA].

During this phase, the complex mass of food is broken down into its elemental units (saṁghāta-bheda) in five groups belonging to the earth group (pārthiva), water group (āpya), fire group (āgneya, taijasa), air group (vāyavya) and ākāśa group (ākāśīya, nābhasa), so that they can appropriately be absorbed into the five elements that are involved in the physical body. This subsequent absorption (śoshaṇa) is due to the action of the 'fires' that are present in the five elemental units (pārthivāgni, āpyāgni etc). The purpose is to build up the primary constituents of the body. This process known as bhūtāgni-pāka is supposed to take place in the fundus of the stomach (adho-āmāśaya) and especially in the liver (cf.*CS*, chikitsā, 15, 13).

It is important to recognize that the body is made up of five primary forms of matter and that the food that nourishes the body is also made up of the same forms of matter. The 'fires' in the body are engaged in breaking down the food into these primary forms (homologues of substances) so that they are rendered fit for being assimilated by the corresponding elements in the body and thus finally nourish the constituents of the body (*SS*, sūtra, 46, 526).

The final phase of digestion (dhātvagni-pāka) consists of metabolic transformations, as the digested food-juice (anna-rasa) is transported through different channels [*see* SROTAS], so as to nourish the seven primary constituents of the body. Responsible for this metabolism is the pitta present in each of the constituents, which manifests itself as the 'heat' (ushmā), resulting from burning fuels in the form of food. The heat in each constituent is responsible for converting the nutrient substance relevant to that particular constituent and found in the general food-juice (anna-rasa), into the nourishing factor (poshaka) for that constituent. This is necessary for the constituent to be built up. There is a channel (srotas) appropriate to each constituent so that the nourishing factor is conveyed to the constituent.

As a result of this metabolism, waste-products (kitta) from each constituent are thrown up: kapha-mala from chyle, pitta-mala from blood, excretions from the ears, eyes, nostrils, mouth, roots of bodily hair and the genital organs from muscle, sweat from bone, the unctuous matter from the eyes, skin and faeces from bone-marrow and ojas-mala from semen [*See* MALA]. The waste products derived from the juice of digested food (anna-rasa) are faeces and urine. [*See also* AVASTHĀ-PĀKA, AGNI, GRAHAṆĪ, PITTA, PRAPĀKA, VIPĀKA, DHĀTU, MALA]

Dinacharyā: [*See* DAILY CONDUCT, HYGIENE]

Discussions (Clinical): Clinical discussions (sambhashā or tadvidya-saṁbhāshā) are recommended by CHARAKA (*CS*, vimāna, 8,15 *ff*). The physician should discuss with other physicians. Such discussions strengthen his desire for knowledge concerning diseases and medicine, brings clarity to his own understanding, generates ability to communicate and provides an opportunity for obtaining recognition. Should one have doubts concerning issues that he has already studied, the discussion would help to remove them. Even if he has no doubts the discussion would deepen his understanding of the issues. He would come to know about many things that he did not know earlier. Further, in the course of discussion it may happen that the knowledgeable physician, when challenged, parts with many a secret that he has learnt from his teacher. Experts therefore recommend such academic discussions.

Clinical discussions fall into two categories; (1) discussions with one's own colleagues, associates, friends and sympathetic folk who are also learned (sandhāya saṁbhāshā); such discussions would be carried on mainly for exchanging views, crystallizing concepts and reaching conclusions, with no ill-will, rivalry, suspicion or prejudice among the participants; and (2) discussions which take the form of disputes (vigṛahya-saṁbhāshā), and where issues are sorted out by arguments, counter-arguments, fault-findings, defence, and so on.

Fault-finding discussions are not recommended by the medical writers. In their view, should one find oneself forced to take part in such a discussion, he should carefully consider even before he speaks (samyak parīksheta) the status of the person whom he is going to criticize and also the nature of the assembly (parishat-viśesha) in which he has to speak. If he is clever, he will then decide whether and how he should participate. CHARAKA offers suggestions for the disputant in such a situation.

The medical assembly (parishat) is mainly of two kinds : (1) assembly of experts (jñānavatī) and (2) assembly of fools (mūdha-parishat). The kinds are again grouped into (a) assembly of friendly participants (suhṛt-parishat), (b) assembly of indifferent people (udāsīna-parishat) and (c) assembly of inimical participants (pratinivishṭa-parishat). Considerations relevant to discussions that go on in these assemblies are: intelligence of the participant, his learning, his ability to remember relevant texts, his capacity to express himself, his moral integrity, his irritability or patience, his brilliance, clarity in his exposition and sense of humour.

Exposition of an issue in an assembly is said to be structured thus: statement of the problem and the enunciation of a thesis (pratijñā), followed by arguments to substantiate the thesis (sthāpanā). The arguments involve reasons (hetu), which are the sources of one's understanding (upalabdhi-kāraṇa), illustrative instances (udāharaṇa), analogical reasoning (upanaya) and conclusion (nigamana). The Nyāya syllogistic form has thus been accepted by CHARAKA. [*For details of the logical technicalities involved in academic discussions and disputes see* HIP. vol.2, pp.373-392.]

Disease: The concept of disease (vyādhi, gada, āmaya, roga, ruk, pāpmā or yakshmā) is dependent upon the idea of health as the prime condition in which the four objectives of life (that is, virtue, wealth, enjoyment, and salvation) are accomplished. Disease is of the nature of obstacle (vighna) for activities towards such accomplishment. It would preclude the opportunity for advancement in life (śreyas), and it might cut short life itself (jīvata) (*CS*, sūtra, 1,15). Health, thus, is a positive endeavour to fulfil the purposes of life and disease interferes with this.

The body by its very nature disintegrates gradually (śarīra is so called because śīryate iti). Ageing, decayingn and breaking down are inevitable processes. When diseases also gain their lodgement in the body, the processes of disintegration are quickened and strengthened. (CHKP on *CS*, ibid, 6). Even as the body needs to be sustained by nourishment and rest, diseases must be avoided by hygiene, preventive measures, and eliminated by medicine, diet and exercise. For disease renders the person incapable of achieving his objectives, and threatens his happiness and even survival. Therefore, human beings are stricken with terror at the prospect of disease (*CS*, ibid, 22).

Health is the balance in the proportions and functions of the several body constituents (dhātus) and the three forces that activate them (doṣhas). Disease is the disturbance of this balance (vaishamya or vikāra), caused by the deficient, excessive, or improper organization of: seasons, modes of consciousness, and objects of sensation (*CS*, ibid, 54) [*See* HEALTH].The aim of medicine is to restore the balance thus lost, for health demands balance (sāmyaṃ prakrtih, *CS*, sūtra,9,4).

These are the main conditions in which disease originates: (1) unsatisfactory association of sense-organs with their objects (asātmyendriyārtha-saṁyoga); (2) errors of judgement (prajñāparādha), resulting in the improper activities of body, mind and speech (karma); and (3) effect (pariṇāma) of seasonal variations (kāla) (*CS*, sūtra, 11,37; also *AS*, 1,22.11). Each of these conditions can again be of three kinds: deficient organization (hīna-yoga), excessive organization (atiyoga), and improper organization (mithyā-yoga). This entire complex of conditions is collectively known as 'improper food and conduct' (mithyāhāra-vihāra), the most important single cause for diseased conditions.

Disease necessarily involves the disturbance of the doṣhas (that is, vāta, pitta and kapha) that move about in the body and activate the body constituents (dhātus). CHARAKA speaks of disease as the imbalance of bodily constituents (dhātu-vaishamya, *CS*, sūtra, 9,4). But VĀGBHATA wants us to understand that he was speaking in a very general and metaphorical way; the body constituents were brought into the picture, not because they were causes of disease but because they were productive of pain which is the concomitant of diseases ('duhkha-kartṛtvād aupachārikaṁ', *Vivarana-siddhānta-chintāmaṇi* of NRSIṀHA-KAVI-RĀJA). It is VĀGBHAṬA'S view that diseases involve the disturbance of doṣhas alone (*AS*, 1,22,10). In this, he follows SUŚRUTA (*SS*, sūtra, 35).

The doṣhas, which are psycho-physiological forces in the body are independent of the body constituents which are capable of being disturbed by the doṣhas (hence called dūshya), for it is the doṣhas that activate them (doshebhya eva dhātūnāṁ pravṛttih, INDU on *AS*, 1, 1, 1). Even as the entire world is a modification of the three guṇas (namely, sattva, rajas, and tamas), all diseases are merely modifications of the three doṣhas, which in their proper measure sustain health and when disturbed produce diseases (ibid, 1,19,43).

The rationale of Indian medicine is that when the doṣhas are disturbed, they in turn disturb the dhātus. The former are aggressive while the latter only react. When the strength of the disturbing doshas is greater, the reaction of the dhātus becomes insignificant and the diseased condition worsens. When the strength of the dhātus is greater, the disturbance of the doṣhas becomes insignificant and the disease gets cured. Treatment involves providing food or drugs that can strengthen the dhātus to resist the aggression of the disturbing doshas. [*See* DOSHA, DHĀTU].

A classification of diseases could be twofold: (1) constitutional (nija) and (2) accidental (āgantu) (*AHṛ*,1, 1,20). The former type of diseases is caused by the disturbances of the doṣhas, which later bring about distress. The doshas in this context would refer to internal causes (antarañga-hetu) and thus include the disturbances of the dhātus also according to *AR* (*AHr*, 1,1,20), though

ARUNADATTA confines the causative role to the three doṣhas only. The accidental type consists of diseased conditions caused by extraneous agents such as wounds, burns, sunstrokes, lightning-strokes, cold, falls and ailments caused by witchcraft and curses. These conditions do not involve any disturbance of the doshas initially, but the distress caused by extraneous agents will in due course bring about a disturbance of the doshas. Both alike trouble the mind, for it is in the nature of disease to be distressing (ARUNADATTA, *AHr*, 1, 1, 20).

Diseases may again be classified into two groups : bodily (śārīra) and mental (mānasa). (*AHṛ*, 1, 1, 21). The bodily diseases are illustrated by fever, haemorrhage, cough and so on, while the mental group includes such ailments as intoxication, fainting, insanity, catalepsy, apoplexy, excessive desires, hatred and so on. The bodily diseases are occasioned by the excitation of the doṣhas and involve directly the bodily constituents, while mental diseases are caused by defective rajas (tendency for over-activity, irritability, excitation, instability) and tamas (tendency for inactivity, laxity, confusion and stupor). *AR* explains that the latter causes are different from the doshas (vāta, pitta, and kapha) which cause bodily ailments, while ARUṆADATTA holds that the same doṣhas are also involved in mental diseases (on *AHṛ*, 1,1,21). CHAKRAPĀṆI-DATTA (on *CS*,1,1,55) suggests that bodily ailments provide the ground for mental ailments, for even the mental ailments must find their locus in the body. He illustrates purely bodily diseases by leprosy, purely mental diseases by excessive desires. Diseases like insanity (unmāda) are said to be both mental and bodily (dvayāśritāh). [*See* MENTAL DISEASES].

The *Charaka Saṁhitā* (sūtra, 11,45) provides a comprehensive tripartite classification of diseases: (1) constitutional (nija, originating in bodily doshas), (2) accidental (āgantu, caused by poison, falls, burns, cuts, attacks, and so on) and (3) mental (mānasa, morbid pleasures and longings such as those caused by the obtainment of what is desired; and distress and dejection caused by the non-obtainment of what is desired). *SS* (sūtra, 1,23) gives a four-fold classification : (1) constitutional or bodily (śārīra) originating in food and drink, and involving the disturbances owing to the faulty organization of vāta, pitta, kapha and blood ; (2) accidental (āgantu), caused by violent attacks and so on , (3) mental (mānasa), caused by desires and aversions (for example, morbid anger, fear, joy, dejection, envy, greed, jealousy, helplessness and passions) and (4) natural (svābhāvika), caused by hunger, thirst, sleep, and the approach of death. All these, according to him, are based both on body and mind.

There is an elaborate classification suggested by SUSRUTA (*SS*, 1,34,4f) and accepted by later medical writers like(VĀGBHAṬA, CHAKRAPĀṆI-DATTA, MĀDHAVA-KARA and so on): (I) diseases which are generated inside the organism (ādhyātmika), comprising of (1) those which are active even from pre-natal stages (ādi-bala-pravṛtta), (2) those which are congenital (janma-bala-pravṛtta) and (3) those which are caused by improper food and conduct (doṣha-bala-pravṛtta); (II) diseases due to adverse conditions which are external (ādhibhautika), comprising (1) those which are caused by physical assaults, accidents, poisonous bites and so on (sāṁghāta-bala-pravṛtta), and (2) those which are brought about by abnormal climatic conditions and seasonal variations (kāla-bala-pravṛtta) and (III) diseases which have their origin in fate, curses, malignant influences (ādhidaivika), comprising of (1) those caused by providential acts, diabolical influences, witchcraft or by natural catastrophes like earthquakes, lightning and epidemics (daiva-bala-pravṛtta) and (2) those which are inevitable functions of time, like sleep, hunger, senility and death (svabhāva-bala-pravṛtta).

Astānga-samgraha (1,22,3) enumerates seven categories of diseases accommodating the above: (1) inherited diseases (saha-janya), like skin diseases, diabetes, (2) diseases occurring in pregnancies (garbha-janya), owing to improper food and conduct of mother, (3) congenital diseases (jāta-janya), occurring at birth or soon after, (4) diseases due to violence (pīḍā-janya), cuts, injuries, falls, fright, anger and so on, (5) diseases due to seasonal changes (kāla-janya), (6) diseases due to supernatural or inscrutable influences (prabhāva-janya), and (7) diseases due to the very nature of the body (svabhāva-janya), hunger, thirst, fever and so on.

However, MADHAVA-KARA narrows down the sources of disease to the troubled malas (body constituents which need to be eliminated from the body, as otherwise they tend to pollute the entire constitution, (malinīkaraṇāt). Diseases are classified into two main groups: those which are brought about by factors which are near (inside the body, saṁnikṛshṭa, like the doshas) and those which are caused by factors that are far removed (viprakṛshṭa, like incompatible food and so on). [*See* MALA].

Diseases are again classified into three groups from the point of view of their manifestation: (1) diseases which are in their early stages (mṛdu), (2) diseases which are neither slight nor severe (madhya) and (3) diseases which are severe and grave (atimātra) (*AHṛ*, 1,22,9). Some diseases are readily amenable to treatment (sādhya); others need to be treated with great difficulty and care (yāpya); still others are impossible to cure (asādhya) but may be suppressed to an extent or for some time.

Despite the classifications, Indian medicine regards all diseases as essentially of the same nature (ēkākārā eva rogāh). The production of distress is the common quality of all diseases. Therefore, disease is one, although its manifestations may be innumerable (asaṅkhya) in accordance with their origination, locus, symptoms, specific distress, influence, spread, and so on (*AHṛ*, 1,22,9).

The course of a disease is traced into two stages, each with three divisions:(1) the initial stage relating to the disturbance of the doshas is accumulation of morbid influences in the body (sañchaya), their excitation (prakopa) and spread (prasāra); and (2) the subsequent stage relating to the manifestation of disease is localization (sthāna-samśraya) and individual or specific manifestation (vyakti) due to which unless properly and adequately treated, the patient would succumb to death (bheda) or life-long suffering.

The concept of secondary disease (upadrava) is significant in Indian medicine. It may occur at the closing phase of a disease or after the disease disappears. It may be caused by the patient's negligence in the matter of diet and conduct or by the physician's ignorance and error. In any case, it becomes itself a disease and needs to be treated [*See* SECONDARY DISEASE].

A disease is identified by its causation (nidāna), premonitory symptoms (pūrva-rūpa), clear manifestation by symptoms (rūpa), verification by the prescription of some drugs, food or regimen with reference to the adaptability (sātmya) and by the development of the disease (saṁprāpti). [*See* PATHOLOGY].

The most frequent classification, which is also a practical one, relates to the gravity of the disease: (1) diseases that are easily cured (sukha-sādhya), (2) diseases that are cured with difficulty (kashṭa-sādhya) including surgical cases (*AHṛ*, 1,1,32), and (3) diseases that are altogether impossible to cure (asādhya, also called pratyākhyeya, or anupakrama). Chronicity in disease is also considered; chronic ailments are practically incurable, but can considerably be assuaged (yāpya), or suppressed for greater or lesser lengths of time (cf. *CS*, sūtra, 10,7-10; *SS*, sūtra, 35,38; *AHṛ*, 1,1,30-32).

Although VĀGBHAṬA (*AS*, 1,2,26) classifies diseases into seven categories according to type, a broad break-up is given as follows: Curable (sādhya) and incurable (asādhya). the former is again divided into two types: easily cured (su-sādhya) and cured with difficulty (kṛcchra-sādhya); the latter likewise into two types: suppressible (yāpya) and impossible to cure (anupakrama).

Symptoms would suggest how easily or whether at all, the diseases can be cured. The physician should be wary to expect success while treating diseases with altogether infavourable symptoms [*See* ARISHṬA]. Treatment would be futile in cases where the life-span of the patient has also drawn to a close; the physician would only lose his reputation as well as practice (*AHṛ*, 2, 5, 4) [*See* Āyus].

Diseases are easily cured when the patient is young, has self-restraint, and has a physical constitution that can withstand treatment; or when the disease has not spread to the vital areas (head, heart, navel); when the disease has slight cause, has been recent, not yet fully developed, and has not been complicated with secondary diseases or by foul blood and vital sap (rasa); such diseases require slight medication and can be cured soon. Diseases that lack the above advantages share to an extent the quality of diseases that are impossibly to cure; they can be treated only with drugs that are strong and methods that are violent (like surgery, cautery); and the diseases take a long time to get cured.

The third variety (yāpya) consists of diseases that are really impossible to cure but which can be held in check for some time. The pain can be mitigated by treatment and complications are avoided. But if the disease is not rooted out, it will trouble the patient all along and take its toll sooner or later. An important aid in such diseases is careful arrangement of diet and conduct (pathya). Treatment in this case is like a prop to a collapsing house. The patient can survive for a time, until his destined end arrives.

The last variety (viz. diseases which are impossible to cure) is the opposite of the first variety. These diseases would have reached their final stage of complications or spread, and no treatment would be able to reverse the process of disintegration that has set in. Unfavourable symptoms (arishṭa) like loss of consciousness, delirium and stupor when the end is drawing near should dissuade the physician from continuing the treatment.

The judgement of the physician is an important factor. He should decide whether the disease is curable or incurable. He should also bear in mind that by an error in diagnosis, absence of nursing or faulty treatment even the curable disease may be rendered incurable. He should examine if the curable disease also has some unfavourable symptoms, for if these symptoms get the upper hand, the disease would no longer be curable. The incurable diseases can never change into curable ones but the curable ones may turn out to be incurable (*AS*, 1,3,36). [*See also* HEALTH. CURE. MEDICINE. RATIONAL MEDICINE. ROGA. TREATMENT. DEATH].

Disease-Courses in Body : Diseases are said to spread in the body along three pathways or courses (roga-mārga): (1) the peripheral system comprising of the body constituents (blood etc.) which are like branches of a tree (hence called śākhā); this is the external course; (2) the vital organs (urinary bladder, head etc.) and bone-joints, including ligaments and tendons (marmāsthi-sandhayah); these constitute the middle course; and (3) the central system (the great channels, stomach, intestines, lungs, heart etc.); these constitute the internal course (*CS*, sūtra, 11,48; also *SS*, chikitsā, 2). [*See* DISEASES. BODY CONSTITUENTS. HEART. DIGESTION. SROTAS].

Disease - Severity of : Patients are afflicted by

diseases which are either severe (guru) or mild (laghu). However, the severity of the disease cannot always be ascertained by appearances. A person suffering from a mild disease may nevertheless appear to be greatly troubled, for his physical constitution may not withstand even that mild affliction and his powers of endurance (sattva-bala, literally mental strength) may be poor. On the other hand, a person suffering really from a grave illness, may appear to be mildly afflicted, owing to his strong physical constitution and great powers of endurance (*CS*, vimāna, 7,3).

The physician should, therefore, not be misled by appearances; he must ascertain the severity of the ailment after proper and careful examination of all aspects of the disease. Otherwise treatment would be either deficient, excessive or wrong; the disease may then be aggravated and the patient may even die. There is a need to understand the entirety (kṛtsna) of a disease before effective medicines are administered; and the entirety of knowledge cannot be obtained by piecemeal information (avayava) (*CS*, ibid., 4 and verses 5-7).

Dosha : The doctrine of the three doshas (vāta, pitta and kapha) constitutes the corner-stone of Indian medicine. It explains normal human constitution (both physical and mental), positive health, abnormal conditions, methods of diagnosis, hygienic measures and therapeutics. It runs through the entire gamut of medicine as the leit motif.

While it bears some correspondence with the humoral theory of the Greeks, it cannot be ascribed to that source (as HAAS attempted to do in *Indische Medicine,* Z.D.M.G., vol. 26, pp. 441). The main argument is to be found even in the *Ṛgveda* (1,34,6,'trir no aśvinā divyāni bheshajā, trih pāthivāni trir udattam adabhyah; ....tridhātu śarma vahatam śubhaspatī'). And we find references to each of the three doshas frequently in the Vedic literature (for example, in the *Yajurveda,* 12,97; 17,6; 19,85; 25,7; the *Atharva-veda,* 1,12,3; 1,24,1; 6,12,7 (1-2); 9,8,10; and 18,3,5). The popularity of the concept among physicians is vouchsafed in the Buddhist period (*Miḷinda-pañho,* p. 379 etc) and even the *Bower MSS* refer to it. All the three classic saṁhitās (*SS, CS* and *AHṛ*) mention the doctrine as an age-old one, and as uniquely relevant to the medical profession.

There is some confusion regarding the expression 'dosha' which literally signifies 'corrupting agent', 'vitiating factor', 'cause of disease' (dūshaṇāt). While the three factors included in the expression (viz. vāta, pitta and kapha) do function as morbific, and are in the background of all diseases, they also function as the three pillars of positive health. They are necessary and sufficient ingredients of the psychophysical constitution in its normalcy and therefore the expression 'dhātu' (which means 'sustaining and supporting factors' dhāraṇāt) would be more appropriate. In fact, the Ṛgvedic hymn already referred to employs the expression 'tri-dhātu' and this appears to have been the earlier usage. However, in due course, the word 'dhātu' acquired a technical flavour and began to be used almost exclusively to refer to the seven body constituents (that is, chyle, blood, muscle, fat-tissue, bone, bone-marrow and semen). And these were liable to be corrupted or vitiated (dūshya) by the disturbances (excess or deficiency) of one or more of the three factors, which, in order to be distinguished from the dhātus, came to be called the 'corrupting agents' or 'vitiating factors' (dosha) (cf. *BPI*).

The outlook of Indian medicine insists that the human constitution is an organization of three units: the doshas (the three fundamental factors), the dhātus (the seven body constituents) and the malas (waste products to be thrown out of the body, like sweat, urine and faeces, for otherwise they spoil the body, malinīkaranāt) (cf. *SS*, sūtra, 28, *AHr*, sūtra 11) [*See* DHĀTU and MALA]. There is nothing in the human body besides these three units. All three in their composition and function comprehend different collocations of the five primary forms of matter (pañcha-bhūta, viz. earth, water, fire, air and ākāśa). *SS* clearly states that there can be no interest for a physician in anything other than the five primary forms of matter ("bhutebhyo hyaparam yasmān nāsti chintā chikitsite"). They are the ultimate reals so far as Indian medicine is concerned. They are modifications of the three gunas: sattva, rajas and tamas [*See* SĀMKHYA] (cf. *AS*, sūtra, 22).

Doshas are the immediate outcome of the collocations of these five, even as the human body represents the organization of these five ultimate reals (with the addition of soul) [*See* PAÑCHABHŪTA THEORY]. Earth (derived from tamas) and water (derived from sattva and rajas together) combine to produce kapha (also called śleshma); fire (derived from sattva and rajas) produces pitta; air and ākāśa (derived from rajas and sattva) together produce vāta. *NiS* identifies vāta with rajas, pitta with sattva and kapha with tamas (on *SS*, uttara, 66.9). The essence of vāta is air, of pitta fire and of kapha water and earth. The three are individualised principles corresponding to the three cosmic principles : moon (soma, cooling agent, kapha in the body), sun (sūrya, heating principle, pitta in the body) and air (vāyu, responsible for all movement, vāta in the body). The correspondence also involves the three-fold preservational framework: 'secretions' (visarga, for body functioning and waste products), 'absorption' (ādāna or metabolism) and 'diffusion' (vikshepa, nervous and motor force) in the body. (*SS*, sūtra, 21).

The three doshas, however, are not mere hypothetical constructs but actual substances (dravyas) in the body, although their presence can only be inferred from their functions (cf. CHKP on *CS*, sūtra, 28). They are not only composed of the five primary forms of matter but in fact they are the forces which produce the body ("deha-saṁbhava-hetavah", *SS*, sūtra, 21), which sustain and nourish the body (and in this sense, they are dhātus) and which comprehend all the structures and functions in the body (*CS*, sūtra, 1, "śārīro dravya-saṁgrahah", cf. also *SS*, sūtra, 21, where 'blood' is added). "The body is borne out by them as a house is supported by pillars, and when they are torn asunder, the body collapses" (*SS*, ibid.). The seven body constituents (dhātu) are produced from these three factors in various combinations, the normal structures and functions of these constituents depending upon the balanced presence of the three factors; when the balance of the factors is disturbed, the impact is immediately felt on the condition of the constituents. That is why the seven body constituents are called 'dūshyas' and the three factors 'doshas'.

All the three doshas are present all over the body in their subtle forms and flow through all the channels (srotas) [*See* SROTAS] (*CS*, sūtra 20, chikitsā, 28 and vimāna 5,50). However, each of them has specific areas in the body as special fields of action: large intestine (pakvāśaya) for vāta, stomach (āmāśaya) for pitta and heart (hrdaya) for kapha. Secondary regions are urinary bladder, pelvic region, the thighs, legs and bones for vāta; blood, sweat and lymph for pitta and head, neck, thorax, joints, upper portions of the stomach and fat-tissues for kapha (cf. *CS*, sūtra, 20, *SS*, sūtra, 21; vāta in lower part, pitta in the middle part and kapha in the upper part, *AHr*, sūtra, 12, ff). It is in these regions that the doshas severally prevail, and that the morbidities of the doshas are likewise manifested. The treatment should also be mainly directed towards these areas. The body is composed of the three doshas, as the universe is composed of the three gunas and all diseases are derived from the three doshas only. Although the doshas are different from each other, in their nature and function and might even be regarded as contrary to each other they can nevertheless cooperate both in maintaining health and causing diseases (*CS*, sūtra, 12, and chikitsā, 26: *AS*, 1,21;). They are also responsible for constitutional peculiarities of individuals, including the susceptibility to particular ailments [*See* CONSTITUTION].

The doshas are specific in their functions: vāta is responsible for circulatory, respiratory, excretory and digestive systems and for enthusiasm, speech, and sense-acuity; pitta for digestion, heat in the body, vision, hunger, thirst, taste, softness of the body, pigmentation of the skin, lustre of the skin, intelligence, cheerfulness and courage; kapha for nourishment, viscidity, solidarity of the body, strength of the joints, sexual vigour, patience, forbearance and fortitude. The separation of limbs and the specificity of their functions even in the womb are due to vata; the strengthening of the limbs is due to pitta and the nourishment of blood and semen is due to kapha.

The three doshas are differentially related to the individual's own developmental stages, to the intake of food from external sources, and to the diurnal and climatic changes in the surroundings.In infancy and childhood, kapha prevails in the body; in youth pitta; and in old age vāta. When one begins to eat food, kapha becomes predominant, half-way through pitta takes over and at the end vāta. In the morning, it is kapha that prevails, during midday pitta and towards evening vāta; likewise, in the first part of the night kapha, at midnight pitta and towards dawn vāta. During the rainy season, vāta is aggravated, during autumn pitta and in spring kapha.

The normal balance and proportion of the doshas are disturbed by articles of food, food-habits, behavioural peculiarities, seasonal influences, aging process and accidental occurrences. The disturbances are manifested by characteristic symptoms. There are three possible conditions in which the balance of the doshas may be disturbed: (a) one, two or all three of the doshas may suffer waning, diminution, reduction (kshaya), (b) one, two or all three of the doshas may increase or aggravate (vṛddhi) in the two stages by acceleration (prakopa) or accumulation (chaya), and (c) a dosha may leave its own area and move on to the area specific to another dosha (prasāra).

When there is a diminution of vāta, the individual feels uneasy, loses consciousness and is in a state of langour. However, when there is an aggravation of vāta, roughness of voice, emaciation of body, darkening of the skin, desire for hot things, throbbing sensation, constipation, insomnia and weakness are the guiding symptoms. In the diminution of pitta, dullness of complexion and reduction of body-heat are the main symptoms. In aggravation of pitta, burning sensations, desire for cold things, yellowish colour in the eyes, skin, faeces and urine, insufficient sleep, fainting fits, and weakness of the organs of sense. When kapha suffers a diminution, dryness of skin, sensation of internal burning, feeling of emptiness in the stomach and other cavities of the body, looseness of joints, thirst, weakness and insomnia are the symptoms. In the aggravation of this dosha, heaviness of the limbs, feeling of cold, drowsiness, excessive sleep, loose feeling of the joints and paleness of complexion are the symptoms.

Treatment consists in aggravating the dosha that has become diminished, diminishing the dosha that has become aggravated, correcting the errant dosha and preserving the doshas that are in a state of balance.

Each of the three doshas is regarded as having five functional varieties, each of which has specific locations (*AHr*, sūtra, 12 and so on).

I. Vāta :
(1) prāṇa is responsible for the respiratory system, the function of the heart, sneezing, swallowing and mental functions. It moves about in the head, throat, chest, ears, eyes tongue and nose.
(2) udāna ('upward-moving') with the tendency to travel upwards, is responsible for vocalizations, articulations, lustre of the body, and also for vivacity, enthusiasm, zealous effort and application. It is located in the chest and moves about around the navel region, and also along the nasal passages.
(3) samāna (equalizing) is responsible for ingestion and digestion of food, absorption of the food essences, excretion of the waste products, regulation of body heat, perspiration and circulation of the other two doshas (viz. pitta and kapha). It is located very near the seat of agni (that is, the digestive tract and the duodenum) and moves about in the entire abdominal region.
(4) vyāna (alround moving) is responsible for all bodily movements (sensory-motor) regulating the related organs and muscles and for circulation of air within the body. It is located in the heart, but moves about in the whole body with great speed, providing energy to the limbs and assisting the circulatory system.
(5) apāna (downward moving) is responsible for the retention and discharge of urine, faeces, semen and also for the regulation of menstrual flow in women; it also helps in the delivery of the baby from the mother's womb. It is located mainly in the duodenum, rectum and the urinary bladder.
II. Pitta :
(1) pāchaka (cooking) is chiefly responsible for digestion of food. It is located in the stomach and small intestine.
(2) rañjaka (colouring) is responsible for the formation of blood by pigmenting chyle. It is located in liver, spleen and stomach.
(3) sādhaka (accomplishing) is responsible for mental alertness, intelligence, cheer, memory and zeal. It is located in the heart.
(4) ālochaka (visual) is responsible for vision (formation of optical images of objects). It is located in the eyes.
(5) bhrājaka (lustre-endowing) is responsible for the colour and lustre of the skin. It is located in the skin all over the body.
III. Kapha :
(1) klédaka ('moistening') is responsible for moistening and softening the food that is ingested and thus helps digestion. It is located in the stomach.
(2) avalaṁbaka (nourishing) is responsible for supporting and sustaining the heart by lubricating and protecting the organ, for nourishing the sacrum (trika) and for providing energy to the limbs. It is located in the heart and the sacrum.
(3) bodhaka (aiding awareness) is responsible for the perception of taste. It is located in the tongue and pharynx.
(4) tarpaka (satisfying) is responsible for supporting and nourishing the sensory functions (organs of cognitions). It is located in the head.
(5) śleshaka (joining) is responsible for protecting the joints of bones, holding them together. It is located in the articulations of bony joints. [*See also* VATA, PITTA, KAPHA, DHATU, PANCHABHŪTA, MALĀ, DISEASES].

Dosha-Bala-Pravṛtta : Also called ādhyātmika-roga , they are the diseases caused by anxiety (ātaṅka), improper food-habits and unhealthy conduct (mithyāhāra-āchāra). They are of two types: those that first appear in the stomach (āmāśaya) and those that appear in the large intestine (pakvāśaya). [*See also* DISEASES].

Drāvaka : They are distilled mineral acids. The usual method of preparing them is to heat several mineral substances or salts in a retort and the distilled fluid thus collected is known as drāvaka. The test to find out if the distilled fluid is proper for medicinal use is to drop a shell (cowrie) into it; if the distillation is proper, the shell will dissolve in the fluid.

There are two kinds of distilled minerals: (1) svalpa-drāvaka, prepared by powdering eight tolas (about nine fluid ounces) each of alum, borax, chloride of ammonium, sulphide of antimony, impurities of carbonates of potash (yava-kshāra) and soda (sarji-kshāra), six tolas of nitre and four tolas of orpiment, mixing them together, repeatedly rubbing with lemon juice, drying in the sun and distilling the mixture in a retort over fire; and (2) śaṅkha-drāvaka, prepared by powdering 32 tolas of sulphate of iron, sixteen tolas of rock-salt, sixteen tolas of alum, and 128 tolas of nitre, mixing them together and distilling the mixture in a retort over fire. The latter is more powerful and should be used with caution, for it may scald the tongue and loosen the teeth even while it is being taken. (*ASM*).

Dravya : Dravya generally means 'substance', but in Āyurveda it is specifically used in the sense of 'drug', a substance employed as medicine. The assumption in Indian medicine is that there is no substance in the world which cannot be employed as a medicine (*CS*, sūtra, 1,26 and *SS*, sūtra 1,41) but that one should know how and when to make use of it and in what measure ("yuktimartham cha abhipretya", *CS*, sūtra 1,26). Indian medicine borrows the concept of dravya from the Nyāya-Vaiśeshika system, which recognizes nine categories of rudimentary and non-specific substances: the five primary forms of matter (earth, water, air, fire and ākāśa), soul, mind, time and space. Of these, the first five (viz. forms of matter) are available for sensory perception, while the other four are not. The entire world has come into being and functions on the groundwork of these substances.

Dravya is defined as the foundation for qualities (guṇa) and actions (karma) and as the combinative cause (samavāyi-kāraṇa) wherein qualities and actions exist. The relation between substances and qualities is inherent, inseparable and perpetual. There can be no substance which does not have quality, and no action exists without substance; quality, therefore, is the associate cause of both substance and action.

The *Suśruta-Saṁhita* (1,40f) and *Rasa-Vaiśeshika-Sūtra* (1,102f) enumerate several features which are both general and medically relevant that distinguish substances from qualities and actions: (1) substances are purposefully and stably organized (vyavasthita), and therefore primary (pradhāna); qualities, although dependent upon substances, are not so organized; (2) substances are permanent (nitya), while qualities are subject to change owing to time, wind, water and so on; it is possible to recognize the substance albeit its form has changed due to time etc; (3) substances do not stray from the genus (jāti) to which they belong; earth-dominated substances, for instance, would continue to be earth-dominated throughout its existential course despite transformations; (4) substances are apprehended by all the five senses (pañchendriya-grāhya), while qualities are perceived by specific senses (like sound by the ear, and form by the eyes).

Among the features that are of significance to medical practice are: (5) substances function as base or ground (āśraya), and qualities and action appear as figures thereon; "substance is of the nature of ground for five factors ('dravyam āśraya-lakshaṇam pañchānām')", namely taste (rasa), quality (guṇa), post-digestive change within the body or organismic transformation of drug (vipāka), potency of the drug for producing medical effects and drug-action (karma) (*RVS*, 1,166); (6) it is only substances that can begin the curative processes (āraṁbha-sāmarthya); (7) textual prescriptions pertaining to the preparation of drugs refer mainly to the substances (śāstra- prāmāṇya) and not to qualities, etc; and become meaningful only on that account; (8) substances are what determine qualities (kramāpekshita); dependent upon the condition of the substances is the nature of the taste; (9) as substances are organized structures consisting of many parts, they are capable of curing ailments by themselves (ekādeśa-sādhya), whereas taste and quality being specific details are not so capable; (10) the attributes of mildness and intensity, which are applicable to taste and quality are not applicable to substance (tara-tama-yogānupalabdhi), because the latter are organized and stable entities; (11) substances are capable of being employed in diverse ways for curative ends (vi-kalpa-sāmarthya); and (12) substances, being concrete structures are not suppressed or supplanted by other substances or qualities (pratīghāta-sāmarthya).

The primacy of the substance is brought out by *Charaka-Saṁhitā* (sūtra, 1,40). "There can be no maturation (pāka) without potency (vīrya), and no potency without taste (rasa); and there can be no taste without substance (dravya). Therefore, substances are primary and most important."

In Indian medicine, 'substance' is specifically defined as constituted by five primary forms of matter (pāñcha-bhautika): earth, water, fire, air and ākāśa. Drugs as substances share this characteristic with the human body-mind complex, which can be diseased. [*See* THEORY OF PAÑCHABHŪTA].

There are several classifications of substances. The nine primary substances (the five forms of matter, soul, mind, time and space) are described as 'causal' (kārana), while the entire world of objects is described as emergent or as effect (kārya). The objects of the world, although constituted by all five primary forms of matter are identifiable by the prevalence of one or the other of the forms (*SS*,1, 41). The guiding principle is:'objects are discrete owing to the excessive presence of one of the forms of matter ("utkarshena tu vyapadeśah", *AS*, 1,17; also *AHr*, 1,9).

Substances are also classified into living beings (chetana, organic) and non-living things (achetana, inorganic). Living beings are equipped with sense-organs while non-living matter does not have this facility. The presence of consciousness is what explains the capability of sensations (sendriya) among the living beings. In the case of non-living matter, consciousness being absent, sensations are impossible (nirindriya). Soul (ātman) becomes conscious only on account of its association with the body and the sense-organs. Living beings are further classified into beings in which consciousness is only latent (antaśchetana, such as plants and trees) and beings in which consciousness is both latent and explicit (bahir-antaśchetana, such as animals and human beings). The former group is also called immobile (sthāvara) and the latter mobile (jaṅgama).

There is another classification based on how substances originate. Substances derived from plants and trees (audbhida or vanaspati-ja) include roots, bark, sap, gum, secretions, leaves, sprouts, flowers, bud, thorns, fruits, bulbs, oil extracts and burnt powders. They are divided into four major groups (*CS*, 1.1); (a) plants and trees which have fruits but no visible flowers (vanaspati): (b) creepers and climbers which grow on the support of a tree or which spread on the ground (vīrudh); and (c) plants the lives of which are over as soon as they yield fruits (aushadhi).

Substances derived from mobile living beings (jaṅgama) include milk, butter, honey, skin, bone flesh, blood, bone-marrow, flesh-marrow, urine, horns, hoofs, nails, hair and excretions. Living beings are classified into four groups: (a) born out of wombs (jarāyuja, viviparous) like animals and humans; (b) born of eggs (andaja, oviparous), like reptiles and birds; (c) born of sweat and slime (svedaja) like worms and insects; and (d) born from the earth (udbhijja) like frogs and fireflies. Substances derived from sources other than the two aforementioned, that is, those obtained directly from the earth (prthivī-janya), like metals, minerals, salts, sand and precious stones, form another sub-group .

The classification of substances into food (āhāra) and drugs (aushadha) is also significant. Articles of food value are taste-dominated (rasa-pradhāna) and are meant primarily to sustain and nourish the body constituents. Drugs, on the other hand, are dominated by intense, moderate or meagre potency (vīrya-pradhāna), and are meant to create new conditions in the body which either maintain health or cure diseases by correcting the malefic influences of vāta, pitta and kapha. [*See* FOOD *and* DRUG]. In case of diseases, it is recommended that drugs must be administered first, and when the diseased condition has been brought under control, articles of food that are suitable for recovery and nourishment of the weakened body constituents need to be indicated. Pharmaceutical preparations (kalpa), therefore, include both drugs and food. The *Charaka-Saṁhitā* and the *Suśruta Saṁhitā* contain elaborate classifications of drugs according to their actions, and food articles according to their morphology.

The three-fold classification of substances in terms of their effects (prabhāva) actually refer to drugs and food articles. Some substances help in eliminating or reducing the malefic influences of the three doshas (dosha-praśamana) [*See* DRUG *and* DOSHA.]. Some, on the other hand, serve to excite or derange the doshas, and bring about disorder in the normal function of the seven body constituents or dhātus (dhātu-pradūshana or kopana). Some substances, however, help maintain normalcy (svastha-hita); they are the articles of food or diet that one is accustomed to take, and those that are conducive to one's well-being.

Substances are also classified in terms of the six taste groups (rasa-skandha) : sweet, sour, saline, bitter, astringent and pungent [*See* TASTE]. Substances are again grouped into eight (heavy, light, cold, hot, coarse, soft, intense and unctuous) or two (cold and hot) groups in terms of drug-potency [*See* POTENCY]. The most elaborate classification, however, is pharmacological (karma). The *Charaka Samhitā* (1, 4) provides a list of 70, and *Suśruta Saṁhitā* (1, 38) 37 groups of substances with their characteristic effects on the organism. [*See* DRUG, GUNA, DRAVYA-GUNA].

Dravya-Guna : An important aspect of Indian medicine dealing with the identification, description and classification of drugs (pharmacology) and also the preparations and administration of drugs (viz. pharmacy, bhaishajya). This aspect has been recognized as the foremost among the eight limbs of the present-day Āyurveda : pharmacology, diagnostics, therapeutics, major surgery, minor surgery, psychotherapy, toxicology and paediatrics (Dravya-guna, Nidāna, Kāya-chikitsā, Śalya, Śālākya, Bhūta-vidyā, Agada-tantra, and Kaumāra-bhrtya). There is extensive literature on this subject both in Sanskrit and in regional languages [*See* NIGHANTU].

The foundation of this aspect is to be found in the concept of 'substance' (dravya) as crystallized in the Nyāya-Vaiśeshika system [*See* DRAVYA]. As far as medicine is concerned, among the categories of existence (padārthas, 6 or 7), substance is the most important, for the other categories are dependent upon it. Substances are known by the properties they possess (guna) and the action they cause in the organism (karma). The science of 'dravya-guna', therefore, inquires into the nature of substances and the medicinal value they have in order to preserve the health of the individual as well as to cure the diseases that he may suffer from. Substances, from this point of view, comprehend both articles of food (āhāra) and drugs (aushadha).

"In a substance are to be found five categories of existence (pañcha padārthāh) : properties (guṇa), tastes (rasa), systemic changes (vipāka), potencies (vīrya), and specific effects (prabhāva), each of which discharges its own function" (*BP*). This aspect of Āyurveda deals with all these details. Broadly, however, three details are recognized : drugs (dravya), their therapeutic properties (guṇas) and their pharmacological actions (karma). The second detail is made to include tastes, systemic changes, potencies and effects. Thus there are seven categories that are treated in 'Dravya-guṇa-vijñāna'. [*See* DRAVYA, GUNA, PHARMACOLOGY, RASA, VĪRYA, VIPĀKA, PRABHĀVA, DRUG, PHARMACOLOGICAL ACTION].

Dream : Three states (waking, dream and deep sleep), have been recognized since the Upanishadic period. The waking state characterized by the awareness of oneself and the outside world and transactions of the former with the latter, signifies the predominance of sattva; and the state of deep sleep, characterized by total withdrawal of the awareness both of oneself and of the outside world and the absence of transaction signifies the prevalence of tamas. The dream state which is neither completely a sleep state nor full wakefulness, is the 'meeting point' (sandhyā-sthāna) of the two states. It is dominated by the mind and its projections; and, therefore, it signifies the dominance of rajas.

SS (śarīra, 4, 30-34) explains sleep as due to the overcoming of the heart (which is the seat of mind) by tamas, and wakefulness as due to the prevalence in it of sattva. The action of tamas in sleep is principally on the sense-organs (including mind), which are the instruments of transaction with the outside world. It is because of this action that the corporeal self (bhutātmā) although never devoid of consciousness, is said to lapse into sleep (*SS*, ibid. 36). However, when the sense-organs continue to be overcome by tamas, but the mind is associated with rajas, it is kept active and there are perceptions of objects, good and bad. These perceptions are of the nature of projections of the mind, based on previous experiences that are bodily (*SS*, ibid, 35).

CS (indriya, 5, 42), however, notes that dreams occur in a state of sleep that is not deep (nāti-prasuptah), and are of the nature of mental perceptions of sensory data in that condition (when the functional aspects of the sense-organs are not entirely suspended by the prevailing tamas). *CS* (ibid., 41) also mentions the 'channels conveying mind' (manovahanam), which are explained by CHKP as signifying 'all the channels in the body' (sarva-śarīra-srotāmsi), especially the ten arteries (dhamanīs) that are found in the heart (for mind is located in the heart, 'hrdayāśritatvān manasah'), as there is no mention of separate 'mind-carrying' channels in the body.

Dreams are classified into seven types : 'seen' (drshṭa', viz. dreams which are mere repetitions of the forms of the things visually apprehended during the waking state), 'heard' (śruta, viz. sounds heard), 'experienced (by the other sense-organs), (anubhūta), 'desired' (prārthita, viz. dreams of the nature of fulfilments of wishes concerning things seen, sounds heard or other experiences), 'imagined' (kalpita, viz. dreams which are neither reproductions of experiences of the waking state, nor 'desired', but spontaneous and exaggerated creations of the mind), 'predictive' (bhāvita, viz. dreams that forebode events that are likely to occur in future), and 'generated by the doshas' (doshaja, viz. dreams that have the derangement of one or more doshas as their source) (*CS*, indriya, 5, 43-44; cf. *also AHr*, śarīra, 6, 61).

The first five of these are without significance (aphalaṁ): like day-dreams and dreams which are excessively prolonged or very brief (*CS*, ibid. 44). The last two of the seven varieties mentioned above have significance, especially when the dreamer is a patient. By the former, the physician understands the prognostic indications, and by the latter, the nature of the dosha that has been vitiated. In the former case, even the prognostic character of the dream may be belied by the patient's conduct soon after he wakes up from the dream (*CS*, ibid. 55-56).

There is a detailed account of dreams that have good and bad prognosis in the classical texts (*CS*, ibid., 6, 27-42 and *AHr*, ibid, 6, 30-58). There are also accounts of characteristic dreams of constitutional types (viz. vāta-prakrti, pitta-prakrti and kapha-prakrti [*See* CONSTITUTION] (e.g. *SS*, śarīra, 4, 63-77; *AHr*, śarīra, 3, 83-104). [*See also* CONSTITUTION, PROGNOSTIC AIDS, SLEEP].

Drug : Substances which have a medicinal property are broadly classified into three groups : (1) articles of food (āhāra), (2) medicinal preparations or drugs (aushadha) and (3) poisons (visha). The basic idea is that besides the actual drugs, food as well as poison can be employed for therapeutic ends. In fact, dietetics is an important aspect of Indian medicine; only when normal articles of food are not competent to correct a disorder, drugs are resorted to. And no serious distinction is made between drugs, food and poison. Food or drug taken when it is not indicated, or in a measure that is not proper, will act like poison and poison, when taken in small measures in the prescribed manner, may be beneficial to the system. [*See* FOOD, POISON].

Drugs listed in the classical pharmacological works include animal products (prāni-janya), substances from the plant kingdom (vanaspati-janya), and minerals and metals (khanija). However, vegetable drugs constitute the bulk of prescriptions in Āyurveda. Drugs being meant to assist the life-force and not oppose it, care is taken to prevent the possible side-effects or unassimilable deposits of the drug in the system. It is therefore that drugs in Indian medicine are not synthetic in character. Further, the main argument of Āyurveda being that diseases are caused by stresses imposed on the individual by his own behaviour, by the food that he has ingested or by the environmental changes and not by germs, microbes or bacillae, the drugs are mostly the substances that share the characteristics of the body and the world around and appropriate to the diseases and seasons [*See* DRAVYA, TRIDOSHA]. Drugs are determined by the differential biological responses to them. [*See* PHARMACOLOGY and DRUG-ACTION].

Drugs of vegetable origin are classified according to the kind of country they are grown in (*CS*, 7, 1, 8). Places of drug origin are of three types : (1) 'Aquatic' or humid (ānupa), where water is abundant (rains are copious, and rivers and ponds abound), trees grow thick and much, winds blow with vigour and speed, and sunlight is scarce. This kind of country is said to be unhealthy, people who live here being stricken with ailments of vāta and kapha (2) 'Arid' or mountainous (jāngala), where water is scarce, sunlight fierce, vegetation meagre and wind strong. This is similar to desert tracts, but is healthy. People who live here are generally free from ailments. And they are distinguished by the predominance of vāta and pitta. (3) 'Medium' (sādhārana), where the characteristics of the above two kinds of land are balanced. People who live here are of average health, their constitution is both favourable and unfavourable to diseases, depending upon other factors (*CS*, sūtra, 25, 36 etc., and *SS*, sūtra, 37).

The soil where the drug is grown is an important consideration. In accordance with the pāñcha-bhautika theory, the soil can be one of five types depending on the predominance of the primary element (mahā-bhūta). The soil which is predominantly 'earthy' (pārthiva) is characteristically stony, hard, black, with thick trees and grass. The soil that is 'watery' (āpya) is smooth, cool, with water in the neighbourhood, whitish in colour, favourable for cereals and soft-wood plants. The soil that is 'fiery' (āgneya) is multi-coloured, full of small gravel and has a few pale trees and grasses. Trees have hollows in them and contain little 'taste'. The soil that is 'windy' (vāyavya) is rough, ash-coloured or grey, has hollows or cavities with few plants. The soil that is distinguished by ākāśa (ākāśīya) is irregular, full of cavities, light blue in colour, soft to touch, has water in it which is tasteless, has lofty mountains and full of vegetation; the trees that grow there have feeble heartwood.

The drug will be most effective if the bhautika-element of the soil in which it is grown is matched with the bhautika element of the disorder. *BPN* (1, 5, 115) makes another classification of the soil in terms of 'brāhmana' (white), 'kshattriya' (red), 'vaiśya' (yellow) and 'śūdra' (black); and suggests that the drugs growing on these soils will be most effective when used by patients belonging to these caste-groups!

While this classification of drugs on the basis of the kind of soil is not taken seriously by the practising physicians at any time, the suggestion of *CS* (7, 1,9) regarding the most effective drugs makes sense. The plants to be used for preparing drugs must have grown either on jāngala or on sādhārana soil, on an even ground which is clean, with source of water in close proximity and open to seasonal rains, sunlight and wind. Plants growing on burning grounds or funerary mounds, or within temple enclosures, or on land that is full of anthills, on the grounds where people frequently assemble (sabhā), on the land that is ploughed or where plants are overshadowed by great trees, are unsuitable.

There are further specifications about the suitability or otherwise of plants for medicinal purposes (*CS*, 7, 1, 10 and *SS*, 1, 37). The plants that have grown in the proper season, that have grown to their normal stature, that have acquired the fullest measure of their taste, potency and smell and that have not lost their smell, colour, taste, etc. due to time, heat, fire, water, wind or animals, are suitable (*CS*). The plants that are attacked by worms, stricken with poison, cut with weapons, dried in the fierce sun or excessive wind, injured by fire or water are unsuitable. The plant that has acquired one taste all over and has grown well, with roots firmly fixed in the earth, is suitable (*SS*).

The plants grown in the northern direction (udīcyam) are said to be specially good (*SS*). The reason for this belief may be because the Himālayas, where precious medicinal herbs abound, are situated in the north or it may be because the guardian divinity of the northern direction is the moon (Soma), who is also the 'lord of the medicinal herbs' (oshadhīnām rājā). While the *CS* does not refer to this belief, it prescribes that the physician should face north while gathering medicinal plants (7, 1, 10). According to this text, the gatherer of the medicinal plants must be good in his conduct (mangalāchārah) and benevolent in his attitude (kalyāna-vrtta); he should purify himself, wear white garments, worship the Aśvins and fast before he sets about collecting the herbs (ibid.).

The parts of the plants that are often utilized in medicinal preparations are roots (mūla), underground stalk or tuber (kānda), leaves (patra), flowers (pushpa), fruits (phala), branches (śākhā), gum-resin and heart-wood (sāra), latex (kshīra), bark (tvak) and wood (kāshtha). Broadly however, the plant is described as 'five-limbed' (pañchānga) : roots, tubers, flowers, leaves and fruits. The *CS* (7, 1,10) prescribes that these parts have to be gathered in specific seasons for best effect. Branches and leaves are best gathered during the rainy season (varshā) or spring (vasanta); roots in summer (grīshma) or late winter (śiśira); bark, tuber and latex in autumn (śarad); heart-wood in early winter (hemanta); flowers and fruits in seasons when they are available (yathā-rtu). *RN*, however, gives a slightly different prescription : tubers in early winter, roots in late winter, flowers in spring, leaves in summer and whole plants (pañchānga) in autumn. The *SS* cites an opinion of early teachers that roots have to be gathered in the early monsoon (prāvrt); leaves in the rainy season (varshā); bark in autumn; latex in early winter; heart-wood in spring; and fruits in summer (1, 37).

The *SS* utilizes the agnī-shomīya theory and says that the herbs related to the Moon (saumya), which are predominantly 'cool in potency' (śīta-vīrya), are to be gathered in the cool months (viz. rains, autumn and early winter), while the herbs related to fire (agneya) which are predominantly 'hot in potency' (ushna-vīrya), are to be gathered in the warm months (late winter, spring, and summer). According to *SaS*, plants grown in the region around the Himālayan ranges are 'moon-related' (saumya) whereas those that grow in the region around the Vindhya mountain area are 'fire-related' (āgneya). The saumya herbs, which are also collected from the saumya soil are supposed to be predominantly sweet (madhura), unctuous (snigdha), and cool (śīta) in property.

SaS, however, offers a more practical suggestion : any part of the plant may be gathered afresh in autumn, except when the parts are required to prepare drugs which are emetics and purgatives (then the parts of the plants must be collected at the end of spring).

With regard to the drugs of animal origin (like honey, milk, urine, blood, bile, marrow, flesh, excreta, skin, horns, hoofs, bone, nails), the seasonal restrictions do not apply. But the parts of the body (blood, nails, bone, etc.) used as drugs must belong to fully mature (adult) animals, while the secretions (milk etc.), excreta and urine must be collected after the food is completely digested in the animal.

There are also instructions in the classical texts regarding the storage of drugs. They must be stored in rooms that are well ventilated and periodically fumigated; they must be kept in cloth-bags or earthern pots which do not reflect the impact of seasonal changes and which are well covered. The place where the drugs are stored must be free from heat, moisture, humidity, smoke, dust, rodents and other pests. It must be equally suitable in all seasons. It is preferable to have the doors of the room where drugs are stored to face north or east.

Indian medicine uses crude drugs as well as various preparations from them. Drugs, when ready for ingestion, must be purified and converted not only into an effective form but also into a form that is easy and agreeable to take. The physical and chemical impurities that the crude drugs may contain naturally must be removed (śọdhana), so that the possible bad effects are eliminated. Especially as this is a necessity where the impurities are inherent in the substance and are capable of toxic effect (like aconitum). Minerals and poisons require an elaborate process of purification before they are used as drugs.

Drugs used in Indian medicine are of numerous forms. The major ones are the following: (1) Extracts (kashāyas) of five kinds: (a) expressed juice (sva-rasa), which is a heavy preparation containing the whole drug, meant for patients who are strong and whose digestive system is good; (b) pounded mass, paste (kalka) of the whole drug; (c) decoction (kvātha); (d) cold infusion (hima) and (e) hot infusion (phāṇṭa). [*See* KASHĀYA. SVARASA, KALKA, KVĀTHA, HIMA, PHĀṆṬA]. The choice of the extract depends upon the general condition of the patient as well as his powers of digestion and upon the sensitivity of the disease. Among the five kinds of extracts mentioned above, heaviness as well as potency decreases in order.

(2) Fatty preparations like clarified butter, ghee (ghṛta) and medicated oils (taila). [*See* GHṚTA, TAILA]

(3) Fermented preparations (sandhāna), like āsavas (where drugs are mixed with

water and allowed to ferment) and arishṭas (where concoctions of drugs are used), both functioning like weak wines but heightening the drug contents, sīdhu (which is fermented product of raw or boiled juices of plants), surā, surā-maṇḍa, medaka etc. [*See* ĀSAVA, ARISHṬA].

(4) Thickened extracts for licking (lehas and avalehas) got from boiling the decoctions down to a thick consistency. [*See* LEHA].

(5) Alkali (kshāra), prepared by the use of caustics and usually of three orders of potency (mild, moderate, intense), and administered internally as drinks (pānīya) or externally as applications (prati-sāraṇīya).

(6) Powders (chūrṇa) containing the whole drugs pounded in the dry state and strained; large pills (guṭika) and small pills (vaṭaka) made by boiling down the decoction to a thick consistency and adding powdered drugs; sweet uncooked pills or bolus (modaka), made by mixing cold syrups to powdered drugs. [*See* CHURṆA, GUṬIKA].

(7) Medicated syrups (śarkara or pānaka) prepared by adding sugar to decoctions of drugs and boiled over mild fire to the needed consistency; confections (khaṇḍa-pāka) where powdered drugs are added to syrup.

(8) Weak decoctions (pānīya); decoctions where the drugs ground into a pulp are boiled (pramatthya); decoctions in milk (kshīra-pāka).

(9) Distilled mineral acids (drāvaka) in two forms: svalpa and śaṅkha-drāvakas. [*See* DRĀVAKAS]. Mercurial and mineral preparations (rasa).

(10) Drugs which take the form of food, like soup thickly mixed with gruel (vilepi), slightly mixed with gruel (peya), a drink of thicker consistency (yūsha), thick gruel (yavāgu), boiled cereal water (maṇḍa), meat-soup (māṁsa-rasa), fermented rice-gruel (kañjikā) and butter-milk (takra).

Drugs are also classified according to the modes of administration (bhaishajya-mārga): (1) oral, like 'gargle' (gaṇḍūsha) and 'paint' (prati-sāraṇa) for local action: 'stimulants' (dīpana), 'digestives' (pāchana), emetics (vamana), purgatives (virechana), etc., for action on the gastro-intestinal tract; inhalation of smoke (dhūmapāna) for action on the respiratory system and oral intake of drugs for general action; (2) nasal, like errhine (nasya) for local action; fumigation (dhūpana) for action on the respiratory system and causing a flow of nasal secretion (śiro-virechana) for relieving cerebral congestion; (3) ocular, like fomentation (seka), eye-drops (āśchyotana), poultice (piṇḍika), cooling applications (tarpaṇa) and applications of paste, collyrium etc to the margin of lids or conjunctiva (añjana); (4) auditory, like washing, fumigation and ear-drops; (5) through the head, by application of oils (śiro-basti) in different ways (parisheka, pichu, abhyaṅga, etc.); (6) through the anus, like enemata (basti-karma), in two kinds (anuvāsana and nirūha) and suppository (phala-varti) to relieve constipation; (7) through the urethra, like uttara-basti in urinary disorders; (8) through the vagina, like fumigation, suppository, swabbing, plugging, etc.; and (9) on the skin, like external applications (lepa) rubbing the body with medicated oils (abhyaṅga), and flooding the surface with a current of medicated oil (parisheka). [*See* BHAISHAJYA, PAÑCHA-KARMA].

Drug administration poses its own problems and this aspect has received attention by the old masters. The major considerations while prescribing a drug are: (a) easy availability of the drug in sufficient quantity, (b) efficacy of the drug in curing the disorder while not bringing about undesirable side-effects, c) capacity for altering the pharmaceutical forms of the drug so that the drugs are conveniently administered and (d) the potency of the drug (rasa-vīrya-guṇa).

In accordance with these considerations, there are (a) substitute drugs (pratinidhi-dravya), (b) postprandial drink (anupāna), pharmaceutical expedients (yoga), and preservation of the potency of the drug by several reinforcing constituents and by suggesting suitable regimen for the patient (pathya). [*See* PRATINIDHI-DRAVYA, ANUPĀNA, YOGA, PATHYA].

It is also regarded as necessary to avoid the physical, chemical or pharmacological incompatibility of the drugs. The physician is asked to avoid prescribing drugs which are incompatible or inconsistent with the climate and soil (deśa-viruddha), seasons (kāla-), the patient's digestive capacity (agni-), the patient's constitution and diathesis (sāthymāsatmya), mode of preparation (saṁskāra), pharmacological details (rasa-vīrya-), condition of the digestive organs (koshṭha-), general condition of the patient (avasthā-), arrangement or order of drug administration (krama-), rules of drug-preparation (pāka-), physical or chemical details (saṁyoga-), the likes and dislikes of the patient (hṛd-) and his normal food habits (vidhi-).

In general, however, drug incompatibility is grouped into three kinds: (1) quantitative (māna-virodha), as, e.g. ghee and honey taken in equal proportions, (2) physical and chemical (guṇa-virodha), when two drugs having opposite properties are mixed (like salt and milk which have opposite tastes) and (3) pharmacological (karma-virodha), viz. antagonisms like the astringent dhātakī (Woodfordia fruticosa) and the purgative danti (Baliospermum montanum)

Dosage of the drug (māna) is an important consideration. Three measures have been used in Indian medicine : measure by weight (pautava-māna), measure by volume (druvaya-māna) and measure by length (payya-māna). As regards the first measure, there are two variant measures in vogue : the Māgadha-māna and the Kaliṅga-māna; the former is regarded as superior to the latter. These measures take 'atom' (paramāṇu) as the smallest unit. (e.g. 30 paramāṇus making one vaṁśī in the Māgadha-scale, while 12 gaura-sarshapas making one yava in the Kaliṅga-scale). The second measure (by volume) takes 'drop' (bindu, a drop that falls from the index finger after its portion upto two nodes is dipped in the fluid) as the unit (8 bindus constituting one sara, etc). The third measure (length) takes 'inch' (aṅgula, the length made by 8 yava-grains being pierced together by a needle length-wise as the unit of measurement (12 aṅgulas making one vitasti, etc). [*See* MEASURES].

The time of drug-administration is another significant topic for discussion in the medical texts. Drug ingestion and food-intake are considered in relation to each other : (1) drugs taken on an empty stomach (abhakta) are said to be most effective for strong constitutions, especially when the disorders are due to aggravation of kapha; (2) drugs taken before meals (prāg-bhakta) are effective in disorders relating to apāna-vāyu, in toning up the intestinal muscles and in reducing fat; (3) drugs taken during meals (madhya-bhakta) are indicated in disorders of samāna-vāyu, especially gastro-intestinal disturbances; (4) drugs taken after meals (adhobhakta) strengthen the upper part of the body; they correct the disorders due to vyāna-vāyu and udāna-vāyu and diseases arising from kapha; (5) drugs mixed with food during meals (sama-bhakta) are recommended for children, patients of delicate constitution and patients who dislike taking medicines; they are also useful in diseases like anorexia and disturbances which have manifested in the entire body; (6) drugs taken between meals, during the day or night (antarā-bhakta) viz. in the afternoon after the midday meal has been digested or in the night after the evening meal is digested, help the patients whose digestion is good and whose diseases are caused by disordered vyāna-vāyu; (7) drugs taken both before and after meals (samudga) are useful in disorders of the upper and lower parts of the body, in diseases like hiccough and convulsions; (8)

drugs taken very frequently (muhur-muhuh) do not bear any relation to the meals; they are indicated in dyspnoea, cough, thirst, vomiting and poisoning; (9) drugs taken with the first morsel of food during meals (sagrāsa) usually take the form of powders, (like hiṅgvashtaka-chūrna) and are effective as appetisers (dīpana) and digestives (pāchana); they are indicated in disorders due to apāna-vāyu; (10) drugs taken between morsels of food during meals (grāsāntara) are useful in diseases due to prāṇa-vāyu, especially heart-diseases; and (11) drugs taken at bed-time (niśā) correct disorders of the head, mouth, ear, eyes, nose and throat.

SaS, however, provides a much shorter list of four times for drug-administration : morning, midday, early night, bed-time and frequent.

Drugs in Indian medicine are usually administered along with some 'vehicle' (anupāna, like cold water, honey, ghee, butter, milk or jaggery) in order that the drug may be assimilated right and to prevent undesirable side-effects that the drug may have. The 'vehicle' is decided on considerations like the nature of the drug; the condition of the patient and the type of disease. [*See* ANUPANA, *also* DRUG-ACTION, PHARMACOLOGY, PHARMACY].

Drug-Action: The major premise of Indian medicine is that the body as well as the drug are constituted by the five primary elements (earth, water, fire, air and ākāśa). [*See* THE THEORY OF PAÑCHA-BHUTA]. The doctrine of the three doshas (vāta, kapha, pitta) as the fundamental fabric of psychophysical constitution also presupposes this premise [*See* TRIDOSHA]. Health is the expression of the normal and balanced functioning of the three doshas and diseases are caused when this balance is disturbed, one or more of the doshas becoming magnified or attenuated. The purpose of the treatment is to tone down the magnified dosha or magnify the attenuated dosha, so as to restore the balance (*CS*, sūtra, 1, 53). The drug that is administered is considered appropriate and effective when the errant doshas are brought under control. The drug is selected by the dominance of a particular element relevant to the disturbance of elements in the patient's body. Thus, there is a close relationship between the 'structure' of the drug and its 'function' in the human body. This relationship is known as 'drug-action' (aushadha karma).

As the drug is ingested, it is first acted upon by the 'stomachic fire' (jāṭharagni) and then 'cooked' by the 'constituent fires' (dhātvagni) and the 'elemental fires' (bhūtāgni) [*See* AGNI]. Thus, the drug gets assimilated into the constituents of the body and into the physical elemental composition of the body (*CS*, chikitsā 15). The action of the drug may be through its properties (guṇa) and 'taste after digestion' in the body (rasa), when the action is said to be local (sthānika); or it may be through the digestive changes in the body (vipāka) and the potency of the drug (vīrya), when the action is called 'general' or 'systemic' (sārva-dehika). Or again, it may be through the 'specific effect' of the drug (prabhāva), when the action is 'specific' (viśishṭa).

The drug-actions are broadly classified as follows :

1. 'stomachics' (dīpana), which stimulate the digestive fire (viz. gastric nerves), but which do not directly help in the digestion of food. Drugs which act as stomachics are predominantly 'fire' and 'air' in their elemental constitution, intense, warm and light in property, predominantly 'fiery' (āgneya) in nature, pungent, sour and saltish in taste and hot in potency. These only increase appetite, like miśi (*Foeniculum vulgare*).
2. 'digestives' (pāchana), which increase the secretion of gastric juices and help directly in digestion of food; but they do not stimulate appetite (*See* ĀMA]. Example is Nāga-kesara

(*Mesua Ferrea*).

3. 'gastric sedatives' (śamana), which tranquillise the excited tissues and nerves in the stomachic region; they pacify the provoked pitta, like amrta (*Tinospora cordifolia*).

4. 'carminatives' (anulomana) which facilitate easy elimination of waste product (mala) through their outlets. They act upon the vāta channels and are soothing in property and hot in potency; like hingu (*Ferula foetida*).

5. 'laxatives' (sraṁsana), which drive downwards the waste matter that remains impacted in the intestines; like eranda-taila (*Ricinus communis*).

6. 'simple and anthracene purgatives' (bhedana), which break the hardened seybala and push it downwards; like katukī (*Picrorrhiza kurroa*).

7. 'drastic purgatives' (virechana), which liquify the excreta and facilitate their expulsion; like snuhi (*Euphorbia nerifolia*).

8. 'emetic' (vamana), which force out (vomit) the bilious matter and mucus, even when the digestive processes are as yet incomplete; like madana-phala (*Randia dumetorum*).

9. 'eliminatives' (Saṁśodhana), which force out the excretory products through the mouth as well as through the anus; like devadāli (*Luffa echinata*).

10. 'expectorant' (chhedana), which, owing to their specific effect, remove from the body the morbid aspect of doshas, especially kapha (hence also called śleshma-hara); like maricha (*Piper nigrum*).

11. 'attenuants' (lekhana), which rarefy the protoplasmic contents of tissue-cells and thus gradually clear the system of its deranged constituents, like vachā (*Acorus calamus*).

12. 'inspissates' (grāhī) which facilitate the absorption of intestinal fluids, because these drugs are predominantly 'fiery' in their constitution; they act as appetisers as well as digestives; they are hot in potency and pungent in taste; like śunthi (*Zinziber*).

13. 'secretions-arresting' drugs (stambhana), drugs which cause stasis and condensation in the tissue-fluids; they are drying, cooling and astringent in their property, and are predominantly air in composition. They increase vāta in the intestines and dry up the liquids. They are not digestive in action; they are cold in potency; like vatsaka (*Holarrhena*).

14 'rejuvenative' drugs (rasāyana) which prevent infirmities of old age and diseases. They strengthen all the body constituents and lengthen the life-span (āyuh-sthāpana); like harītakī (*Terminalia chebula*) and guḍūchī (*Tinospora cordifolia*).

15. 'aphrodisiacs' (vājīkaraṇa) which reinforce and increase sexual appetite and potency; like nāgabalā (*Sida spinosa*).

16. 'semen-promoting' drugs (śukrala), which increase the secretion of semen; like sugar and śatāvarī (*Asparagus racemosa*).

17. 'subtle' drugs (sūkshma), which can penetrate into the minutest parts of the body; like honey and salt.

18. 'decomposing' drugs (vyavāyi), which initially diffuse through the entire body and then get dissolved (digested); like ahiphena (opium) and vijayā (*Cannabis indica*).

19. 'relaxing' drugs (vikāśī) which initially rob the body constituents of their vigour (ojas) and then relax the ligaments, joints, etc. of the body; like betelnut.

20. 'poisons' (visha), which deprive the body of its vigour (ojas) and cause loss of life; like aconite and opium.

21. 'churning' drugs (pramāthi), which owing to their potency churn up the morbid matter (secretions, excreta, etc.) in the channels of the body and throw it out; like maricha (black pepper) and vachā (*Acorus calamus*).

22. 'irritants' (vidāhī), which cause eructations and acidity in the stomach and thereby generate abnormal thirst and heart-burn, like sarshapa (*Brassica campestris*) and laṅkā (red pepper).

23. 'drugs which obstruct the channels of cir-

culation' (abhishyandi), owing to their heavy and slimy properties, retard lymphatic circulation and arrest secretions in the channels of the body; like curds. They tend to increase *kapha*.
24. 'vehicular' drugs (yoga-vāhī); which, as they are digested, facilitate the action of other drugs which are taken at the same time; like honey, ghee, mercury and alkali.
25. 'analgesics' (vedanā-sthāpana), which remove pain and stabilize pleasurable feeling; like opium and aconites. Because of their unctuous property, they increase kapha and facilitate sleep. They are 'hot' in potency and excite the vāta element.
26. 'nutrients' (jīvanīya), which facilitate health, vitality and life; like milk and vidārī (*Ipomea paniculata*).

There is also a classification of drugs according to their actions on the body's several systems, like digestive, respiratory, nervous, circulatory, etc. [*See DGV*, I,pp.246-303].

Drug-properties: The physical properties of substances listed in *CS* and *SS* [*See* DRAVYA-GUNA] are relevant not only for the constitution of the human body but also for the composition of drugs. Each of these properties has a nature of its own, a specific rôle in the human body both in health and in sickness, a characteristic action on the body constituents (dhātu), on the doshas, and on the waste-products (mala). Selection of the drug takes all these details into consideration.

Twenty of these properties are listed in the *CS*, and three more are added in *SS*.
1. 'Heaviness' (guru): contributes to the gravity of 'earth' as well as 'water'; tends to make the body bulky and strong, and nourishes the body constituents; it increases the quantity of waste-products; it renders the 'fires' in the body sluggish; it makes one feel heavy, dull and fatigued. Examples are māsha (*Phaseolus mungo*) and muśalī (*Chlorophytum tuberosum*).
2. 'Lightness' (laghu): opposite of the above, it is the property of ākāśa and it contributes to the upward movement of air and fire; it tends to make the body emaciated and weak; it starves the body constituents; it diminishes the quantity of waste-products; it quickens the 'fires' in the body to help digest the food; it makes one feel energetic and active. An example is mudga (*Phaseolus radiatus*).
3. 'Cold' (śīta); its support in the physical world is 'water'; it is also a property of air; it reduces heat in the body; it facilitates vāta and kapha but acts against pitta; it contributes to the enrichment of body constituents; it impedes the flow of blood; it makes for pleasurable feeling; it cools down the disturbances of pitta, like thirst, burning and fainting. An example is chandana (*Santalum album*).
4. 'Hot' (ushna): opposite of śīta. It is a property of 'fire' and therefore increases the heat in the body, and brings thirst; it facilitates pitta but acts against vāta and kapha; it impedes the nourishment of the body constituents, but favours the flow of blood; it promotes the production of urine, excreta and sweat; it stimulates appetite and digests food; but an excess of it results in fainting, thirst and burning sensation, and induces mental unrest. An example is chitraka (*Plumbago zeylanica*).
5. 'Unctuous' (snigdha): it is the special property of 'water', and therefore it makes things wet and unctuous; it produces oiliness, softness and wetness in the body, and also increases the strength and colour of the body constituents; it acts against vāta, but facilitates kapha; it helps eliminate the waste products from the body and it favours sexual appetite. An example is ghrta (ghee).
6. 'Dry' (rūksha): opposite of the above, it is the special characteristic of 'air' and, therefore, it can dry things up; it makes for dryness, hardness and coarseness in the body; it acts against kapha but facilitates vāta; it har-

dens the faecal matter and impedes its elimination and also diminishes the sexual appetite. Example is yava (*Hordeum vulgare*).

7. 'Slow' (manda): it is the property of 'earth' and 'water'; it acts slowly and little; but when it enters the body it pacifies the errant doshas; it provokes kapha and works against pitta; it increases the body constituents and makes for bulkiness of the body; it impedes the process of elimination of waste-products from the body. An example is gudūchi (*Tinospora cordifolia*)

8. 'Sharp' (tīkshṇa): opposite of the above, it is the property of 'fire' and therefore, facilitates pitta and acts against vāta and kapha; entering the body, it cleanses the system (śodhana), but works against the body constituents and emaciates the body; it encourages the elimination of waste-products from the body; it contributes to restlessness of mind. An example is jayapāla (*Croton tiglium*).

9. 'Stable' (sthira): it is the property of 'earth', and assists in rendering the body constituents stable, strong and resistant; it makes the roots of hair, teeth and nails firm; it stabilizes nerves and semen; it arrests the easy elimination of waste-products from the body; it increases kapha. An example is prthukā (grain?).

10. 'Mobile' (sara): opposite of the above, it is a property of 'water' although in its action it is dominated by 'air'; it facilitates vāta; it provokes in the body the formation and elimination of waste-products; it emaciates the body constituents. An example is svarnapatrī (*Hoya viridiflora*).

11. 'Soft' (mrdu): it is the property of 'water' and ākāśa, and is illustrated in the body constituents like muscle, blood and marrow, and organs like liver, spleen and intestines; it contributes to the soft texture and the fragile character of some parts of the body; it enhances kapha, retards vāta and pitta; it softens the waste products. An example is eranda-taila (*Ricinus communis*, oil).

12. 'Hard' (kaṭhina): opposite of the above, it is a property of 'earth' and makes for hardness and firmness of the body; it renders the body constituents hard and firm; it hardens the waste-products; it facilitates vāta. Examples are pravāḷa (coral) and muktā (pearl).

13. 'Pellucid' or 'Clear' (viśada): it is a property of 'earth', 'air', 'fire' and ākāśa, and cleanses the interior of the body, also keeps the organs and their functions distinct and well-regulated; it helps in the emaciation of the body but heals the wounds; it facilitates vāta. Examples are nimba (*Azadirachta indica*) and kshāra (alkali).

14. 'Slimy' (picchila): opposite of the above, it is a property of 'water', and makes things slimy and stringy; it increases the body constituents, contributes to body weight and to the integration of the organs of the body; it also helps unite broken bones and heal ruptured parts; it facilitates the elimination of waste; it promotes kapha. An example is isabagola (*Plantago ovata*).

15. 'Gentle' or 'Smooth' (slakshna): very similar to the above, it is a property of ākāśa (according to *CS*), of water (according to *SS*), and of 'fire' (according to Nāgarjuna); it increases the body constituents and facilitates elimination of waste-products; it provokes kapha. An example is milk.

16. 'Coarse' or 'Rough' (khara): similar in action to pellucid (viśada) and opposite of the above, it is a property of 'air' and 'earth' (according to *CS*), of 'air' and 'fire' (according to *SS*); it diminishes the body constituents and emaciates the body; it retards the formation and elimination of waste-products, hardens them; it provokes vāta. Example is karkoṭaki-fruit (*Momordica mixta*).

17. 'Fine' or 'Delicate' (sūkshma): it is a property of 'fire', 'air', and ākāśa; it can enter even into the minute parts of the body, and by pervading the entirety of the body it keeps the channels in the body in good shape; it dries up the waste-products; it facilitates vāta. Example is madya (alcoholic drink).

18. 'Thick' or 'Gross' (sthūla): opposite of the above, it is a property of 'earth' and tends to increase the body's bulk; while it facilitates the growth of body-constituents, it impedes the flow of fluids within the body channels; it helps eliminate the waste-products from the body; it increases kapha. Examples are pishṭaka (flour cake; pounded sesamum seeds) and dadhi (curds).
19. 'Compact' or 'Solid' (sāndra): it is a property of 'earth'; entering into the body, it helps in making the organs of the body compact and well-knit; it facilitates the growth of the body constituents and thickens the waste-poducts; it provokes kapha. An example is butter.
20. 'Fluid' (drava): opposite of the above, it is the property of 'water'; it pervades the entire body, making the parts wet and connected; it facilitates the growth of some body constituents like chyle (rasa) and blood (rakta); it increases the quantity of watery waste-products (like urine) and facilitates their elimination; it provokes kapha and pitta. Examples are water and milk.
21. 'Decomposing' (vyavāyi): it is a property of 'air' and ākāśa; upon entering the body, it diffuses all over the body even before it is assimilated, and later gets assimilated. Examples are bhaṅga (*Cannabis sativa*) and ahiphena (opium).
22. 'Blowing' (vikāśi): it is a property of 'air'; upon entering the body, it spreads all over, diminishing the vitality (ojas), weakening the body constituents and slackening the joints. An example is betelnut (*Areca catechu*).
23. 'Quick-acting' (āśu-kāri): it spreads easily and fast in the body; like oil in water, and accomplishes its action.

Dūshī-visha: This is the name given to poisons that are weak in effect and slow in action. Poisons that may be fatal when fresh, may be rendered quite tame when they become old or when they are exposed to the sun and breeze or when caught in wildfire. Some poisons would not possess all the ten properties that are normally to be found in visha, and therefore would not prove fatal [*See* POISON]. Introduced into the human body, poisons may be weakened by several factors like place (marshy), weather (cloudy, rainy, windy), food (wine, sesamum etc.) and sleep during day time, which serve to aggravate kapha, which in turn would 'cover over' the poison and mitigate its effect. Under 'food', however, are included other factors like physical exercise, sexual congress, violent emotions (anger, etc.). But the poison would remain in the body for many years before it is eliminated, and although not fatal, it may continue to vitiate the body constituents (hence its name dūshī-visha, viz. 'yasmād dushyati dhātūn').

The expression is also used for the toxins generated in the body owing to exposure to the eastern breeze and cold wind, indigestion, habitual sleeping during daytime, improper food etc. These toxins adversely affect the body constituents (dhātu) (cf. also *SS*, kalpa, 23, "constant use of some particular time, place and diet as well as constant and regular day-sleep tends to poison the fundamental root-principles of the body").

It is usual for these slow and weak poisons to get aggravated in cold weather and on rainy days. Among the symptoms that forebode the effect of these poisons are sleepiness, heaviness of limbs, uncontrollable yawning, feeling of loosened joints, body pain, and hairs standing on end. Subsequent symptoms include sense of intoxication after food is eaten, indigestion, loss of relish for food, round patches on the skin, urticaria, spells of fainting, debility, swollen face, ascites, nausea, discolouration of skin, epileptic attacks, excessive thirst and high fever. Insanity may also be brought about in many cases. Atrophy of hands and legs, stuttering, leprosy, incontinence and involuntary discharge of semen are some of the other possible consequences. Among the side-effects are ailments like fever, burning sensation, hiccough, diarrhoea, loss of consciousness, tremor, and pain in the heart.

The course of these poisons in the body is helped by the combined action of vāta and kapha when the poisons enter the stomach, and by the action of vāta and pitta when the poisons reach the intestines. Thereafter, systematic disorganization begins, and the person appears like a bird whose wings are severed (*SS*, kalpa, 19).

Treatment for the disturbances due to slow and weak poisons commences with fomentation and cleansing by emetics and purgatives, and is followed by the administration of the anti-poison drug known as 'dushī-vishāri' (cf.*AHṛ*, Uttara, 35) [*See* POISON, TOXICOLOGY].

E

Ego: [*See* AHAṀKĀRA].

Embryo: Known in Sanskṛit as 'garbha' and defined as "the soul, confined in the uterus, alongside the parental sperm and ovum, the ingredients of nature (prakṛti) and the modifications thereof" (*SS*, śarīra, 5,2), or as "a conglomeration of the five primary forms of matter functioning as the ground for the soul or consciousness" (*CS*, śarīra, 4,6), this topic has merited an elaborate consideration in the classical texts of Indian medicine (*CS*, śarīra, chapters 2 to 5; *SS*, śarīra, 3 and 4) [*See* FOETUS]. The vital factors (prāṇāh) that are essential to the formation of the embryo are: 'fire' (agni, i.e. pitta), 'moon' (soma, i.e. kapha), 'wind' (vāyu, i.e. vāta) (which are the three doshas), sattva, rajas and tamas (which are the three guṇas), the five cognitive organs (viz. their essential possibility) and the individuated soul (bhūtātmā) (*SS*, śarīra, 4,2). The last mentioned factor is the soul (ātman) that enters into the womb, composed of the five primary forms of matter, as a result of past actions. This individual soul (jīva) descends into the zygote (produced from the union of the sperm and ovum) in the uterus, along with the mind, which carries with it the influences of major actions done in previous states of existence (*CS*, śarīra, 3,3). This is the womb which grows, being nourished from the food-juices (of the food ingested and assimilated by the mother) and protected by proper regimen. It develops all the organs, limbs, abilities, strength, complexion and compactness inside the womb, until it is finally delivered in the ninth or tenth month of gestation (*CS*, ibid.)

The efficient cause of the womb is the integration of the sperm from the father and ovum from the mother (śukra-śoṇita-saṁyoga). The material cause is the group of twenty-four aspects of nature (eight-fold, prakṛti, mahat, ahaṁkāra, five tanmātras) and their modifications (sixteen-fold vikṛti). The organizing cause is the individual soul (ātmā), whose presence is indispensable for the formation of the womb as well as for its development (*CS*, śarīra, 4,42).

For the womb as an organism to get formed, there are six determining factors: (1) soul (ātmā) (2) contribution from the mother (3) contribution from the father (4) wholesomeness (sātmya) (5) food-juices assimilated and contributed by the mother (rasa) and (6) mind (sattva) conveying the influences of the main actions performed in previous states of existence (*CS*, ibid., 3,3 and 4,4). They are likened to the several substances that go to make a house come into being, or to a cart being fashioned (*CS*, ibid.,14).

The Indian view is that the womb is derived ultimately from the soul, which continues to be present in the individual all through his life as the 'inner spirit' ('garbhātmā hy antarātmā yah', *CS*, ibid., 8). The involvement of the individual soul in the womb is mysterious but real (*AHr*, śarīra, 1,3). It is because of this involvement that the individual is conscious, has a life-span, has a mind, has sense-organs, can breathe in and breathe out, acquires a definite form, possesses complexion etc., exerts himself, has intentions, experiences pleasure and pain. The soul enters into the womb along with mind (sattva), which carries with it the imprint of the past actions. It is this that makes for individual differences among human beings with regard to temperament, mental ability, feelings, emotions, tastes and aspirations (*CS*, ibid., 10).

The contribution from the mother includes the basic material for the formation of such body details as the layers of the skin, blood, muscle, fat-tissue, large and small intestines, stomach, heart, liver and spleen, bladder, colon, rectum and anus. The contribution from the father includes hair on the head, face and body, nails, bones, teeth, blood vessels, ligaments and sperm. 'Wholesomeness' means the conditions that are favourable to one's own growth and the conditions include the state of general health, energy at one's disposal, clarity of sensory functions, effective vocalizations, complexion, sexual vigour and pleasurable feelings (or contentment, santosha) (*CS,* ibid., 3,11). The organism that is represented by the womb is fed by the food that has been assimilated by the mother, and this becomes the source for the formation and growth of the physical body, nourishment, satisfactions, vital connections and energy for work (*CS,* ibid., 3,12).

Of these six determinants, four (viz. soul, father, mother and mind) are responsible for the initial formation of the embryo, while the other two (wholesomeness and food-juices) contribute to the later growth of the foetus and can function only when the four are present.

The nature of the womb is determined by the sperm and ovum that have provided the basic material, the season in which the womb is formed, the condition of the mother's uterus, the food habits and conduct of the mother, and the nature of the five primary forms of matter that go to form the physical aspect of the womb. Whatever dosha is dominant at the time of the womb's formation will be the characteristic constitution of the individual that develops in due course. Some are vātala (vāta-dominated), some pittala (pitta-dominated), some śleshmala (śleshma- or kapha-dominated), some belong to mixed types (samsrshta), and some have balanced doshas (sama-prakrti) (*CS*, vimāna, 8,15). [*See* CONSTITUTION, TEMPERAMENT, also FOETAL DEVELOPMENT].

Epidemics: Known as 'janapadoddhvamsanīya', epidemics are diseases that afflict people simultaneously despite dissimilarity in their physical constitution, nature, strength, homologation, age, intelligence, food habits, etc. Responsible for such simultaneous affliction are factors that are common to those people, viz. air, water, locality and season. They lead to the simultaneous manifestation of a particular disease in the same set of symptoms in large numbers of people residing in close proximity, and thus destroy whole communities of people (hence called 'janapada-ud-dhvamsanīya') (*CS*, vimāna, 3,5-6).

Air, in epidemic diseases, will be inappropriate to the season, unusually violent or quiet, very dry, hot, cold, rough or humid; turbulent with cross-currents, cyclonic, smelling foul, and carrying gases, sand, ashes and smoke. Water will be foul-smelling, of bad colour and bitter taste; sticky and unpleasant. Aquatic birds will avoid such water, and animals like fish and tortoise will not survive in it. The earth where epidemics thrive will have unpleasant smell, colour, taste and touch, will be very sticky, will be covered with wild vegetation, will abound in reptiles, mosquitoes, locusts, rodents, vultures, owls and jackals, and will not favour growth of edible vegetation; and animal behaviour will markedly change to the worse in such a land. The atmosphere there will be agitated, eery, dark and fearsome. The land invites meteorites, thunderbolts, tremors of the earth, etc. Seasons will have unusual and abnormal characteristics (*CS,* ibid., 7-11).

.Even when all these factors are operative, not all individuals will be afflicted and not all of those who are afflicted will die, provided proper medical treatment is provided. Of the therapeutic methods, elimination (emesis, purgation, enema, errhines) is recommended. Alongwith the drugs and these therapeutic methods, rejuvenation therapy is indicated; and it is necessary to maintain the physical strength of the patients (*CS*, ibid., 12-15).

Errors of judgement: Pathology in Indian medicine regards 'errors of judgement' (prajñāparādha) as one of the three main factors that bring about disease (unhealthy association of sense-objects with organs of sense and seasonal variations being the other two) (*CS*, sūtra, 11,37) [*See* DISEASE]. This is also called the insufficient, excessive, or improper organization of actions (karma) (*AHṛ,* 1,19)

Error of judgement is by its nature an improper ascertainment (vishama-vijñāna), and, in its manifestation, an impulse to an improper conduct (vishama-pravartana) (*CS*, sarīra,1,109). Both aspects are mental, being functions of intelligence (buddhi). Thus, this source of pathology works at the level of the mind (manaso gocharam), although improper thoughts will lead to improper speech and improper conduct.

Mind works in close association with the five cognitive sense-organs; the sensory-data are organized by the mind. Mind not only endows the meaning on sensations, but makes resolutions on the basis of which the organs of action begin to function. The expression 'judgement' (prajñā) signifies the twin aspects of organizing the sensory data and resolutions with regard to conduct.

Judgement has three modes: intelligence (dhī), will (dhrti), and memory (smrti) (*CS*, sūtra 1,98). Intelligence is the general ability to know things as they are and to discriminate between what is proper and what is not. To take the improper as proper, or the proper as improper is the error of intelligence ('the straying of intelligence', buddhibhramśa) (ibid.99).

Will is resolution to do the proper things, after intelligence has discriminated and ascertained the nature and effect of things. It is also to restrain the mind from temptation to do improper things and to strengthen its decision to do the right thing. Lack of will leading to indecision and consequent wrong conduct is the error of will (ibid. 100). Memory is to recollect relevant previous experience and to be vigilant. Inability to recall and profit by previous experience, either owing to excessive activity or to sluggishness is an error of the memory (ibid.,10).

Whatever improper action is done by one from whom intelligence, will and memory have strayed is regarded as 'the error of judgement'. It is principally due to the qualities of rajas (fickle-mindedness, instability, excessive activity, passion, strong aversion, intoxication, pride, fear, sorrow, worry etc.) and tamas (sloth, resistance, inertia, delusion, depression etc.). As a consequence, all the doshas are excited and are thrown out of balance.

Error of judgement may pertain to the bodily actions, mental processes, or modes of speech. Again, each of these groups may be further classified into insufficient, excessive or improper organizations. Illustrations are inactivity, excessive exercise, suppression of bodily urges when they arise, forcing the discharges before their time, exertion in the sun, exposure to heat and cold, over-indulgence of sex, unnatural contortions of the body, etc. (pertaining to bodily actions); mental inertia, overwork, prolonged excitement, fright, intense anger, greed, jealousy, looking for lapses, pride etc. (pertaining to mental processes); speaking loudly or inaudibly, continued silence, talkativeness, fault-finding, falsehood, slander, untimely talk, quarrel, abusive language, unpleasant talk etc. (pertaining to speech). [*See also* DISEASE].

Eshana: [*See* NORMAL PURSUITS]

Examination: Treatment of a disease involves examination of the patient. The purpose of examination is to get at the truth concerning the diseases (sat). This is done by four ways: (1) 'instructions by competent elders' (āptopadeśa), (2) observation (pratyaksha), (3) inferences (anumāna), and (4) use of reason (yukti). There cannot be any method of examination other than these four (*CS*, sūtra, 11,17).

(1) The competent elders are sages whose instruction is authoritative, whose competence is derived from penance and wisdom and those whose knowledge is valid for all three aspects of time (past, present and future); they are characterized by unprejudiced consideration for the suffering folk (āpta), gentle and cultured manner (śishta) and enlightenment (vibuddha). Their words cannot be doubted for they have no motivation for being untruthful. The scriptures (Veda) come under this category; as also other works based on them, composed by worthy ones in accordance with the traditional framework (śishtānumata), and prompted by a desire to help humanity (lokānugraha). (*CS*, ibid., 18 and 19).

(2) observation is a mental process which emerges when the soul, sense-organs, mind and the objects of sensory apprehension come together (sannikarsha); it is experience that is immediate and contemporaneous with the events outside (tadātve) (*CS*, ibid., 20) [*See* PRAMĀṆA].

(3) Inference depends upon and follows observational data and it pervades all three segments of time (tri-kālam). Examples are: deducing the presence of fire from observing smoke (present), presupposing the act of copulation from observing pregnancy (past), and inferring the future plant from observing the seed (future) (*CS*, ibid., 21-22). [*See* PRAMĀNA].

(4) Use of reason is where the intellect can perceive the occurrence of events (bhāva) as the result of the concatenation of a multiplicity of causes (bahu-kārana-yogaja), and by means of which all the three goals of life (virtue, wealth, and pleasures) can be accomplished. It is valid for all time. Examples are: knowing that the foetus occurs as a result of the interplay of all the six constituents (shad-dhātu-samyoga), knowing that fire comes into being as a result of the interplay of fuel, ignition etc., and deciding the treatment where the four props of therapy (physician, patient, medicine and nurse) would eliminate the disease [*See* YUKTI].

Exercise: Physical exercise (vyāyāma) is commended as indispensable for health. It is invariably included in the prescriptions for hygiene and preventive medicine. A medical poet claims that being habituated to two excellent norms, which are moderate food (mitāhāra) and sufficient physical exercise (vyāyāma), he does not need any medical care whatever.

Exercise is defined as "action that facilitates the natural processes in the body" (vegakṛdvyāpāra) (*CS,* sūtra , 15). It is described as the movement of the limbs calculated to bring about fatigue of the body (śarīrāyāsa janana-karma) (*BP*,II,4). *SS* recommends walking (chaṅkramana) as the best exercise, as it does not excessively tax the body (chikitsā, 24). Running as a form of exercise is to be avoided, for 'death runs after one who runs'. *CS* would confine exercise to the body; the comm. explains that during exercise, mind must be relaxed (*CS*, sūtra, 7,34). Further, physical exercise needs to be something that one relishes (ishta) (ibid.).

Among the benefits of exercise, the following are listed: lightness of body (laghutā); capacity for work (karma-samarthya); firmness (sthairya); endurance of annoyances (kleśa-sahishṇutā); elimination of constitutional imbalances (dosha-kshaya, 'dosha', here means, according to comm., śleshman, or alternately all the three doshas because the next benefit involves digestive power); and increase of digestive power (agni-vṛddhi); (*CS*, sūtra, 7,32); overall invigoration of the body (dehaṁ vimṛdhnīyat samantatah); development of the body (śariropachaya); proper proportion of limbs (gātrāṇām suvibhaktatā); lustre (kānti); and absence of sloth (anālasya) (*SS*, chikitsā, 24); perfect digestion of food even when the food is improper; reduction of fat (medasah kshayah, *AHṛ*, 1,2,10; sthaulyāpakarshaṇa); prevention of premature aging and freedom from ailments (*RVN*). An additional verse in Yogīndranāth Sen's edition of *CS* (*NS* edition,p.51) states that exercise is characterized by sweating, increased respiration and enhanced activity of the heart. The main purposes of exercise are to facilitate proper elimination of waste products from the body (malanihsāraṇā), to increase the digestive power (agni-dīpana), and reduction of fat (medo-nāśa).

Exercise is not indicated for young children, old people, people who suffer from excess of vāta and pitta, people who are constipated and people who ail from cough, dyspnoea, asthma and wasting diseases. Exercise is harmful soon after food, after sexual congress, when one is thirsty, or when wounded.

Excessive exercise is harmful even for healthy people. One must consider one's own bodily condition, age, strength, climate and place, and wisely determine the suitable measure of exercise (*RN*,2). Otherwise, exercise may lead to physical exhaustion (śrama) shown in shortness of breath and palpitation of heart, depression (klama), wasting of body-tissues (kshaya), inordinate thirst (tṛshṇā), fever (jvara), cough (kāsa), vomiting (chhardi) or nausea, haemorrhage (raktapitta), asthma (tamaka) (*CS*, op.cit.; *RN*).

CS, indicates that the 'proper measure' (mātrā) of exercise for each individual is to be determined insofar as it is not detrimental, when it brings about the benefits mentioned above, without causing the disturbances just enumerated (comm., sūtra, 7,31). It is recommended that the exercise must not be more than half the capacity of the individual (ardha-śakti) (*AHṛ*, 1,2,11). *CS* explicitly states that even the proper exercises must not be resorted to beyond this limit (ibid., 34). *SS* explains that the measure of exercise (where only half of one's energy is expended, balārdha) should be until the air (vāyu) that is settled in the heart gets disturbed (viz. until the onset of palpitation) and comes to the mouth, or until the body starts perspiring, especially on the forehead, on the nose, and in the arm-pits and limb-joints.

The months in which exercises may be done in this measure are winter (hemanta, generally November-December), the cool months (śiśira, generally January-February) and spring (vasantha, generally March-April). The measure of exercises must be reduced in other months, for summer is the time when bodily strength is sapped, rains tend to increase vāta, and autumn stirs up pitta.

The benefit of exercise is said to be enhanced when exercise is followed by a massage (mardana), including rubbing, anointing, and shampooing.

Exercise is especially helpful to those who suffer from diabetes and spermatorrhoea. It should be avoided by patients who suffer from asthma, consumption, haemoptysis ulcer, loss of body weight, emaciation, or from diseases caused by an excess of vāta and pitta. Exercise is not indicated for old people and children (under sixteen years of age). Those who habitually drink water at dawn should also avoid an excess of physical exercise.

Expressed juice: One of the five decoctions (pañcha-kashāyas) [*See* DECOCTIONS], sva-rasa (expressed juice, *succus* in Latin, *afsurda* in Persian, *asir* in Yunāni medicine) is the natural juice of a herb, obtained by pounding the selected parts of fresh plant in a mortar (*CS,* 1,4). The plant selected must be still green, free from worms, and not injured by the inclemencies of weather. It is then washed in clean water, cut into small pieces, and pounded in the mortar with a stone pestle. The juice is then strained through a piece of cloth. The technique of 'expression' is meant to separate the medicinal juices and oils from other non-medicinal parts of the plant.

When, however, fresh and green plants for the purpose are not available, selected portions of the dried plant are cut into tiny bits or pounded and soaked in water (in the proportions of two parts, or according to another view eight parts, of water to one of the herbs) in an earthern vessel and left for a day-and-night (aho-rātraṁ, viz. twenty-four hours) (*SaS,* II,1,5). That would be as good as the expressed juice from fresh plants. [*See* PREP ARATIONS]

F

Foetal Development: The manner in which the foetus (garbha) is formed is explained thus (*SS,* śarīra, 3,3). During copulation owing to the friction of the sexual organs, heat (tejas) is generated, and this is aggravated by the local wind; the wind and the heat together manage to dislodge semen from its sac in the male partner; and it enters the uterus of the woman through the vaginal canal and there it combines with the ovum (ārtava), dislodged and secreted by the same cause. The combined ovum and semen are then confined in the uterus, the receptacle for the foetus (garbhāśaya).

This is a material mass: the male contribution having the qualities of 'moon' (saumya) and the female contribution having the qualities of 'fire' (āgneya). However, all the primary forms of matter (viz. earth, water, fire, air and ākāśa) are present in it, and they are mutually beneficial, mutually supporting and mutually fusing. Into this mass enters the soul (kshetrajña, whose nature is inscrutable) owing to fate (daiva-samyogāt) and takes hold of this complex of primary forms of matter (brought into being by impregnation) enlivening it. It then assumes a subtle shape, marked by the three aspects of prakṛti (viz. sattva, rajas and tamas), and led by the wind. It is this entrance of the conscious principle that makes it possible for the foetus to get formed and grow.

The living foetus represents the primary state of the three doshas: vāta (the cosmic vāyu), pitta (the mother's ovum), and kapha (the father's sperm). These three engender the three gunas, the five faculties, and the specific individuality that is incorporated and that grows (bhūtātmā or karma-purusha). After conception, the 'air' structures the three doshas and forms the seven body-constituents (dhātu) together with the organs (aṅga) and limbs (pratyaṅga) in due course.

The 'fire' element sets the stage for metabolic changes. The 'water' element makes the foetus soft and humid. The 'earth' element stamps it with the peculiarities of the species; and the 'ākāśa' element provides the space and scope to grow.

Development of the foetus inside the body of the mother is accompanied by specific symptoms in the mother's body, mind and behaviour. The presence of the foetus becomes available to nāḍī-examination of the mother [*see* NAḌI and CLINICAL EXAMINATION] in the first two months of pregnancy: there will be distinct changes in the pulses representing pitta and vāta. There are dietary, behavioural and psychological prescriptions for the mother that facilitate normal foetal development (cf. *SS*, śarīra, 3,16-17; *CS*, śarīra, 8,21-23).

The foetus will be in the form of a gelatinous substance (kalala) in the first month of gestation. It is an amorphous (unstructured) mass of all the material ingredients (substances and properties) mixed indistinguishably ('avyakta-vigraha', *CS*, śarīra, 4). According to *Garbhopanishat*, the gelatinous shape is acquired the night after conception; it becomes a 'bubble' (budbuda) after seven nights, and the womb (piṇḍa) is formed after a fortnight and it gets hard in a month's time. Although by this time, the foetus contains in a seed (unmanifest) form all the organs and limbs, all the body-constituents and individual characteristics (prakṛti), it will neither be solid nor watery. It is after a month that it becomes hard, and begins to grow.

The second month transforms this gelatinous mass into an identifiable foetus, which grows in size because of the fresh accretion of the five primary forms of matter (derived from the mother's body) under the influence of the three doshas inherent in the foetus. The sex of the child to be born is indicated by the form of the foetus: male if spherical and female if elongated.

In the third month, five small lumps (protuberances) are formed on the foetus representing the five major organs (aṅgas), (viz. two hands, two legs and head) and also many extremely small papillae to represent the rudimentary limbs (pratyaṅgas). The human form is clearly distinguishable at this stage.

According to *CS* and *AS* the heart (consciousness) is also formed during the third month and the foetus thus enters into a transaction with the surrounding, becoming aware of comfort and discomfort (*AS*, śarīra, 2,16); and all the organs emerge simultaneously (yaugapadyena) including the sense-organs (*CS*, śarīra, 4,14). It is at this stage that the living foetus becomes endowed with movement (spanda) and intentions (prārthanā) (*CS*, śarīra,4,15). According to *SS*, however, the heart (consciousness) is formed clearly during the fourth month (śarīra, 3,21).

In any case, during the third and the fourth foetal months (till the fifth according to *AS*, śarīra, 2,17) the mother is described as 'possessed of two hearts' (dauhṛdini) and as full of longings (longings of the foetus manifested through the mother). These longings are said to reflect the experiences of the previous lives of the child to be born, and the future child's first responses to the awareness of the surrounding through the rudimentary sense-organs in the foetus. If these longings are unfulfilled, there is risk of the foetus becoming tense and defective.

In the fourth month, the organs and limbs of the foetus become more pronounced (better structured), and consciousness (called chetanā in *AHṛ*, śarīra, 1,57) becomes crystallized as intentions ('hṛdayam pravyaktataro bhavati'...indriyartheshu karoti', *SS*, ibid.,3,17).

In the fifth month, the foetus becomes endowed with an explicit mind ('manah pratibuddha-taraṁ', *SS*, ibid.,30, also *AS*, śarīra, 2). The interpretation of the expression 'prati-buddha' (*SS*, ibid.) is given as 'waking up from a state of unconsciousness'.

AS (śarīra, 2,23) adds that the blood and muscle of the foetus are also nourished during this month.

The sixth month is distinguished by the appearance of intellect (buddhi). Also, hair on the head, body hair, nails, ligaments, strength, complexion etc. appear (cf. *AS*, śarīra, 2,24 and *AHṛ*, śarīra, 1,57).

In the seventh month, all the organs and limbs are clearly and almost completely formed and distinguished; and this may be apprehended by touch. If, due to any reason, delivery takes place during this month, the baby will survive, provided proper care is extended. But, owing to premature delivery, the individual may not be healthy or long-lived.

In the eighth month, the vitality (ojas) will be maturing and getting firmly established in the heart. But the process involves periodical movement of vitality from the foetus to the mother's body and its return to the foetus. If delivery takes place during this period, there is danger both to the foetus and to the mother, owing to the unsettled condition (asthira, *SS*, ibid., 38 anavasthitatvāt *AS*, ibid. 27) of the vital force.

It is usual for the delivery to take place in the ninth month; but it may be prolonged till the eleventh or twelth month. Abnormal delay in delivery calls for medical treatment or surgical intervention (cf. *SS*, śarīra, 3; *CS*, śarīra, 8; *AS*, śarīra, 2, and *AHṛ*, śarīra, 1).

There was a difference of opinion among the ancient experts about the organ that first gets structured in the foetus (cf. *SS*, śarīra, 3,32). According to SAUNAKA, the head (śirah) develops first, for that is the organ on which all the other organs and limbs depend. KṚTAVĪRYA, on the other hand argued that the 'heart' (hṛdaya) gets formed first, since that organ is the seat of mind (manas) and intellect (buddhi). PĀRĀŚARYA held that it was the umbilicus (nābhi) that develops first, for it is through this organ that the foetus derives its nourishment from the mother's body. The view of MĀRKAṆḌEYA is that the extremities (pāṇipādaṁ, hands and legs) are formed initially for all movement (viz. activity) of the foetus presupposes them. SUBHŪTI-GAUTAMA thought that the trunk (madhya-śarīra) gets formed first, for all the other organs are attached to it.

DHANVANTARI, however, rejects all these views, and holds that all the organs and limbs develop simultaneously (yugapat), although in the earlier stages of foetal development they cannot be discerned owing to their minute character (*SS*, ibid., 41-42).

There is an account of the contributions to the foetus from the mother and the father: muscle, blood, muscle-fat, heart, umbilicus, spleen, liver, intestines, anus and all other soft portions from the mother; and hair on the head, on the face, and on the body, bones nails, teeth, veins (sirā), ligaments (snāyu), arteries (dhamanī), semen and other hard and steady portions from the father. The 'soul' (ātmā) that enlivens the foetus is responsible for the emergence of the sense-organs, consciousness (jñāna) and knowledge (vijñāna), for the life-span, pleasures and pains. The three guṇas (sattva, rajas and tamas) and the qualities of the mind (manas). The innate physiological conditions (sātmya) provide the foetus with such factors like strength (vīrya), health, stamina (bala), complexion, intellect etc. The assimilated food that sustains the foetus (rasa) is responsible for the growth of the body (śarīropachaya), stamina, complexion, integration (sthiti) and disintegration (hāni) in the foetus (*SS*, ibid., 19).

Foetal developmint is gradual and depends upon the life-force (prāṇa-śakti), which consists of the following aspects: 'fire' (energy in the form of heat, viz. thirteen types of agni: the five forms of pitta, seven 'fires' in the body-constituents, dhātvagni, and the power of speech as the thirteenth 'fire'), 'moon' (soma, cooling and nourishing, of six kinds viz. the five forms of kapha, coolness in the body which is a power, and the power of the mind), 'air' (vāyu, the bodily winds in five forms), sattva, rajas, tamas (three characteristics of all nature), sense-organs (indriya, five faculties of perception), and 'incorporated soul' (bhūtātma, motivated by consciousness and mind, actualizing the behaviour modes, and experiencing pleasures and pains).

Food: The three main props (upastaṁbha) of life are : food, sleep and sex (*AHṛ*, 1,7,52); and of the three, food is the foremost for all living beings, inasmuch as it is the foundation (mūla) for strength (bala), appearance (varṇa) and vitality (ojas) (*SS*, 1,46). It is natural, therefore, that Āyurvedic texts discuss at great length the details of the food that maintains and promotes health. They also discuss the problem of food habits and the diseases that are caused by unwholesome food and wrong food habits.

The main intake of food (meal) is to be resorted to only twice in twenty-four hours: once in the day (after the expiry of the first quarter of the night time) and once in the night (after the expiry of the first quarter). Eating food inbetween (antarā-bhojana) is injurious to health, unless one is oppressed by hunger. Eating when the food eaten earlier is as yet not completely digested puts an extra load on the digestive mechanism. Skipping the two prescribed times for food is also injurious as it deprives one of strength (bala-kshaya). These restrictions, however, apply only to healthy adults, and not to patients or children (under sixteen years of age) (RJN).

It is wise to follow the directions of the stomach: to eat only when one is hungry. Hunger is felt when the chyle (rasa) is digested, when the doshas of the body are pacified and when the waste products are eliminated from the body. Whenever one feels hungry, it should be regarded as the proper time to eat food. It is an important detail of personal hygiene that one should not eat when one does not feel hungry (adhyaśana defined as "ajırne bhujyate yat"). As man is a creature of habit, the time when one gets normally hungry more or less clearly gets fixed. Taking food before the usual time or long after it, is described as 'untimely food' (akāla-bhojana) and is classed under 'unbalanced or improper food' (vishamāsana, which also includes eating too little or in excess). Before the usual time (aprapta-kale), the food will result in various diseases, as the normal course of digestion is interfered with, long after the usual time (kāle atīte), the food eaten will excite the vata in the abdomen and impairs the digestive power.

Food eaten must be what one is used to (sātmya), clean (śuchi), wholesome (hita), lukewarm and oily (snigdhoshṇa). Food that has become cold, stale and dry must be avoided and it is harmful to the system if the food once hot and cooled is heated again (ushṇīkṛtam punah). Also to be avoided are the food articles that are very hot, or those that contain much salt. Food eaten at a sitting must include different kinds of ingredients and must normally comprehend all the six tastes (sweet, sour, pungent, bitter, saline and astringent), but predominantly sweet (madhura-prayam). Food must be relished and eaten in pleasant company (ishtam ishṭais saha); neither too fast nor too slowly (nāti-druta-vilaṁbitaṁ) (*AHṛ*, 1,8,35-38).

An important detail to be considered is the proper measure of food (matrā) to be eaten. While the proper measure is a relative term, depending as it does upon the type of the food, the needs of the person, his digestive power, his work, his habits, time, place, and so on, it gets more or less well-defined for each person. Āyurvedic texts insist that one must eat according to his measure (mātrāśī syāt *AS*, 1,11,3), for it is the measure that will properly impel the digestive power (agneh pravartikā).

But the measure which is proper is not only

much less than the point of satiety (ati-sauhitya) but also less than the point of gratification (sauhitya or tṛpti), or the full appeasement of hunger and thirst. (*CS* vimāna, 2) prescribes that the stomach must be figured as composed of three parts; the first part must be filled with solids, the second with liquids, and the third with the three doshas; "one that eats thus will never come to grief caused by over or under-eating". *AHṛ* (1,8,46), however, would divide the stomach into four parts and suggest that two parts thereof must be filled with solid food, one part with liquids, and the other part be left alone, for being the field of operation (āśraya) for the doshas, viz. vāta.

There are also certain well-defined indications for the proper measure of food to be eaten. The measure is proper when hunger and thirst are just appeased, and the sense-organs are satisfied and invigorated. One must stop before he feels any pressure in the stomach, discomfort at the sides, heaviness in the belly and choking sensation in the heart. The proper measure of food will not prevent him from, sitting, standing, lying down or walking at pleasure, nor from continuing pleasant conversation with people around him. Food eaten in the morning must sustain him till night, and the food eaten in the night must sustain him till the next morning. And the food eaten must nourish the body constituents, and help eliminate the waste-products from the body (*AS*, 1,11,5).

If the food eaten is short of the proper measure (hīna-mātra), it will not tend to provide strength for the body and sustain vitality; it will, on the other hand, cause diseases which are predominantly disturbances of vāta. The body begins to degenerate, longevity is threatened and the mind gets gradually feeble. If the food eaten is in excess of the proper measure (ati-mātra), it will agitate all the three doshas at the same time, and bring about several ailments (such as indigestion, loss of appetite, tympanites and cholera) (*AHr*, 1,8,3-4).

Another consideration while taking food is that it should not be an unwholesome combination of different kinds of food-articles, especially ingredients that are antagonistic in character (viruddhāśana). Each of the ingredients may be harmless by itself but when they are taken together or several times on the same day, the effect will be injurious to health. Examples are: milk with fish, meat or any food which is sour in taste; fish with butter, ghee, milk, meat or sweets; meat with milk, oil, or fish; plantain fruit with butter-milk or palmyra fruit; butter and ghee with fish or oil. Meat of more than one animal should not be eaten on the same day. Honey, ghee, milk, oil and water should not be taken together. Such food operates like deadly poison (māraka-visha) or secondary poison (gara, dūshī-visha). Also included in the category are restrictions like not keeping butter, ghee or coconut water in bell-metal containers, not heating again the decoction of herbs or food once prepared, not taking honey, ghee and oil together in the same measure, not drinking rain-water even after honey and ghee are taken in unequal measures, not drinking milk after eating radish or garlic or not taking milk preparations with thin gruel (*CS*, 1,26,84).

Such mutually contradictory combinations of food articles are said to cause several diseases like vitiation of blood, obstructions in the channels of circulation, constipation, diseases relating to blood, toxic conditions, tremor, epilepsy, diphtheria, scrofula, aggravation of doshas, diarrhoea and loss of sensory acuity (*CS*, 1,26,82-84).

However, the mutually antagonistic articles of food taken together will not harm those who habitually take physical exercise, whose body is oily, whose digestive power is good, who are youthful and strong, who are habituated to such food, and who normally eat only little food (*AHr*, 1,7,47).

Drinking water while taking food is still another topic that is discussed at length in Āyurvedic texts. Drinking much water interferes with the digestive process; not drinking at all is equally harmful. Water must, therefore, be drunk in small quantities frequently while food is being eaten, but never much; this will stimulate the digestive fire ('vahnivivardhanāya muhur-muhur-vāri piben na bhūri'). If water is drunk at the commencement of eating (viz. before half the quantity of the meal is consumed), the digestive powers are weakened, and the person tends to be lean and lanky, owing to inadequate assimilation of food. If water is drunk at the end of the meal, kapha is aggravated, and the tendency to obesity is facilitated. The best period to consume water is in the middle of the meal (viz. just after half the quantity of the meal is consumed). Water will then keep the digestive power active and will assist the proper assimilation of food.

It is also a rule that one should not drink water when he is hungry (for he will then be a victim to dropsy), nor eat food when thirsty (for he will then be stricken by phantom tumour or gulma). The hungry man should drink water only after half the quantity of the meal is consumed; the thirsty man should eat food only after the thirst is quenched.

Chewing betel leaves and areca nuts along with selected spices is recommended after the meal, for it will cleanse the mouth, encourage the flow of saliva necessary for digestion, and remove foetid odours; it will also pacify the three doshas. [*See* TĀMBŪLĀ].

After the meal, bathing, physical and mental exercise, running, travel by vehicles (yāna), fighting, sexual activity, singing and study are to be avoided for at least forty-eight minutes (a muhūrta). One should also not lie down or sleep immediately after taking food; but slow walking with measured steps for a while ('hundred steps', śatapatha) is beneficial to the digestive process.

Indigestion, which is the root-cause of many diseases is caused by drinking too much of water (atyambupāna, viz in excess of what is required to quench the thirst), eating unwholesome and untimely food (vishamāśana), suppression or long delay in answering the calls of nature (sandhārana), and perverted habits of sleep (svapna-viparyaya, viz. sleeping in daytime and keeping awake during night). The food eaten, even when it is timely, accustomed and in moderate quantity, will not get digested, owing to these factors. [*See* INDIGESTION].

Eight factors are listed as determining the value of food (*CS,* vimāna, 1,21): (1) inherent nature of the food-articles (prakṛti); (2) the method of processing of food or preparation (karaṇa), involving a transformation of the inherent qualities of the food by dilution, heating, cleansing, churning, flavouring, storing etc.; (3) combination of two or more substances (saṁyoga), thus producing characteristics not present in each of the ingredients; (4) quantity of food (rāśi); (5) habitat (deśa) of the articles of food (locality, climate etc); (6) time (kāla), viz. day or night, seasons, condition of the individual, age of the individual etc; (7) dietetic rules (upayoga-samsthā) (such as taking food neither too hurriedly nor too slowly, masticating properly before swallowing, not eating until the previously eaten food has been digested, etc), largely based on the digestive conditions; and (8) the individual who eats (upayoktr), on whom alone depends the wholesomeness of the food by the habitual intake (okasātmya). These factors are responsible for the good or bad effects of the food eaten; and they are interrelated. The wise man should understand the significance of each of these factors, and should not be under the influence of ignorance (moha) or negligence (pramāda), and succumb to the temptation to eat the food which is apparently pleasant although harmful in the long run (priyamahitam) (*CS,* ibid., 23).

To sum up, food that is beneficial to the system should be warm, (ushṇam), unctuous (snigdham), in proper measure (mātrāvad), and free from contradictory potencies (vīryaviruddham). One should take care not to eat before the food eaten earlier has been digested (jīrnah). One should eat in a place that one likes best (ishte deśe), and surrounded by things that he desires (ishta-sarvopakaranam). He should eat neither too fast (nāti-drutam), nor too slowly (nāti-vilambitam). One should be mindful while eating (tan-manāh), concentrating on the things to be eaten and relishing the taste thereof. He should not indulge in irrelevant and continuous talk (ajalpan) nor in loud laughter (ahasan) while eating. Finally, one should eat with confidence that what he eats will nourish him well (ātmānam abhisamīkshya) (*CS,* vimāna, 1,25,1-9).

Four Props of Medical Practice : Medical practice is said to be 'four-legged' (chatushpāda), i.e. supported on four props: physician (vaidya or bhishak), drugs (dravya or bheshaja), nursing attendant (parichara or upasthātā), and the patient (ātura, vyādhyupasprshta or rogī) (*CS,* sūtra, 9,5 to 10; cf also *SS,* sūtra, 34,15-24; and *AHr,* 1,1,27 to 29).

Of the four, the physician is said to be the chief (pradhāna), with the other three as aids. The analogy provided by CHARAKA (sūtra, 9,11 and 13) is that of a cook being assisted by utensils, fuel, and fire; or that of the commander of the army being helped by the terrain, army and weapons or that of the potter utilizing clay, the rod, and the wheel. SUŚRUTA concedes that all four are essential to the course of treatment, but without a competent physician, the other three are useless, even as the priest who chants the Sāman hymns (udgātr), the priest who recites the rk hymns (hotr), and the priest who renders the yajus portions (brahman) would be, without the officiating chief priest (adhvaryu or master of ceremonies, who is well-versed in all the three hymnal collections), in a sacrifice. The physician guides, regulates, and instructs the other three 'props'. But the four together make medical practice a total affair, even as four quarters of anything constitute a whole. Even grave diseases can thus be cured (*SS,* sūtra, 34,16).

Effective contribution from each prop would render the treatment successful. Therefore, the texts prescribe necessary qualifications for each of them, so that the contributions are properly complemented.

1. The physician must be well-informed and learned (śruta); he must have a thorough acquaintance with the medical texts, and must have profited by apprenticeship with master (tīrthārtta-śāstrārthah); his medical knowledge must be profound and clear (paryavadāta). He must have watched carefully how patients are treated for different ailments, medicines of many kinds prepared and variously administered (bahuśo drshtakarmatā). He must himself have practiced (svayam krtī). If a surgeon, he must be deft with this hands (laghu-hasta), and he must be brave (śūra), and not easily rattled. He must also be quick in thinking and resourceful (pratyutpanna-mati). He must be honest and pure in his purpose and conduct (śaucha); his main interest must be to help the patient. And he must be competent (dākshya); i.e. he must be clever (chatura), quick (patu), industrious (udyogī), soft-mannered (peśala), and himself healthy (svastha). *SS* (sūtra, 34,18) adds that even if the other three props are absent or inadequate, a clever physician will be able to manage by himself.

2. The drug must be of adequate quantity (bahutā); it must have plentiful of medicinal quality (bahuguna). It must be suitable to counteract the disease (tatra-yogyatva); and proper also for the time, place and the patient. The drug must be capable of being made available in many forms (aneka-vidha-kalpanā) such as expressed juice (svarasa), decoction (kvātha), infusion (kasāya), and powder (chūrna) to suit different patients and different disease-conditions. The drug

must also have preservative value (sampat); it should not lose much of its potency even when attacked by insects etc. or made wet by water etc. The herb must have grown in a good place and gathered at an auspicious time (*SS,* sūtra, 34,22); it must also be pleasant to take.

3. The nursing attendant needs to be intelligent (buddhimān) and knowledgeable (upachārajñatā). He must be competent (daksha) and he must be pure-hearted (śuchih); his main interest must be to help the patient. He must have a sense of loyalty and regard for his chief, viz. the physician (anurāgah bhartari). He must be friendly and pleasant (snigdha); he must not find fault and should be obedient; he must not be easily tired (*SS,* ibid., 4,24).

4. The patient must be willing to follow fully the instructions of the physician (nirdeśa-kāritva), he must confide in the physician and entrust himself to his hands (bhishag-vaśyatā). He must be hopeful and not yield to despondency (abhīrutvam); he must be confident that he will be well again (sattva-vān; āstika). 'Oftentimes, the disease will grow worse when the patient is scared' (Chkp. on *CS,* sūtra, 9,9,). He must be frank and honest (satyavān), and able to recognize and remember his troubles and symptoms and communicate them to the physician (jñāpakatva). An additional trait that is helpful in successful treatment has been mentioned, *SS* (ibid. 21) and in *AHr* (1,1,29): the patient must have people to care for him and must have money to spend (ādhya; dhanavān). SUŚRUTA adds that he must be endowed with long life (āyushmān, ibid, 21).

The four props are mentioned in a meaningful order. The physician is mentioned first, for he is the most important factor. The determination of the drug is due to him; the nursing attendant is instructed by him and the patient's health is dependent on him. After him comes the drug, for that is the thing that figures prominently in treatment (pradhāna-kārana). Next in order is the attendant, for the preparation and administration of the drug (bheshaja-prayoga) are his responsibility. Last of all comes the patient. Although it is for the sake of the patient that the other three are active, he is not counted as the most important factor, for unless the other three are active, he will merit little consideration. Further, his role is but passive, being the recepient of the benefit (upakāri) which the other the three confer on him. (CHKP *CS,* sūtra 9,3)..

Nevertheless, treatment as an activity will not be complete or successful even if one of the factors is inadequate, improper, or if the patient or attendant refuses to cooperate. The four factors are collectively the cause (kāraṇam) in eliminating the ailment, and in this capacity are necessarily 'involved' (vyāpriyamāṇā) in the effect, viz. the cure. The four factors are distinguished from each other as four different kinds of activities of treatment ('pravṛtter bhedam puraskṛtya chikitsāyāh kriyārūpāyāh kathanaṁ', (CHKP).

However, there is no rule that a disease will not be cured without these props; for we do find in actual life that some diseases are cured independent of the physician, drug or the attendant (*CS,* sūtra, 10,4). The rule is merely that the physician etc. will be causes for the elimination of the imbalances of the bodily constituents ('vikāra-śamane kāranam eva iti niyamah'). [*See also* HEALTH PHYSICIAN].

G

Gada : Disease, sickness. It refers to the condition which makes one disabled (gadyate).

Usually the term is employed to describe the diseases that have multiplicity of causes (aneka-kārana-janyatva). [*See* DISEASE].

Garbha : Derived from gṛbh ('to conceive'), the word signifies foetus or embryo. When the unimpaired sperm of man and the unafflicted ovum of woman come together at a favourable time, they get lodged in the uterus (garbhāśaya). The soul (jīva) along with the mind (sattva) descends into this complex and thus the foetus is formed. It grows when the wholesome rasa (assimilated food in the mother's body) nourishes it and when the mother maintains a favourable regimen. In due course, organs (sensory and motor) get formed, and individual characteristics (like strength, complexion, temperament, body-build etc.) begin to appear (*CS,* śārīra, 3,3).

The foetus is properly formed owing to four factors: impregnation at the proper time (rtu), the healthy condition of the uterus (kshetra), wholesome diet of the mother (ambu), and the suitable sperm and ovum (bīja) (*SS,* śarīra, 2,33; cf. also *CS,* ibid., mentions five factors responsible for the foetus: mother, father, soul (ātmā), wholesomeness (sātmya) and assimilated food in the mother's body (rasa); mind (sattva) is also added as the connecting link (aupapāduka). The foetus is formed from these factors, even as a house is constructed from several substances or a chariot is fashioned by several ingredients (*CS,* ibid.,. 14). [*See* FOETAL DEVELOMENT].

Grahaṇī : A part of the abdominal cavity (koshṭha) above the umbilicus (nābhi) and between the stomach (āmāśaya) and the large intestine (pakvāśaya) where the pitta-dhāraka-kalā, mainly involved in digestion of food, is located. It is called grahaṇī, because it receives and retains the food during the digestive process ('annasya grahaṇāt', *CS,* chikitsā, 15, 56 also CHKP on it). It is described as the seat of the 'stomachic fire' (agnyadhishṭhāna-nāḍī, *CS,* ibid. and *SKD*). [*See* AGNI]. The integrity of this organ depends upon the digestive fire; when the 'fire' is disturbed, the organ also becomes defective and when the organ is impaired, the 'fire' also becomes disturbed (*SS,* uttara, 40, 169; and *AHr,* śarīra, 3, 50-53).

The main function of the grahaṇī is to support the pitta (pāchaka-pitta), which is the main factor responsible for digestion of food as it is brought to this part of the abdominal cavity on its way to the large intestine (pakvāśaya). Located on the way to the large intestine, it retains the food till it is digested: it helps in the separation of the nutrient portions (kiṭṭa), before sending it (viz. the nutrient portion) down to the large intestines. (*SS,* uttara, 40, 169-70).

The identification of this structure in the light of present-day knowledge of human anatomy and physiology has not been firmly established. But it may roughly be taken to correspond with the region of small intestine (adho-āmāśaya or pachyamānāśaya), which extends from the terminal end of the stomach (ūrdhva-āmāśaya), which in turn extends from the cardiac sphincter to the pyloric sphincter, where in fact food in the stomach is retained during gastric digestion or, in other words, from the pyloric antrum to the ileo-cecum (uṇḍuka). (cf. DWARAKANATH, *DMA,* pp.38-39).

(2) The name is also given to a disease, chronic diarrhoea or sprue syndrome. [*See* GRAHAṆĪ-ROGA and also AGNI, PITTA, DIGESTION].

Guṇa (1) : There are few words that are used as frequently in Indian writings as this word. Its employment as a technical expression is as wide as its use in popular parlance. But it is a word of uncertain origin, and has a variety of shades of meanings: 'quality', 'secondary', 'strands of the rope', 'bow-string', thread', 'to increase', 'to invite', 'deliberation' (especially in a royal assembly) , 'merit' and sense-organ'. Indian medicine which relies on these two systems for its philosophical position, has borrowed freely from the discussions concerning the concept of guṇa.

But the two systems differ in their basic approach to the problem of guṇa. In the Vaiśeshika system, guna is a category of existence (padārtha), but is different from substance (dravya). It is a quality that is inherent in a substance. The list of twenty-four 'qualities' that is given here includes the perceptible properties of material things (number, measure, separateness, contact, disjunction, belonging to a genus, or species), the qualities of the soul (knowledge, pleasure, sorrow, desire, aversion, effort), and an odd assortment of qualities that was appended later (heaviness, liquidity, oiliness, elasticity, samskāra, merit, and demerit). CHARAKA refers to these qualities. [*See* VAIŚESHIKA].

The Sāṁkhya system, on the other hand, does not regard the guṇas as abstract properties in this sense, but as real entities or ultimate and irreducible subtle substances, although they do not have their own independent existence. Things do not possess properties (or qualities), as the Vaiśeshika school supposes, but they manifest themselves as modes of modification, which are what the guṇas signify. Guṇas, thus, are manners or modes in which substances exist, act or react. These modes are continually in a state of flux, involved as they are in groupings and regroupings, unlike the constant and changeless 'soul'. In this sense, the guṇas are 'secondary', i.e., not primary like the soul (apradhāna). All things in the world (material objects as well as mental processes) are but manifestations of these guṇas, which, however, in their actuality are not available for sensory apprehension. The real nature of the guṇas are revealed only by intuitive wisdom (prajñā).

The guṇas are infinite in number but they can be conveniently grouped in three categories, in accordance with the major manifestations of the subtle substances: (a) Sattva, intelligence stuff, self-luminous, plastic; (b) rajas, 'energy-stuff', units of activity and (c) tamas, 'mass-stuff', heavy, obstructing. These 'reals' (S. N. Dasgupta) combine in varying proportions, thus bringing into being a variety of things and their modes of manifestation. They act upon each other and react to each other; while they unite, they also oppose.

The original condition of nature (prakṛti), which however is a hypothetical construct, is a perfect balance of these gunas (sāmyāvasthā); an equilibrium in which the guṇas contend with each other so well that no guṇa (or class of guṇas) can stand out or apart. It is a condition which is altogether incoherent, indeterminate and without meaning. It is a state which cannot be described as 'being' or 'non-being'. But when the gunas are thrown out of 'balance', they begin grouping themselves in accordance with the modes of manifestation, and in varying proportions. This is what the Sāmkhya system calls 'evolution' or the development of new categories of existence due to sequential changes (vṛttyantara-pariṇāma).

The guṇas, which function like 'strands of rope', are responsible for the intricate web of existence of life; they project themselves and 'bind' the Purusha. But they are also capable of withdrawing themselves, and thus liberating the Purusha. [*See* SĀṀKHYA YOGA].

The doctrine of guṇas is thus fundamental to the Sāṁkhya school of thought. But it was not until the 16th century that the concept was crystallized into a theory of 'reals'; Vijñāna-bhikshu, the author of *Sāṁkhya-pravachana-bhāshya,* is credited with this important contribution. Earlier to this, the guṇas were looked upon as factors which occurred and operated in a variety of proportions, and which, by their periodical increase and decrease, brought about the external world, as well as the human personality. And even before this teaching gained ground, the guṇas were regarded as nothing more than different kinds of mental states, good and bad. For instance, this is the outlook on guṇas that we find in the Sāṁkhya account given by Charaka and by Pañchaśikha.

It has been supposed that the doctrine of guṇas emerged from the nucleus of thought concerning 'bhāvas', which were merely the moral and psychical properties of the principle of transactional consciousness or buddhi (cf. *Mahābhārata,* 12, 187 and 239-40). Scholars like Johnston and Frauwallner have argued that the conception of bhāvas was the fore runner of the guṇa-theory. Bhāvas are essentially psychical processes or modifications ('chitta-vṛtti'), which engender activity in the body, sense-organs, and mind. The processes are broadly three-fold : sattva, rajas and tamas, (*SKD*). Relevant in this context is the notion of 'nature' (sva-bhāva), which determines the individual's action in the world and his reactions to the world.

Ayurveda, proceeding on the general framework of the Sāmkhya and Vaiśeshika schools of thought, has sought to reconcile the two viewpoints regarding guṇa. The physical and mental aspects of the individual, being composed of the five material elements [*See* PAÑCHABHŪTA THEORY], each element is distinguished from the others by characteristic qualities, physical, chemical, physiological and pharmacological. Charaka also gives a list of other 'substances' (dravya, self, mind, time and space), having their own 'qualities'. There are two lists of qualities that he provides : one beginning with 'heavy' (gurvādi) and the other beginning with 'distance' (parādi). The details of the former list are uncertain, but the details of the latter are spelt out : distance (para), proximity (apara), selection of drugs (see YUKTI); number (sāṁkhyā), contact (samyoga), division or dysfunction (vibhāga), difference or separateness (pṛthaktva), measure in weight (parimāṇa), production of new qualities (saṁskāra), and habit (abhyāsa) (*CS,* sūtra, 26, 27-29). These belong to substances which are living as well as to substances that are inert. While the 'qualities' are drawn from the Vaiśeshika system, Charaka provides new connotations to each of them, so that they become relevant in the medical context. For instance, the expressions 'para' (which in the Vaiśeshika framework means only physical distance or remoteness) and 'apara' (proximity or nearness) are interpreted here as meaning 'superiority' (with regard to place, time, age, measure, digestive fluid, potency and taste) and 'inferiority'. It is important to note that in the medical context, guṇa does not mean merely a property, quality or attribute, but physical, chemical and biochemical relationships that obtain between substances (dravyas).

The theory of five material elements is also in the background for the doctrine of the three doshas that figures prominently in Indian medicine (*See* DOSHA]. It also bears an intimate relationship with the three-guṇa theory of the Sāṁkhya system (sattva, rajas and tamas). Each of the doshas has its own characteristic guṇa-complex, like form, action, difference (bheda), and location (sthāna).

In the field of pharmacology, taste (rasa) is an important consideration and while taste itself is a quality of a substance (dravya), the six tastes (*See* TASTE) are described with reference to the chemical and physiological properties they have. Here, guna is viewed not merely as an incidental attribution but as a subtle substance itself, in keeping with the Sāṁkhya thought. Substance (dravya) and quality (guṇa) are distinguished in this context as 'ground' (aśraya) and form (aśrayī), which is characteristically a Vaiśeshika view (*CS,* sūtra 1, 50). Guna is thus intimately associated with substance (dravya) and action (karma). While referring to the potency (vīrya) of a drug, it is indicated that such potency is a resultant of the guna inherent in the drug (ibid., 26, 68).

Guṇa (2)

The word in its etymological sense signifies that our attention is forcibly drawn to the substances by the qualities that inhere in them (guṇyate, āmantryate iti), as if by so many ropes (guṇākhyā rajjavo yathā). The substances and their qualities are related invariably. There can be no substance without qualities and there can be no action without a substance; therefore, qualities are co-operative causes (sahakāri-kāraṇa) for both substances and actions. Dependent upon substances, and constantly related to them, the qualities however are inactive (niś-cheshṭa) in their causation. Actions, like qualities, inhere in substances; but they do not inhere in qualities. Likewise, qualities abide in substances, but do not abide in qualities. Thus, the quality (guṇa) is defined as without quality (nirguṇa) and devoid of action (nishkriyā). It becomes a cause only when associated with substances for the purpose of producing action. However, the action in substances is possible only because of the qualities inherent in substances. And the qualities inherent in substances can be inferred only by the actions. The qualities are impossible to be perceived as such, or in isolation. They become meaningful only when considered in the form of substances. This is why in Indian medicine, substances are sought to be understood in terms of their constant and inherent qualities. Substances, in fact, imply practically their qualities.

Substances and qualities are similar only inasmuch as they bring into being other entities of their own kind (sajātīya āraṁbhakatva) : substances produce other substances, and qualities produce other qualities. The outlook of Āyurveda with regard to the causative character of qualities is slightly different from that of the Vaiśeshika school, which denies the possibility of causative inseparable inherence (samavāyi-kāraṇa) for the qualities.

Qualities differ from other categories of existence (like substance, taste, potency) in being multi-dimensional in characterization (viśva-lakshaṇa, *RVS,* 1, 168). Substance (dravya), being the ground for sound etc., is limited to this characterization; taste is limited to differential gustatory perception; potency (vīrya) is limited to the various actions of the drug; digestive transformation (vipāka) is limited to changes within the organism. But quality is not limited to specific characterizations in this manner. It is comprehensive and diverse in its characterization.

The three fundamental qualities (mahā guṇa) are sattva, rajas and tamas (*AS,* 1, 1, 41). From them arise all the qualities that are of significance in medicine and pharmacy. (*CS,* sūtra 1,49 f) enumerates 41 qualities in four groups ; qualities of the sensory objects (sārthah, 5), physico-pharmacological qualities (gurvādayah, 20), psychological qualities (buddhih-prayatnāntāh, 6), and para-pharmacological qualities (parādayah, 10). *Chkp* suggests a three-fold classification; specific sensory qualities (vaiśeshika or viśishṭa which is the sārtha group of *CS*), general qualities (sāmānya, comprehending gurvādi and parādi groups of *CS*), and psychological and symbolic qualities (ātmaguṇā, which is the same as in *CS*). There is a more inclusive classification : objective (ādhibhautika) and subjective (ādhyātmika), the former comprehending the first two groups of *Cpd,* and the latter representing the third group of *CS* and *Chkp*.

Twenty qualities that *CS* and *SS* listed under physico-pharmacological group are common to articles of food and drugs. They are also qualities that are to be found in the bodily constitution of living beings. They are, therefore, called bodily qualities (śarīra-guṇas, Gaṅgādhara). They are arranged in ten pairs of mutually opposite qualities. The qualities are significant as determinants of characteristic ('karmaṇya-guṇā', *RVS,* 3.

111). Each quality represents a primary action-mode.

(1) 'Heaviness' (guru) is a quality that is constituted by the physical element, of earth and water, and its main action is providing satisfaction (tṛpti) and increasing the bulk of substances (bṛmhaṇa). Its effect is seen primarily on kapha and secondarily on the vāta, among the doshas. It represents the dominance of the fundamental guṇa, tamas. It is illustrated by the drug māshā (Phaseolus mungo). 'Lightness' (laghu) is its opposite quality, composed of fire, air and ākāśa elements, having the main function of bulk-reducing (laṅghana). The effect of this quality is primarily on vāta and secondarily on kapha. It is illustrated by the drug mudga (Phaseolus trilobus).

(2) 'cold' (sīta or hima) is a quality that is predominantly composed of the water element, and that has as its main function 'pleasing' (hlādana) or 'cooling' (staṁbhana). It pleases by eliminating the distress caused by heat. The Sanskrit expression 'staṁbhana' actually means "stoppage"; this quality helps stop the flow of substances like blood when they are flowing out of the body. It also conquers thirst, burning and fainting. Its effect is primarily on vāta and kapha and secondarily on pitta. Illustrating this quality is chandana (Santalum album).

'Heat' (ushṇa) is its opposite quality, composed predominantly of the fire element, and its main function is producing heat, (i.e., sweating, svedana) and cooking (i.e., ripening of wounds etc, pachana). It helps the formation of pus etc., which can be eliminated from the body. Its effect is on all three doshas. This quality is illustrated in the action of agaru (Aquilaria agallocha).

(3) 'Unctuous' (snigdha) is mainly made up of the water element and its main function is moistening (klédana), or lubrication. It also strengthens the system and provides complexion. Its effect is mainly on kapha, and secondarily on vāta.

Its opposite is 'Dry' (rūksha), 'parched up'; composed predominantly of the earth, the fire, and the wind elements, it acts on vāta and kapha. Its main function is to absorb (śoshaṇa). It arrests the elimination of urine, faeces, etc., and renders substances rough, hard and coarse. It is illustrated by the action of the drug yava (*Hordeum vulgare*).

(4) 'Slow' (manda) is mainly made up of the earth and the water elements, and acts on kapha and pitta. Its major function is to slow down (mandaṇa) the errant constituent forces in the body, and help preserve health. Hemādri describes it as pacification (śamana) of the doshas. It is illustrated by the action of curds.

Its opposite is 'sharp' (tīkshṇa), which is predominantly the fire element, and therefore, distinguished solely by the guṇa rajas. It acts on pitta and kapha. Its main function is to sharpen the substances (tejana), and help throw out the malefic influence of the errant doshas (śodhana, according to Hemādri). The action of the drug chitraka (*Plumbago Zeylanica*) illustrates this function.

(5) 'Stable' (sthira) is composed principally of the earth element and has its impact on kapha. Its function is to stabilize (dhāraṇa) the physiological structure and functions. The action is illustrated by the drug musalı *(Chlorophytum tuberosum)*.

Its opposite is 'mobile' (sara), made up of the water element and has its impact upon kapha. Its main function is to provoke the doshas into action (prerana). It also helps eliminate the errant vāta and faeces. Its action is represented by the drug Senna (*Cassia tora*)

(6) 'Soft' or 'tender' (mṛdu) is a quality which is composed principally of the water and ākāśa elements and acts on kapha. Its function is to loosen (ślathana) stiffness and prevent oozing out of liquids from the body (asrāvaṇa). Its action is seen in the way fats work when taken in.

'Hard' (kaṭhina), on the other hand, is

composed mainly of the earth element and its action is principally on vāta. Its function is to 'harden' (dṛḍhīkaraṇa): it renders the body strong and resistant. The action of calcium is given as an instance of this quality.

(7) 'clear' or 'pellucid' (viśada) is made up of the earth, fire, wind and ākāśa elements predominantly and its effect is mostly on vāta. Its function is to cleanse (kshālana) the inner organs and constituents of the body, as alkali does.

Its opposite quality is 'slimy' or 'slippery' (picchila), which is essentially water element, and acts upon kapha. Its main action is to anoint (lépanā) and lubricate the inner structures. It joins the severed parts (sandhāna) and makes for the continuance of the life principle (prāṇadhāraṇa). The action of the drug isafgol is given as an illustration.

(8) 'gentle' or 'smooth' (ślakshṇa) is predominantly composed of the fire element, and acts upon pitta. It heals the wounds in the body (ropaṇa), and functions similar to the 'slimy' or 'slippery' quality (picchila). The action of dugdha-pāshāṇa (talc) is given as an example.

Opposite to this quality is 'rough' or 'coarse' (khara), which is mainly the wind element, and which acts upon vāta. Its main function is 'scraping' (lekhana), similar to the work of tuttha (copper sulphate).

(9) 'fine' or 'delicate' (sūkshma) is made up of the fire, the wind and the ākāśa elements mainly, and acts upon vāta. Its chief function is to 'pierce' (vivaraṇa), i.e. enter into even the minute channels inside the body and make its presence felt, like alcohol. The quality is pleasurable (sukhānubandhi).

'Gross' or 'thick' (sthūla), on the other hand, is mainly made up of the earth element and it acts on kapha. Its function is to 'obstruct' (saṁvaraṇa) the flow or entry into the channels, as cakes are supposed to do.

(10) 'compact' or 'solid' (sāndra) is composed predominantly of the earth element and it acts on kapha. Its function is to 'solidify' (prasādana), to bind substances together, to provide mass or bulk (upachaya). It is also associated with the cleansing action (sattva-guṇa). Butter is the example of the substance that is distinguished by this quality.

Its opposite is 'fluid' (drava), composed predominantly of the water element and acting upon kapha. Its main function is to liquefy (vilochana) or melt. It helps dripping or flowing. The action of milk is illustrative of this quality.

SS (1, 46) adds 'decomposing' (vyavāyī) and 'blowing' (vikāśī) as independent qualities. However, the former is taken by Indu and others to be only the heightened form (prakarsha) of 'mobile' (sara), and the latter the heightened form of 'sharp' (tīkshṇa). *AS* (1, 1, 39 and 40) lists the twenty qualities after *CS,* and adds 'the objects of sense-organs, vyavāyī and vikāśī as other qualities (apare guṇāh). Decomposing (vyavāyi) is defined here as "that which pervades in its raw condition the entire body and gets ripened (pakva) as it enters the blood and the cavities". Alcohol and poison provide examples of this action. 'Blowing' (vikāśī) is illustrated when substances pervade the entire body in their raw state and loosen the fine connections within the system, thus bringing about a feeling of expansiveness. The action of opium or dhattūra is suggested as an example.

Besides these two, *SS* also introduces qualities like 'quick acting' (āśu-kārī), 'pleasant odour' (sugandha) and nauseating odour (durgandha). 'Quick-acting' is also mentioned by BHELA in the sense that whatever enters the blood-stream acts quick. While twenty is the standard number of the qualities listed under this group, it is conceded that the qualities may be more numerous; but they can all be accommodated among the twenty. [*See* DRUG-PROPERTIES].

The second list of ten qualities commencing with 'para' (parādi, *CS,* 1, 1, 26) are para-pharmacological, having relevance to pharmacy and medicine. They are distinguished from the list of twenty qualities mentioned above, which are both physical and physiological, qualities alike of drugs and of bodily constituents. The present list, however, consists of abstract qualities, more principles than characteristics; they have been borrowed from the Vaiśeshika system of thought.

(1) and (2) 'Preferable' (para) and 'not-preferable' (apara) constituting a pair, the former being superior and the latter inferior, when considered in relation to place, time, age, potency and other details pertaining to the drug.

(3) The rational approach (yukti) involved in the preparation of medicine which must take into account the doshas. Preparations lacking this approach will prove futile or disastrous, though they are medicines.

(4) Enumeration (saṁkhyā) of ingredients, etc. to achieve precision and effect and to avoid duplication and waste.

(5) and (6) Conjunction (saṁyoga) of ingredients which by themselves are different and discrete, so that their combined effect is desirable. Three kinds of conjunctions are recognized : (a) conjunction arising out of two interacting ingredients (dvandva-karmaja or ubhaya-karmaja); (b) conjunction where only one ingredient is active (eka-karmaja or anyatara-karmaja); and (c) conjunction of all the ingredients which are already active and organized (sarva-karmaja or saṁyoga ja-saṁyoga). Disjunction (vibhāga) is not merely the absence of conjunction but a positive process (bhāva-rūpa) of separation, or dissolution of conjunction. This also is three-fold as above.

(7) Isolation (pṛthaktva), or ascertaining the separateness of each object. This can be one of three types: (a) isolation of objects which can never combine or come under a common concept (asaṁyoga-lakshana); (b) isolation of things which have dissimilar characteristics, although they can come together; (vailakshaṇya-rūpa); and (c) isolation of individual things belonging to the same class (anekatā-rūpa).

(8) Weights and measures (parimāṇa), according to conventional norms.

(9) Preparation or processing (saṁskāra) of things or collection of things so that a new quality that is desired is generated. The concept of 'saṁskāra' in the Vaiśeshika system, however, is different from the sense in which the concept is construed in *CS*.

(10) Regular use (abhyāsa) of a thing, or constant consideration of a thing in accordance with the synonyms, etc current among the people.

The list of psychological qualities (buddhih prayatnāntāh) enumerates: (1) buddhi (organismic awareness or general consciousness) which includes intelligence (dhī), persistence (dhṛti), memory (smṛti), and ego (ahaṁkāra); (2) intentions (icchā); (3) aversions (dvesha); (4) pleasurable feelings (sukha); (5) distressful feelings (duhkha); and willed efforts (prayatna). These are styled subjective qualities (ātma-guṇāh) in the sense that they are not to be found either in the physical objects or in the physiological process. They are strictly details of the individual's own experience.

The qualities of the sensory objects (sārthāh) which constitute one group are: (1) sound (śabda) as the object of audition, (2) touch (sparśa) as the object of kinesthesis; (3) form (rūpa) as the object of vision; (4) taste (rasa)as the object of gustation; and (5) smell (gandha) as the object of olfaction. [*See also* DRAVYA-GUṆA].

Guṭika : Meaning a small ball or pustule (resembling a pearl) it means a medicinal preparation in the form of pills. [*See* PILLS].

H

Health : Of the two terms used for health in Indian medicine, svāsthya and ārogya, the former means 'positive well-being', while the latter signifies 'diseaselessness'. Although the two expressions are used interchangeably in the medical manuals, svāsthya (literally "abiding in oneself") approximates more closely to the Indian conception of health. 'Diseaselessness' (ārogya or arogatā) is a condition that is relevent to the practising physician: it is the state prior to the onset of disease and it is the state that is restored by the removal of disease. In diagnosis, prognosis, medication and nursing it is this condition that provides the practical framework.

But health is not defined as merely an absence of disease. The expression svāsthya connotes a state of well-being of body and mind, a condition in which one is not dependent on other human beings or on any drug for his own physical and mental welfare. It is defined as the state of body and mind which provides the foundation for vigour and strength ('balādhishṭhānaṁ') expressed in wholesome living involving pursuit of the values of life (purushārtha).

Health has been regarded right from the Vedic times as an essential requisite not only for the accomplishment of the three common objectives of life (viz. virtue, .wealth and enjoyment) but also for the liberation from the miseries of phenomenal existence which is the ultimate good. The religious manuals have insisted that good health needs to be preserved in order to be able to perform the prescribed rituals and austerities. Health has been extolled as the most precious of gifts that the gods can bestow on man.

Āyurveda, as the science and art of integrated and meaningful life, is as much concerned with the maintenance and promotion of health as with curing the illnesses that have arisen. [*See* HYGIENE, PREVENTIVE MEDICINE]. Health in this context is an independent and positive idea.

CHARAKA lays down: "One must always manage to maintain health (svāsthya), so that the disturbances (vikāra) that have not arisen may not arise" (*CS,* sūtra, 5,13). Health, here, is defined by his commentator thus : "the condition in which one abides (avatishṭhate) well (sushṭhu), i.e. without any disturbances whatever (nirvikāratvena) (CHKP). CHARAKA'S prescription has two aspects : the causes that promote (poshaka) health, and the causes that interfere with (vighātaka) health. The former is the balance (or equilibrium) of the bodily constituents (dhātu-sāmya) while the latter is the imbalance thereof (dhātu-vaishamya). Imbalance excites and disturbs.

The maintenance of health is accordingly regarded as two-fold (1) The body, which is constantly being worn out and liable to be thrown out of balance, must be nourished and maintained by good food and correct conduct like a flame being tended by pouring oil to the lamp and by trimming the wick. (2) The body must also be protected from disturbances, internal and external, by appropriate medication and curative methods, like the flame being guarded from breeze, insects, etc. The latter, viz. disturbances, are brought about by internal factors (e.g. the doṣhas being excited by careless or thoughtless conduct), over which the individual has control, or by external factors (for example seasonal variation, occurrences in nature, ageing) over which he has little control.

Health, thus, is a dynamic concept; it is constantly being subject to factors of disturbance and needs to be restored as often as it is disturbed. It is a continuous process of integration (yoga) of time (kāla), sensory objects (artha) and actions (karma) (*AHṛ*, 1,1,19). Time refers to seasonal variations: cold, heat and rain. Sensory objects are physical stimulations: sight, sound, touch, smell and taste. Actions are threefold: bodily (physical reactions), mental (thoughts, fears, wishes etc) and vocal (speech and expressive behaviour). These encompass the substances constituting reality that Charaka spoke of (*CS*, sūtra,1,47) (the three units of time; the five primary elements; direction, mind and soul). Perfect integration (saṁyag-yoga) of the three factors (time, sensory objects and actions) is the single causative condition of health. Imperfect integration or association of the same three factors brings about disease.

Association of the three factors could be deficient (hīna-yoga), excessive (ati-yoga) or improper (mithyā-yoga), when disease is occasioned [*See* DISEASE]. If the weather is proper (cold in cold season, hot in the hot season, and raining in the rainy season), if the sensory objects are just and adequately presented for sensory experience (viz. not straining the sense-organ either by insufficient stimulation or by excessive or unpleasant stimulation) and if the work done by the body and mind is in keeping with the natural demands of the body and the normal needs of the mind, there can be no disturbance whatsoever and disease cannot arise. This is the condition to health.

Integration is further explained in terms of the equilibrium of the doshas, bodily constituents, the digestive fire and the elimination of waste products (*BP*):

"sama-doshah samāgniś cha sama-dhātu-malakriyah, prasannātmendriya-manāh svastha ity abhidhīyate".

The above definition, which is a standard one, also includes the quiet and clear functioning of the sense-organs and the mind.

Diseases are twofold: bodily (śarīra) and mental (sattva or mānasa). Body is the ground for the former while the mind is the ground for the latter. An absence of bodily diseases is bodily health and absence of mental diseases is mental health. Thus the balanced functioning of the body and mind is the basis for health in general, which is experienced as 'happiness' or 'well-being' (śukha-saṁjñakam ārogyaṁ', *CS*, sūtra, 9,4). The balanced functioning (yogah samah) involves the integration of the constituents, viz. the three doshas (vāta, etc.); the seven body-constituents (dhātus) or ingredients of the physical frame (rasa) and the three guṇas (rajas etc). It is in this context that health is described as 'prakṛti' (nature), borrowing the Sāṁkhya idea of undifferentiated balance of guṇas in the primal condition ('prakṛtir guṇānām sāmyāvasthā' CHKP on *CS*, sūtra, 9, 4).

A pragmatic definition of health is that it is the condition when the digestive fire is nourished ('ārogyaṁ vahni-vardhanam', *RN*, 20). Good digestion is regarded as symptomatic of good health, for digestive disturbances are at the root of most of the ailments. It is in order that the digestive fire may be kept in good shape (viz. neither dull, manda, nor fierce, ati) that the daily regimen of diet, exercise etc, and the conduct appropriate to seasonal variations are prescribed.

A legend makes the god of medicine, Dhanvantari, assume the form of a bird, and chirp thrice the question 'Who is healthy ?' (ko'ruk ?), in order to test the wisdom of the physicians. Vāgbhata is said to have answered, "He is healthy, who eats what is good, eats moderately and eats only when hungry" (hita-bhuk, mita-bhuk, kshuta-bhuk), to the satisfaction of the god. [*See* DAILY ROUTINE, DHĀTU, DOṢHA, HYGIENE, MALA, PREVENTIVE MEDICINE, SEASONAL CONDUCT, YOGA].

Heart : The importance of the heart (hrt, hrdayaṁ) as the central organ is brought out both in *CS* (sūtra, 30,3-8) and in *SS* (sarira, 4, 30-31). The recognition of this importance goes back to Vedic literature, where the organ is recognized as the secret seat of the soul (viz. consciousness, chetanā) and of the mind (manas) (e.g. *BU,* 2,1,19-20; 5,5,3; *CHU,* 3,12,7; *Kau. U,* 4,19; *Mait. U,* 7,11,2; *KU,* 6,18,16; *SuU,*3,17,20). The medical tradition in India has followed this lead but has attached significance to its practical aspects rather than the mystical.

The heart is defined as the chief seat of consciousness ('viseshеṇa chetana-sthanaṁ', *SS,* sarıra, 4,30), which , in fact, pervades the entire body. That it is an organ has been recognized by the description that it resembles a lotus-bud with its apex hanging down (*SS,* ibid., 31), and by the identification of its location: "to its left below are the spleen (plıha) and lungs (pupphusa) and to its right liver (yakrt) and pancreas (? kloma)". Its expansion and contraction are also mentioned: while one is awake it spreads out (vikasati), but when one is asleep, it folds itself up (nimilati) (*SS,* ibid., 31).

It is said to be formed out of the essential and nutrient portions of blood and kapha ('sonita-kapha-prasadajaṁ', *SS,* ibid, 30) and all the blood-vessels which carry the vital principles of the body ('prana-vahāh dhamanyah', ibid) depend upon it. All the organs of the body (viz. the two upper limbs, the two lower limbs, trunk, head, the viscera), the sense-faculties, the five sensory objects, mind and the objects of the mind, consciousness and the soul (with its phenomenal properties like happiness) are all located in the heart (*CS,* sutra, 30,3). Location here is not to be construed as actual physical placement, but as their dependence upon the heart for their functioning. If anything could be imagined as localized in the heart, they are consciousness, mind and soul. But the entire body rests on the heart as "the wooden framework of a house rests upon the central beam or girder". (*CS,* ibid., 3-4). When the heart is injured, all these organs are affected. Even a small injury to it (up-aghātāt) results in loss of consciousness, while a serious injury leads to death (ibid.).

Its significance consists in its being the seat of vitality (para-ojas). Attached to the heart are the ten vessels that carry this vitality and pulsate all over the body. Vitality is the essence of all the seven body constituents [*See* VITALITY], and is likened to the honey produced by the bee from the essences of various flowers (*CS,* ibid., 30, and sūtra, 17,75). It is this vitality that keeps all beings refreshed and there can be no life without it. In fact, it marks the beginning of the embryo; it is the nourishing fluid that enters into the heart even when the embryo is getting formed (*CS,* sutra, 30,9-11).

A word of uncertain origin, bukka, is sometimes used for the heart (*Trikaṇḍa-śesha*). It is defined as "a special kind of muscular structure in the interior of the breast-region" ('vakshobhyantara-maṁsa-visesha', SKD). There is also an opinion that the heart-proper is the frontal portion of this muscular structure (agra-maṁsa).

There are two synonyms for hṛdaya used in Ayurvedic texts: mahat and artha (*CS,* sutra, 30,6-7). The former word is of Sāṁkhyan origin and refers to the unsurpassed generative principle (of consciousness); and the word is used for the heart because of the overall biological importance of this organ. The latter word strictly means 'object', or 'meaning', and as a synonym of hṛdaya it signifies the excellence of the organ, for when that organ is destroyed, life itself goes out and during life all the organs are 'established' upon the heart alone ('pratishṭh-artham hi bhavanam eshāṁ hrdayam ishyate', *CS,* sutra, 30,4).

An ancient view (ascribed to Kṛtavirya) which is cited in *SS* (sarıra, 3,41), defines heart as the structure for consciousness and mind (buddher manasas cha sthanatvat). In philosophical literature, buddhi and mahat are synonyms, and the expression artha is used interchangeably and thus the view concurs with that expressed by *CS*. But there is a discussion in recent times about the identifi cation of hṛdaya with heart. Gaṇa-nath Sen, for instance, argues that employment of the word 'hṛdaya' in *SS* actually refers to the brain and not to the heart, because the dis cussion of 'hṛdaya' in *SS* follows the account of the head, and because sleep is described as dependent upon the 'hṛdaya'. But the textual description of the organ, of its diseases, and of its location in the breast region leave no doubt that what the ancient meant by 'hṛdaya' was the heart and not the brain. The ancient texts do not describe the brain as an organ of the mind or of consciousness, although 'brain' (mastishka) was known even to the Vedic poet as an organ in the head (cf. *RV*, 10,163,1) [*See* BRAIN *and also* DISEASES OF THE HEART].

Hima : [*See* COLD INFUSIONS].

Hygiene : Indian medicine is preoccupied more with positive health and prevention of diseases than with curing the diseases when they occur. Therefore, there is a well developed branch of study inquiring into the conditions of health, and the methods by which the state of health is maintained or enhanced. This branch of study is called 'svastha vṛtta' (conduct conducive to health), and includes daily routine (dina charya) and seasonal conduct (ṛtu-charyā).

Ancient Indian treatises, medical as well as non medical, praise health as the best possession, for it is only when one is in sound health that all other things in life can be enjoyed. Life would still be worthwhile and enjoyable, with the blessing of good health, even if there are deficiencies by way of wealth, comfort, children, occupation and so on. The objectives of life (viz. virtue, wealth, enjoyment and liberation) are attainable only on the foundation of good health. Therefore, even religious manuals and law-books (smṛti and dharma śāstra) invariably contain rules of conduct by following which good health is maintained. Religious prescriptions concerning food, bath, dress, sex, conduct, rest interpersonal behaviour, social conduct and spiritual practices are essentially hygienic. The garb of religion has helped the general (almost universal) acceptance of these rules.

Medicine is thus not divorced from morality; 'good' conduct (sad vṛtta) is also 'con duct for health' (svastha-vṛtta). Being dev out, clean, honest, hard-working, pleasant, generous, compassionate and moderate in all things, one can hope to make his body and mind adequate instruments for realizing the highest goal in life. The body is not considered as evil, or as an impediment to spiritual welfare. It is inherently neutral, like a knife; it can be used for advantage or for harm. It is therefore , necessary that the individual must understand fully the instrumental value of the physical constitution, and keep it efficient in order to be advantageous.

The same rule applies to the mind. Mind can bind or liberate, in accordance with how it is maintained, trained and used. In Indian thought, distinction between body and mind is neither absolute nor practically real. They together constitute one unit: psychophysical complex ('body-mind'). Even as religion and ethics do not envisage the independent functioning of either body or mind, Indian medicine also regards the two as intimately associated with each other.

Hygiene in India, therefore, contains rules for maintaining physical as well as mental health. Prescriptions of food, for instance, take into consideration not only the nutritive value of the articles of food, the needs of the body, the condition of the 'digestive fire', the time of eating, the quantity of food that is most desirable and the manner of preparation, but also details like the purity of the food (places where it is grown, gathered, cooked, and served), the ethical impact of the food on the human temperament (the sattvik or tamasik element in the food article, the person who has prepared the food, the manner in which it is eaten, the activities immediately prior to eating and soon after, the company in which food is eaten, etc.) and the general approach of the individual towards the necessity and relish involved in eating food.

Likewise, regulations regarding evacuation of bowels, cleaning the teeth, bathing, wearing dresses, resting, exercise, indulgence in sex and earning a livelihood are all directed towards making both body and mind efficient and strong. Health viewed in the context of psychophysical well-being and hygiene has the same approach.

That is why in the Indian medical books, there are suggestions to keep one's passions under control and free oneself from greed, envy, anxiety, possessiveness, cruelty and sloth in order to maintain health. Exercising control over the mind (sattvavajaya) is an accepted method of treatment (*See* MEDICINE). Qualities like piety, humility, modesty, fearlessness, softness in speech, moderation in conduct, hospitality and friendliness are recommended not so much as spiritual requirements but as hygienic prescriptions. They enable the mind to gain an upper-hand in the body-mind complex and thus maintain health in its most satisfactory and productive level. [*See also* PREVENTIVE MEDICINE, DAILY ROUTINE, SEASONAL CONDUCT, FOOD, HEALTH].

I

Infusions : Infusions are of two varieties: (1) cold infusions (hima or śīta-kashāya) and (2) hot infusions (phāṇṭā). Both of them are classed under decoctions (kashāyas), where selected drugs are mixed with water in the ratio 1:4, 8 or 16.

(1) Cold infusions (hima; khusanda or julāl in Yunāni) are prepared from drugs which are cold in property and in potency and which are aromatic, mostly to pacify the aggravation of pitta. The method of preparation is to steep one part of the drug, well pounded and powdered, in six parts of warm or cold water for an entire night, and to strain the fluid through a piece of cloth in the morning (*SaS*, II,4,1). The suspension of the drugs in water is an important detail.

There are several varieties of cold infusions such as (a) panaka (śarbat in Persian and Yunani), where citrus fruits are steeped in cold water, with sugar and pepper added; (b) śarkarā (syrup), where the selected drugs are steeped in cold water with sufficient quantity of sucrose to preserve them and to render the drink tasty; sometimes, syrups are also prepared by boiling over a slow fire and by straining the fluid through a piece of cloth; (c) arka (aquae or distilled water), concentrated aromatic waters which are prepared with weak and simple solutions of volatile oils [*See* ARKA]; (d) taṇḍulodaka (rice-water; ab birañja in Yunani), which is cold water in which rice has been steeped (in the proportion of 8:1) for four to six hours (or for an entire night) and then macerated [*See* BHAVANA]; (e) avakledana, which is the method of steeping a drug in alcohol (or any other menstruum) without application of heat; (f) mantha (emulsions), where one part of the drug, finely powdered,is mixed with four parts of cold water. Sometimes the last variety is classed under hot infusions (phāṇṭā) (*SaS,* II, 3,9).

(2) Hot infusions (phanta, also chūrṇa-drava; nakia in Arabic, khisanda in Persian, mankuā in Yunāni) are watery solutions, prepared by steeping one part of coarsely powdered or bruised drugs (crude) in eight parts of hot (boiling) water in a covered vessel (earthern vessel preferred) for a specified duration (or for the entire night), and then decanted. The drug is squeezed in hot water, so that the active principles of the drug get into the water. Honey, sugar or jaggery may be added to the strained fluid (*SaS, II, 3, 2*). [*See* PREPARATIONS].

Impulses : Called vega in Sanskrit, they denote bodily urges like evacuation, yawning, sneezing, hunger, thirst etc., the non-satisfaction or delay in satisfaction of which may lead to disturbances and diseases. [*See* SUPPRESSION OF URGES, VEGA, HYGIENE]

Indriya : Literally 'belonging to Indra' (as in *RV,* 1,107,2 and *AV,* 19, 27,1), the word is employed to signify powers or faculties that belong to the Indra in the body, viz. the ātman (soul); they are what suggest the presence of the ātman ('atmano liṅgam anumāpakam'). They are instruments of perception and action that evolve out of the principle of self-formulation (ego or ahaṁkara), mainly out of the sattva-dominated aspect thereof (vaikārika). [*See* SĀṀKHYA].

The organs of perception (jnānendriya) are ears (presided over by space, dik), eyes (Sun), nose (the Asvins), tongue (Prachetas), and skin (Vāyu). The organs of action (karmendriya) are: hands (Indra), feet (Vishṇu), speech (Agni), anus (Mitra), generative organ (Prajāpati). In addition to these there are four others, collectively called the 'inner organ' (antar-indriya), to distinguish them from the above ten which are external, bahir-manas (mind), buddhi (individuated consciousness), ahaṁkāra (ego or self-formulation), and chitta (memory), presided over by Moon, Brahman, Śiva and Vishṇu respectively (*SS,* śarīra 1,7). [*See* SENSE-ORGANS].

J

Jāṭharagni : One of the thirteen 'fires' in the body (*See* AGNI), and the most important among them, the 'stomachic fire' (jātharagni) is obviously a figurative expression for the heat in the organism which digests food, maintains health, endows strength and growth (ushmā tejo-mayaṁ). The stomachic fire, in particular, is said to be located in the navel region (nābhi-sthāna), or between the stomach (amaśaya) and duodenum (pakvasaya) (*AHr,* 1,12,10). It is also called 'bodily fire' (kāyāgni) or 'internal fire' (antarāgni (*SS,* 1,21,17), 'fire in the intestinal cavities' (koshṭhagni) and 'the digestive fire' (pāchakagni).

The prevalent view is that it is the same as pitta, for there can be no 'fire' in the body other than the pitta (*SS,* 1,21,9). Pitta, one of the three doshas [*See* DOSHA], is 'fiery' (āgneya) in nature; although composed of all the five primary forms of matter [*See* PAÑCHABHUTA], because of the predominance of the qualities of 'fire' (taijasa guṇodayāt, *AHṛ,* ibid.) it fights against the cool characteristics (soma-guṇa), and with the aid of wind dries up liquidity (tyakta-drava-svabhāva). That pitta is the 'fire' referred to in this context becomes evident by the fact that the treatment of deficient pitta consists of 'hot' drugs, meant to increase the digestive 'fire', and the treatment of aggravated pitta consists of 'cold' drugs, meant to decrease the vigour of the digestive 'fire' [*See* PITTA, DIGESTION].

The function of the stomachic fire is mainly to help digest the food. The food (composed of the five primary forms of matter) needs to be transformed into a state in which the five material aspects of the food are utilized by the bodily constituents (dhātus). This involves the separation (vibhajate) of the essential or nutritive portion of the digested food (sāra, prasāda) from the waste products (kitta) to be eliminated (*AHṛ*, 1,12,11). [*See* DIGESTION].

The stomachic fire is directly correlated with the 'fires of the body constituents' (dhātvagni) and tissue metabolism (dhātupāka) (cf. *AS*, 1,14,26). If the stomachic fire is excessively active, there is also an increased activity in all the tissues; if the stomachic fire is dull (manda), the activity in the tissues is also weakened. The increase or decrease in the body constituents is dependent upon the strength or weakness of the stomachic fire.

All the other 'fires' in the body (viz. all functions of the pitta) are dependent upon (anugraham) the stomachic fire (*SS*, 1,21,10; *AHr*, 1,12,12). When this 'fire' is kept normal, the individual is healthy and his longevity is assured. When it is abnormal, diseases are caused; and when it fades, life is extinguished.

There is an attempt precisely to describe and locate the 'stomachic fire' : above the navel (nābhi), which is the heating centre (jyotih sthāna), about two inches to the left (for men, and to the right for women) shines this 'fire of the stomach' (agnir jātharah); it is about the size of a grain of paddy (vrīhi), but its light and heat pervade the entire body (ushmā vyapṛtah, sarva-dehe). Sometimes, it is described as the vaiśvānara-flame, (like a nīvara-śūka), yellow in colour and extremely subtle, in the centre of the 'heart-lotus'. Whatever the description, it is what digests the food that is eaten (jīṛṇa-kārī); it surges up like a spring from the belly (kukshi), and acidic in taste (amla-rasa). The strength of the individual depends upon this 'fire' (agni-mūlam balam). It is because of this 'womb-heat (garbhoshma), there is blood circulation, and because of the blood circulation the individual lives and moves about (cf. Bhela-saṁhitā, 'ushmā hy atrā-gneś cha karma dehe'). [*See also* AGNI, DIGESTION]

Jīva: Derived from jīv ('prāne' , 'to live'), the word signifies the unseen factor that is responsible for an individual having come into existence and being alive. It is the principle of life, and is usually referred to as the personal soul. It is said to descend into the uterus of the mother at the time of the initial formation of the foetus (*CS*, śarīra, 3,3).

Regarded in the medical texts as synonymous with ātman (although in philosophical literature it is carefully distingushed from the latter) it is the principle of cognitive organization in each individual (jñāna-pratisandhātā, CHKP on *CS*, sūtra, 1,42) [*See* ĀTMAN]. It is what holds life in the body (asu-dhāraṇa), and makes all bodily functions possible. More importantly, however, it is the main subjective framework for which even bodily functions and all experiences, sensory and motor, are objects of awareness (kshetrajña, vedayitā). In this sense, it is the eternal, 'witness' (sākshī), who enters into the womb to constitute an individual and departs from his body at death (srashtā, gantā). It is also called purusha (the individual soul) (*SS*, ibid., 4). [*See* ĀTMAN, PURUSHA].

Jīvana (Jīvita) : Meaning life (from jīv, 'to live'), it is defined as the organization of the physical body, sense faculties, mind, and the soul ('śarīrendriya-sattvā-tma-saṁyoga', *CS*, sütra, 1,42). The expression is also used to denote whatever supports life (prāna-dhāranam), viz. water (*Āryā-sapta-śatī*,

463), air (*Haṭha-yoga-pradīpikā,* 2,3), bone-marrow (majjā, *RN*), and Vishṇu (*Mahābhārata,* 13,146,112). [*See* LIFE].

K

Kalā : The word etymologically means 'a tiny fraction', 'a small part', 'an aspect'. It is generally employed in the sense of a phase of the moon ("one sixteenth part"), or in the sense of a small unit of time. In Indian medicine, however, it is used to denote extremely minute anatomical structures ('cellular tissue and fascia of body').

SS (śarīra, 4,5) defines kalā as fine structures that separate the primary constituents of the body (viz. the seven dhātus) from their physical locations (āśaya, 'receptacle', places where they are contained, avasthāna-pradeśa, *NiS*), and describes them as situated at the extreme borders (forming encasement and support) of the various physical constituents. "As the duramen or core of a piece of wood or stem becomes exposed to view by cutting into it, so the root principles (dhātus) of the body may be seen by removing the successive layers or tissues of its flesh. These kalās are extensively supplied with snāyus (fibrous tissues), bathed in mucous, and encased in a membranous covering" (ibid., 5-6, tr. Bhishagratna, vol II, p. 145-146). They are the substrates of the primary body constituents.

They are seven in number: (1) 'māṁsa-dhara-kalā' (fascia-bearing), depending on which the veins (sirā), fibrous tissue (snāyu), arteries (dhamanī) and the other capillaries (srotas) are spread out in the flesh, even as the lotus-stock planted in slimy water spreads out all-around (*SS,* ibid., 7-8); (2) 'rakta-dhara-kalā' (bearing vascular tissue of blood), supported by which are the blood-vessels inside the flesh, and especially in the veins (sirā), in the liver and in the spleen (yakṛt, plīha); even as milky juice is exuded when the plants containing latex are pricked (ibid., 9-10); (3) 'medo-dhara-kalā', bearing fat or adipose tissue, which supports the body constituent of that name (medo-dhātu), present mainly in the abdominal region of all animals as well as in the cartilages or cavities in the shafts of the long or small bones mixed with blood, and also the other body constituent marrow (majjā, found in the large bones) (ibid., 11-12); (4) 'śleshma-dhara-kalā' (mucosal cells, synovial tissue), present in all the joints of bones (sandhi), and lubricating them so that movements are easy, silent and free from friction, comparable to the greasing of an axle so that the wheel turns smoothly (ibid., 13-14); (5) 'purīsha-dhara-kalā, (faeces-bearing), which occupies the abdominal region (koshṭha), extending from the liver (yakṛt) to the intestines, small and large (antra), and whose function is to separate the nutrient portions of the food (sāra) from the undigested or indigestible food residues (kiṭṭa), which is kept in the lower intestines (uṇḍuka) (ibid., 15-16); (6) 'pitta-dhara-kalā' (bile-bearing) occupying the part of the abdominal cavity known as 'grahaṇī' (stomach, *See* GRAHAṆĪ) and providing the digestive juices (pāchaka-pitta) so that food brought to this region is well digested (by retaining the food in this region for the duration of the process of digestion, and the separation of the nutrient substances from the waste-products, before it moves on to the large intestines or pakvāśaya) (ibid., 17-18); and (7) 'śukra-dhara-kalā' (semen-bearing), pervading the entire body (like fat in milk, or sugar in the sugar-cane juice) but principally located in the testes (vṛshaṇa) and phallus (śepha), and supporting the production and flow of semen (ibid., 20-22). [*See also* SROTAS, DHĀTU].

Kāla-Bala-Pravṛtta: Diseases that have their origin in time, viz. due to seasonal changes like cold, hot, wind, rains. Such diseases are of two types: those that are due to unexpected and unnatural changes in the weather (vyāpannartu meaning 'disordered season'), and those that are due to normal changes in the weather (avyāpannartu). [*See also* DISEASES].

Kalka : [*See* PASTE].

Kaṇḍara : Described as 'gross ligaments' (snāyu) (CHKP on *CS*, chikitsā, 15,17), these are tendons of the body, responsible for movements like extension, contraction etc. They are sixteen in number, four in the legs (pāda), four in the hands (hasta), four in the neck (grīva) and four in the back (pṛshṭha).

The tendons of the extremities cover the region of the thighs and shoulders and extend till the roots of the toes and fingers (called prarohas or sprouts). The tendons of the neck cover the region of the chest (viz. heart, hṛdaya), and extend on one side to the head and on the other to the penis (its prarohas). The tendons of the back extend to the ball joints of the shoulders above and the buttocks below (*SS*, śarīra, 5,10). [*See* BODY (HUMAN)].

Kapha: Etymologically signifying emanation from water ('kena jalena phalati'), this word stands for one of the three doshas in the body which are responsible for good health when normal and diseases when morbid. The dosha is also called śleshman (from the root ślish, 'to embrace' 'āliṅgane'), meaning the 'uniting' principle. It is composed of all the five primary forms of matter, but principally of water (representing the combination of sattva and tamas of the three guṇas), together with earth (representing tamas). Therefore, it is tamas in its general orientation (as vāta is rajas and pitta is sattva).

The significance of this detail will be understood when it is realized that vāta which provides the direction and motivation for all physiological functions, and pitta which provides the heat and energy for the efficient accomplishment of these functions would fail to achieve normalcy unless balanced by a restraining force which is provided by kapha (which is tamas, viz. inertia, causing obstruction to both sattva and rajas). It is also to be remembered that kapha is made to correspond with the moon (soma), as vāta with the air (vāyu) and pitta with the sun (sūrya). The air as well as the sun dry up and make way for disintegration (ādana and vikshepa), while it is the moon that softens and integrates by the cooling influence (visarga). Thus, the balance is maintained among the three doshas.

Of the two primary forms of matter that enter into the composition of this dosha, earth provides stability (sthairya), strength (bala) and solidity (saṁghāta), and water makes for unctuous nature (snehana), flooding (hlādana), moistening (kledana) and binding (bandhana). Together, they contribute the protective quality to kapha. The physical properties of this dosha are mainly: viscid, sticky and slimy, heavy, cold (to touch and in action), sweet in taste, inert, soft (to touch), and white in colour.

Among the main functions of this dosha in its normal condition are: contributing stability, solidity, compactness, strength, and heaviness to the body, generating unctuous character within the body, making the joints firm and efficient, rendering vitality to persevere and forbearance to grow, and causing courage and generosity to appear. Resistance of the body to diseases and the ability to recover normal health are due to this dosha. Minor errors in the body-function are corrected without drugs or regimen, as a result of the healing power of kapha (which corresponds to moon, who is described as 'the lord of the healing herbs').

This dosha is principally located in the chest (urah), but its field of action includes throat, head, oesophagus (kloman), joints (parvāṇi), stomach and small intestine (āmāśaya), chyle (rasa), fat-tissue (medas), nose, and tongue. The stomach is also the seat of the 'sweet' taste (madhura-rasa); the dosha, therefore, is sweet in taste, when 'uncooked' (avidagdha), but becomes saline (lavaṇa) when it undergoes the process of 'cooking'.

This dosha is aggravated by eating sweet, heavy, sour, cold and unctuous articles of food, over-eating, drinking much water, much use of curds, sugar, fruits, sleeping during daytime. The disorder is manifested by paleness of skin, coldness, heaviness of body, itching, constipation, unctuousness, sticking of excreta in different orifices of the body, the feeling of being covered with a wet cloth, feeling that some external thing is sticking to the body, swelling, excessive exudation, delay in action and response, drowsiness, nausea, aversion to food, and feeling of old age.

It is naturally aggravated in winter and in spring. It tends to increase during the forenoon and just after a meal. In child-hood it is on the ascendant.

Treatment of the disorders of kapha includes prescription of diet and drinks which are alkaline, astringent, bitter and pungent, physical exercises (walking, jumping, swimming, etc), keeping awake in the night, exposure to heat and sun's rays, emetics, inhalation therapy, fomentation, application of hot ointments and so on.

It is said to be 'strength' (bala) when in its normal measure, and 'waste product' (mala) when the balance is tipped. It is 'vitality' (ojas) in the body, and it is also called 'pāpmā' (viz. excessively tamas-oriented) (*CS*, sūtra, 27).

Kapha is five-fold in its function:

(1) klédaka-kapha ('moistening'): This aspect of the dosha is chiefly located in the stomach (including small intestine, āmāśaya), produced there as foamy secretions, according to *SS* (sūtra, 21), where the food is moistened, broken down to its component parts and liquified, with the assistance of prāṇa-vāyu, samāṇa-vāyu [*See* VĀTA] and pāchaka-pitta [*See* PITTA]. While the main function of this aspect is to soften the food, it nourishes the other four aspects by its humid properties. The disorders of this aspect include impairment of digestion, dyspepsia and the whitish colour of urine and faeces.

(2) avalambaka-kapha ('clinging'): The principal seat of this aspect is chest (urah, thorax), to which it clings, and the sacrum (trika), which it supports. It nourishes the heart by lubricating it with the food-juices (rasa) which have now become humid and watery (*SS,* sūtra, 21 'hṛdayāvalambanam karoti'). It protects the heart from excessive heat by cooling it. If the former aspect (kledaka) is the source of kapha, this aspect represents the store-house of the dosha : for, on it depends the nature and efficiency of the other aspects of kapha. Textual descriptions suggest that the body-water is mostly this aspect of kapha. It also provides energy to the limbs. Disorders of this aspect include disinclination to work and heaviness in the joints.

(3) bodhaka-kapha ('aiding perception') : Located in the root of the tongue (jihvā-mūla) and throat (pharynx), it moistens (by salivation) any substance placed on the tongue before it descends through the oesophagus to the stomach and in the process helps perception of the taste of that substance. It also helps increase appetite. When this aspect is disturbed, the sense of taste is affected.

(4) tarpaka-kapha ('satisfying')· Located in the head (śirah), it nourishes the sense-organs by cooling them, and keeps them in

good shape. Disorders of this aspect include impairment of sensory functions, loss of memory and diseases like meningitis.
(5) śleshaka-kapha ('joining'): Located in the joints (articulations of bony-joints), it is responsible for the smooth functioning of the joints by lubricating them and protecting them against excessive heat by its viscid property. It keeps the joints firm and united (sandhi-samślesha). Disorders of this aspect include heaviness and pain in the joints, and impairment in the function of the joints. [*See* DOSHA].

Karma: Literally meaning 'action', the word has acquired a specific connotation signifying actions done in the previous states of existence but yielding their results in the current. (*CS* śarīra, 6,116) describes it as 'fate' (daiva), and points out that it may be the cause of many diseases. Such diseases (karmaja-roga) cannot be cured by normal therapeutic procedures (kriyāghnāh); they subside only when the influence of these past actions are spent (*CS*, ibid, 117).

The very birth of the individual is explained as due to this factor. The soul enters the womb of the mother and becomes responsible for the formation and development of the foetus owing to the influence of 'fate' ('daiva-saṅgāt', *SS*, śarīra, 3,4); prompted by past actions ('karmaṇā choditaṁ'), the being is subjected by necessity to certain experiences; the foetal development follows a natural course, but the merits and demerits of the foetus are determined by the past actions, good or bad (*SS*, ibid. 46). For, it is only when guided by past actions that the soul transmigrates from one body to another, along with the four primary forms of matter with the help of the mind (*CS*, śarīra, 2,31).

The soul, whose nature is pure consciousness, cannot by itself transmigrate through the bodies. It can do so only when it gets associated with it ('sattvam aupapādukam' *CS*, śarīra, 3,3). The association of mind with the soul is determined by the past actions. The vital factors (prāṇa) that enters into the constitution of the embryo include the 'bhutātmā' or the 'elemental soul' (i.e. consciousness that gets involved in the five primary forms of matter, in accordance with past actions) which organizes the other factors (viz. 'fire' or pitta, 'moon' or kapha, 'wind' or vāta, the three guṇas, and the five senses of cognition) (*SS*, śārīra, 4,2)..

It is thus that 'fate' (daiva) enters into the framework of the individual. "Fate (daiva) is the influence obtaining from actions done in previous states of existence, but effort (paurusha) is what is relevant in the present state. The former is responsible for diseases, while the latter may lead to health" (*CS*, śarīra, 2,44).

CS (vimāna, 3,33), however, points out that while a strong 'fate' (daiva, viz. past actions) invariably overcomes 'effort' (purushakāra, viz. present actions), weak 'fate' can be overcome by strong 'effort'. The expression of a strong 'fate', however, awaits favourable time and situation (kālaniyata). Both the factors together determine the life-span of the individual (*CS*, ibid., 36). But the life-span is not predetermined, and one can prolong or cut short his life with his effort or negligence (*CS*, ibid.).

Karmendriya: Organs of action: hands (for prehension), feet (for locomotion), mouth (for speech), anus (for elimination) and generative organs (for procreation and pleasure). They evolve out of the principle of 'self-formulation' (ego, ahaṁkāra) [*See* SĀṀKHYA]. There are two views about its origination: one view is that along with the five cognitive organs, these arise from the sattva-dominated (vaikārika) ego with the co-operation of the ragas-dominated (taijasa) aspect, while the other view is that these originate from the rajas-dominated aspect, as distinguished from the cognitive organs which originate from the sattva-dominated aspect. [*See* INDRIYA, ORGANS]

Kashāya: (1) astringent flavour [*See* TASTE]; (2) decoction where one part of the drug is boiled with four, eight or eighteen parts of water until one quarter of the whole remains. [*See* DECOCTION]

Kaumārabhṛtya: Name for paediatrics, it is one of the eight branches of Indian medicine, where details of birth, development from the neonate stage till the stage when the child can eat solid food, care of children, the value of good milk and breast-feeding, bodily diseases of children, the curative measures as well as the treatment for mental diseases (graha-samuttha) are discussed (*SS*, sūtra, 1,5).

Kāya-chikitsā: It is one of the eight branches of Indian medicine, and the most important among them. It deals with the causes, conditions, symptoms, progress, and cure of ailments afflicting the body (kāya, viz. all the limbs, 'Sarvāṅga-saṁspṛshṭānāṁ vyādhīnāṁ') like fever, dysentery, cough, dropsy, epilepsy, skin diseases, diabetes, etc. (*SS*, sūtra, 1,3).

It is described as the therapeutic procedure employing such preparations as decoctions, powders, pills, and methods such as purgation, sweating, etc. to alleviate and eliminate diseases pertaining to the cavities (koshṭha) (Atri-Saṁhitā,2).

Therapy under this head falls into three types: (1) use of herbal decoctions, powders, emetics etc. (mānushī, 'human'); (2) use of surgical instruments e.g., cautery etc. (āsurī, 'diabolic'); and (3) use of alchemic preparations of mercury and metals (daivī, 'divine') (*BR*).

Kiṭṭa: The word (probably from kiṭ, 'gatau', 'to go') means waste-products, secretions in the body, unusual impurities that need to be expelled, in order to maintain health. Mainly, they are the undigested or the indigestible portions (residual) of the food that is ingested, as they are separated from the nutrient portions (sāra) in the organ known as grahaṇī [*See* GRAHAṆI]. These are pushed into the large intestine (*pakvāśaya*), propelled by samāna-vāyu.

Metabolism involves the production of specific secretions in each of the body-constituents (dhātu): kapha in chyle, pitta in blood, excretions of the ears, eyes, nose, mouth, roots of hair and the genitals in muscle, sweat in fat-tissue, hair and nails in the bone, the unctuous secretions of the eyes, faeces and skin in bone-marrow, and vitality in semen. [*See* DHĀTU]. Not all these, however, can really be called waste-products, for some of them are needed for body structure and functions. [*See* DIGESTION, MALA].

Kshāra: [*See* ALKALI]

Kvātha: Also known as śṛta or niryūha, it is decoction, prepared by boiling one part of the drug (selected parts of fresh plants) with sixteen parts of water (or eight parts of water if the substances are dry) until one quarter of the water remains. Before being added to water, the drugs are coarsely sliced or powdered. The boiling is done on a slow fire (mandāgnau), and in an uncovered vessel (apidhānamukhe pātre). The decoction is strained through a piece of cloth. While being administered, rock-salt, honey, sugar, alkalis or some medicinal powders may be added (Cf. *SaS*, II,2,1-2). [*See* DECOCTION, PREPARATIONS.]

L

Lavaṇa: [*See* SALTS]

Leha: [*See* AVALEHA]

Life: Called in Sanskrit āyus (or jīvitam), life is regarded as an organization (saṁyoga) of the body (śarīra), the sensory faculties (indriya), the mind (sattva) and the soul (ātmā) (*CS*, sūtra, 1,42). The body is composed of the five primary forms of matter (earth, water, fire, air and ākāśa), and is the field of individual experiences (pleasure and pain) for the soul. [*See* BODY]. The sense-faculties are instruments of transaction with the outside world. They are ten in number, five for cognition (visual, auditory, olfactory, gustatory and tactual), and five for action (prehension, locomotion, articulation, excretion and procreation); and thus the entire range of human behaviour is covered [*See* SENSE ORGANS]. Mind is the internal organ, without which the sense-organs cannot function, and sensory experience cannot be organized or regulated. [*See* MIND]. The soul is the core of life (and hence called jīva); and without its involvement, the foetal development cannot occur; without it, life is impossible. It is of the nature of consciousness, and it enlivens the body-sense-mind complex [*See* ATMAN, JĪVA, PURUSHA].

Life is likened to a tripod (tridaṇḍa), consisting of mind (sattva), soul (ātmā) and body-complex (śarīra). (*CS*, sūtra, 1,46). Although it is mainly consciousness (chetanā), transaction requires the organization of twenty-four constituents (mind, ten sense faculties, five objects of sense-perception, and eight-fold prakṛti, viz. five primary forms of matter, buddhi or consciousness, ahaṁkāra or ego, and the avyakta or the unmanifest soul). (*CS*, ibid., 16-17; cf. also *SS*, sūtra, 1, 'pañcha-mahābhūta-śarīri-samavāyah purushah').

Life is further described as the sequential occurrence of consciousness (chetanānuvṛtti), the act of living (jīvitam), the continuum of several states of existence or units of living (anubandha), and the condition which supports the psychophysical complex preventing it from disintegration and decay (dhāri) (*CS*, sūtra, 30-22).

Life can be four-fold in general orientation: 'favourable' (hita), 'unfavourable' (ahita), pleasant (Sukha) and unpleasant (dukha) (*CS*, sūtra, 1,41). Among the conditions that make the life 'favourable' are: balanced pursuit of the three goals of life (virtue, wealth and pleasures) without one interfering with the other (trivargam parasparānupahatam), careful consideration before resorting to any action (parīkshyakāri), mindfulness (apramatta), self-restraint with regard to the urges like love, anger, envy, pride etc. (suniyata-rāga-rosha-īrshyā-mada-māna-vega), concern for the welfare of fellow-beings (bhūtānām hitaishī), honesty (satya-vādī), modesty (śama-para), disinclination to appropriate the property of others (parasvad uparata), generosity (vividha-pradāna-para), spiritual knowledge and practice (adhyātma-vid-tat-para), and recognition of both the worlds, here and hereafter (lokam-imam-amum-chāvekshyamāṇa). The 'unfavourable' life is characterized by traits contrary to all these (*CS*, sūtra, 30,24).

The life that is 'pleasant' is made possible by the absence of bodily and mental ailments (śarīra-mānasābhyāṁ-rogābhyāṁ anabhidruta); possession of youthfulness (yauvana), bodily strength (bala), enthusiasm (vīrya), celebrity (yaśa), and courage (paurusha); general knowledge and textual knowledge (jñāna-vijñāna); efficiency of sense-function (indriyārtha-bala); possession of adequate wealth and enjoyment of normal pleasures, effort towards and accomplishment of life's objectives (samṛddha sarvāraṁbha); and opportunity to move about at will (yatheshta chārī). Absence of these factors renders the life 'unpleasant' (*CS*, ibid).

The life-span of an individual (āyuh-pramāṇa) is determined by the nature of the physical constitution (deha), temperament (sāra), and personality type (prakṛti), and peculiar characteristics or symptoms (lakshaṇa) (*CS*, vimāna, 8,111 and 8,96) [*See* JĪVANA]

M

Majjā: Translated as bone-marrow, this is counted as the sixth of the body constituents (dhātu), derived from bone (asthi) and generative of sperm (śukra). The action of 'wind' (vāta) in the bones creates sponginess in the internal portions which get filled from the unctuous and soft material obtained from fat (medas). This oleating material, which also fills the cavities and pores of the bones, is called bone-marrow ('asthnah śuddha-sneha-bhāgah').

When the bone gets 'cooked' in its own 'fire' (asthy-agni), and its essential part or the tough juice (sāra) becomes frozen and separated like perspiration, this bone-marrow is generated. It is especially located in the interior of the big bones (sthūlāsthishu viśeshena). Its main function is to give strength to the body by contributing viscidity. It also nourishes sperm (śukra), which is the final constituent.

Derived from bone-marrow is the hair on the head as a secondary constituent (up-dhātu).

Among the diseases of bone-marrow are included pain in the finger-joints, giddiness, fainting spells, loss of consciousness, and deep-seated abscess of phalanges. [*See also* DHĀTU].

Mala : The term, derived from the root mṛj ('to clear out', 'to purify', 'to cleanse', mṛjyate śodhyate iti), is usually translated as waste-products of body metabolism which need to be eliminated. But its employment in the context of the main triad of life and health (the three doshas, the seven dhātus and the malas), suggests a wider connotation. It is an essential ingredient of the living organism, an indispensable activity in the living body, viz. production not only of material which needs to be eliminated from the system (for which the expression kiṭṭa is used) but also of material that can be utilized to support the body (hence called dhātu).

It is also usual to refer to mala as 'polluting agents' (malinīkaraṇāt), which, unless expelled from the body, would render the body impure (viz. unhealthy, diseased). But it is important to recognize that what are called mala are actually by-products of the digestive process, and that as long as they are in proper proportion they do not cause any disorder in the body, but, on the other hand, sustain the body and facilitate its efficient functioning. It is therefore that they are called 'mala-dhātu', which may sound paradoxical. Each of the seven bodily constituents has its own specific byproducts: phlegm from chyle, bile from blood, urine from muscle, sweat from fat-tissue, faecal fat from bone, faeces from bone-marrow, secretion of genitalia from sperm or semen. These are called 'dhātu-mala'.

The process of digestion (in terms of body metabolism or dhātupāka) is principally a matter of separating the essential tissue-nutrients (prasāda) from the waste-products (asāra), and of expelling the latter (kiṭṭa, from the root kit, 'gatau', 'to go'). The body-building process (anabolism) is suggested by the expression 'prasāda-pāka', and the process of breaking down (katabolism from the Greek root katabole, 'to throw down') by 'kitta-pāka'. All by-products (including waste-products) that arise in the course of body metabolism (dhātu-pāka) are collectively known as 'mala-dhātu', because they are all necessary to sustain life, some by utilization and others by elimination.

As a result of the action of the 'fire' in each of the seven body constituents, the supporting material for the subsequent constituent is generated (called poshaka-dhātu), like 'blood' in chyle, 'muscle' in blood, 'fat-tissue' in muscle etc, [*See* DHĀTU], which is then circulated all over the body through an appropriate channel [*See* SROTAS]. Thus, it is absorbed and assimilated. The undigested portion is then eliminated from the body as waste-products (kitta). This includes discharges, secretions, excretions, some solid, some semi- solid, some liquid in form, some gaseous (vāta), and some hard (like the keratin of the nail).

The seven body-constituents (dhātu) are said to generate seven groups of by-products which need to be eliminated from the system. (1) From chyle, the mucoid excretions of phlegm as waste-product (kitta-kapha); (2) from blood, bile-pigment as waste-product (kitta-pitta); (3) from muscle-tissues, waxy excretions of the ear (karna-mala); mucous excretions of the eye (akshi-mala), nasal discharges (nāsikā-mala); the discharges from the mouth (āsyamala), excretions from the hair follicles (loma-kūpa-mala), and excretion from genitalia (prajanana-mala); (4) from fat-tissue, sweat (keśa), hair on the face (śmaśru), body-hair (roma), and keratin of nails etc (nakha); (5) from bone-marrow, the unctuous substances in the eye (akshi-sneha), in the stools (vit-sneha) and in the skin (tvak-sneha).

But usually, mala refers to three excretions: faeces (śakṛt), urine (mūtra) and sweat (sveda) (*AHr*, 1,1,13). Their proper elimination is necessary for the maintenance of health. They must also be in proper proportions: an excess in the discharge or a deficiency in their production is regarded as an abnormal condition, and generative of ailments.

Faeces are the refuse of food as also substances eliminated from the tissue-cells of the body. It is the portion of undigested food in the large intestines (pakvāśaya) dried up by the heat and transformed into lumps. It is recommended that one should evacuate faecal matter twice in twenty-four hours; and that one should avoid the suppression of the urge to evacuate. Improper elimination of faeces results in diseases in the gastro-intestinal tract and other parts of the body. Among the diseases caused by improper evacuation are lumbago, rheumatism, sciatica, paralysis, bronchitis, asthma and different kinds of intestinal worms. When the formation of faeces is deficient, there will be pain at the sides and in the region of the heart, and flatus accompained by the rumbling sound around the region of liver and intestines (*SS*, sūtra, 15,11). When the formation is excessive, there will be distention of the abdomen and colic pain in the loins and intestines (ibid. 19).

Through urine, many body wastes are thrown out. Normally, the healthy person passes urine about six times in twenty-four hours, and it is recommended that one should take sufficient quantity of water for this purpose. If the formation of urine is deficient, there will be aching pain in the bladder, causing urine to dribble or come out in thin and scanty jets (ibid., 11). If the formation is excessive, there will be constant urge for micturition and distention of the bladder accompanied by a gnawing pain (ibid., 19).

Sweat or perspiration is the result of proper physical exercise, some therapies like fomentation, and the intake of some drugs.

Along with sweat, many waste-products of the body are thrown out. When there is deficient perspiration, numbness about the hair-pores is felt and the skin is dry (ibid., 11). When there is excess of perspiration, there will be itching, and the skin emits a bad odour (ibid., 19).

Māṁsa : Enumerated as the third among the seven body constituents (dhātu), flesh (including muscles, peśī) is derived from blood and chyle (the second and the first constituents). As blood is 'cooked' in its own 'fire' (śoṇitāgni), and condensed or coagulated by the wind within the body (vāta), its subtle aspect transforms itself as flesh. [*See* DHĀTU]. It gets formed in the first eight months of foetal life.

Its main functions are to provide physical strength, to cover the bones, and nourish the fat-tissue which is the next constituent in order. It contributes to the bulk of the body and resists the action of the 'wind' within the body.

It acquires various forms in accordance with the different locations in the body. Although muscles are actually innumerable, broadly 500 of them have been counted (*SS,* śarīra, 37-40): 400 in the four extremities (two legs and two arms), 66 (or 60 according to GAYADĀSA) in the trunk (koshṭha), and 34 (or 40 according to GAYADĀSA) in the region above the clavicles (head and neck). "The ligaments, veins, bones and joints etc. of a human body, derive their strength from the fact of their being supported by or covered over by the muscles" (*Bhishagratna,* II, p. 170). Females are said to have 20 extra muscles: 10 in the two breasts, 4 about the parturient passage (or vagina), 3 in the lowest extremity of the spine and 3 along the passages of ovum and sperm. (*SS,* ibid., 42).

The muscles, composed of all the five primary forms of matter, are predominantly 'earth'. When 'cooked' in its own 'fire' (māṁsāgni), its subtle aspect, viz. fat-tissue (medas) becomes the causative factor for the succeeding constituent. Derived from muscle are muscle-fat (vasā) and the six layers of the skin as secondary constituent (upadhātu).

Among the diseases that mainly involve muscle are cervical adenitis, goitre, granuloma, tumour, warts, tonsilitis, gangrene, uvulitis and some skin diseases. [*See also* DHĀTU].

Manas: [*See* MIND].

Mandāgni : Meaning 'slow fire', it refers to the digestive condition being poor, the 'digestive fire' (jāṭharāgni) being inhibited to a smaller or greater degree by the prevailing influence of kapha. It is caused by drinking much water, improper food habits, suppression of natural urges, sleeping during daytime, and keeping awake in the night. In this condition even normal food when properly taken, cannot be digested and metabolized. Associated ailments include heaviness of the abdomen, heaviness of the head, cough, dyspnoea, emesis, weakness of the body, and other disturbances due to kapha. [*See* AGNI, JĀṬHAPĀGNI, DIGESTION, KAFHA].

Mantra-Chikitsā: Treatment of diseases by incantation of appropriate mantras under specified conditions, is indicated where the unseen factor of past actions (daiva) is overpowering human effort (paurusha). [*See* DAIVA-VYAPĀŚRAYA].

Marma: Vital points or spots in the body which are sensitive and vulnerable ('mortal spots' 'mārayantīti', from the root mṛ, 'to die'). They are described (*SS,* śarīra, 6,15; *AS*) as places where flesh (māṁsa), veins (sirā), arteries (dhamanī), ligaments (snāyu), joints (sandhi) and muscles (peśī) unite, or are intimately associated (sannipāta); and , therefore, life abides there especially . An injury to this spot (by a cut, incision, blow, burn, or puncture) would result in permanent deformity of that organ or death.

It is also defined as the spot where the vital forces are concentrated (jīva-sthānaṁ, *RN*); 'they sustain life' ('jīva-dhāraṇī', *SaS*, 1,5,39). The reason why they are mortal spots is that they are the primary seats of the activating air (vāyu), the cooling moon (soma) and the warmth-endowing heat (tejas); and also of the three fundamental aspects of all existence, viz. sattva, rajas and tamas. The five sensory faculties are also located there; these are called twelve prāṇas. It is natural, therefore, that the 'embodied self' (bhutatma) resides in these spots (*SS*,ibid., 85).

Such spots are 107 in number: 11 in the muscles [*See* PEŚĪ], 41 in the veins [*See* SIRĀ], 27 in the ligaments [*See* SNĀYU], 8 in bones [*See* BONE], 20 in the joints (sandhi) (*SS*, ibid., 4). Another enumeration has: 11 in each extremity, 12 in the abdominal and thoracic regions, 14 in the back and 37 in the region above the clavicles (ibid., 5). The spots are named after the veins (sirā), ligaments (snāyu), flesh (māṁsa), bones (asthi) and joints (sandhi). Although in each such spot all these are located (because, by definition, a vital or mortal spot is where all these are intimately associated), the factor that occurs predominantly gives the spot its name. The arteries (dhamanī) are not separately mentioned here, because as instruments of circulation of the vital currents, their role is indispensable in all kinds of marmas (*SS*, ibid.). There are no mortal spots in the body apart from these, for there are no concrete things in the body besides veins, ligaments, flesh, bones and joints.

The mortal spots are classified into five types, according to the risk involved: (1) causing immediate death or death within a day or week (sadyah-prāna-hara) when the spots are injured, for in such spots (19 in number) prevail the quality of 'fire' (āgneya) and as soon as the 'fire' is put out, life goes out; (2) causing death after some interval, viz. after a fortnight or a month after injury (kālāntara-māraka), for these spots (33 in number) prevail in the combined quality of 'fire' and 'moon' (saumyāgneya), and even if the 'fire' is put out, the life-giving 'moon' would linger on for a while; (3) causing death as soon as the foreign body (śalya, viz. any substance that is unwanted by the body, that enters the body with violence, and stays inside producing undesirable effects and disturbances, local or systemic) is extracted (viśalyaghna), for such spots (three in number) are mainly of the quality of 'air' (vāyavya), and life would endure as long as the opening (made by the foreign body piercing through) continues to be covered by the foreign body, thus preserving the 'air' within; (4) causing permanent loss of the limb, or deformity of the organ (vaikalya-kara), for such spots (44 in number) prevail in the quality of the 'moon' (saumya), which nourishes and cools, and thus the injury would not be fatal; and (5) causing intense pain in the affected region (rujā-kara), for such spots (8 in number) abound in the qualities of 'fire' and 'air' (vāyvagni-bhūyishtha), both of which are pain-producing (*SS*, ibid., 11).

Injuries to the first kind of marmas (immediately fatal) are attended by debility of the sense-organs, loss of consciousness, confused state of mind, and different types of pain. Injuries to the second kind are attended by loss or diminution of bodily constituents (dhātu) and supervening diseases (upadravās), which lead to death in due course. The other kinds, which are not by themselves fatal, but result in deformity of organs or loss of limbs are to be handled skilfully, for otherwise they may prove fatal (*SS*, ibid.,37-41).

Injury to any part of the body other than these fatal spots would not spell certain death or deformity of the organ. Injury to the fatal spots may be slight or serious, resulting in deformity in the former case and death in the latter. But there can be no injury to these spots which involves risk of a lesser nature (*SS,* ibid., 43). If any disease originating in another part of the body spreads to these fatal spots, cure becomes difficult (*SS,* ibid., 44).

The knowledge of mortal spots in the human body is essential for the surgeon, and in fact this topic comprises half the scope of surgery (*SS*, ibid., 33). Even if the spots, injury to which would cause immediate death are injured, a clever surgeon might manage to make the patient survive, albeit deformity of that particular limb would not be avoided (*SS,* ibid., 34). [*See* BODY].

Mātrā : Measure of medicine that is sufficient for counteracting the disease, without any deleterious side-effects ('anapāyi-parimāṇa', *CS,* sūtra, 1). The measure depends on such considerations as diet, time of the day, season, constitution of the patient, the potency of the drug, and the form in which the drug is administered (powder, paste, decoction, etc). There were two principal measures that were widely employed, Māgadha and Kaliṅga, the former being regarded as superior.

Matter : [*See* DRAVYA].

Medas : Translated as 'fat-tissue' or 'adipose-tissue', this is counted as one of the seven body constituents (dhātu), after flesh (māṁsa) and before bone-tissue (asthi). [*See* DHĀTU]. Derived from flesh, as its essential portion, during its 'cooking' in its own 'fire' (māṁsāgni), the subtle aspect of flesh is responsible for nourishing this constituent. In its turn, when 'cooked' in its own 'fire' (medogni), the subtle aspect of fat is transformed into bone.

Its chief locus is the belly (udara). Its primary function is to support the body, lubricating the structure and contributing to its firmness. Its specific function is to nourish the bones. It also cools the system, causing perspiration. It is heavy by nature, unctuous and providing bulk. Excess of this constituent manifests itself as obesity, especially around the belly. And it is associated with loss of strength.

Derived from this constituent (upādhātu) are the nervous tissues or ligaments (snāyu), which along with the veins (sirā) help fleshy organs tied to the bone structures. There are 900 ligaments in the human body, of which 600 are in the four extremities (legs and arms), 230 in the trunk (koshṭha), and 70 in the head and the neck. They are of four types: branching (pratāna-vatī in the extremities and joints), circular (vṛtta, large ligaments or kaṇḍaras), thick or broad (pṛthu in chest, back, sides and head) and perforated (sushira) in stomach, intestines and bladder (*SS,* śarīra, 5,30-35) [*See* SNĀYU]

Among the diseases involving these constituents are thirst, dryness of mouth, palate and throat, burning sensation in the body, especially hands and feet, numbness of limbs, increase in excrements of the body, increased discharges from the orifices of the body, lack of energy, sweet taste in the mouth, and matting of hair. [*See also* DHĀTU]

Medical Discussions: Known as 'tadvidyā-saṁbhāshā' ('conversation with a student of that very science'), medical debates are recommended as one of the three methods of acquiring medical wisdom (the other two being study and teaching) (*CS*, vimāna, 8,6).

The physicians must meet with each other and discuss, so that practical application of each ones knowledge may be promoted, and new knowledge obtained by academic debates (saṁharsha). Such discussions lead to clarity in understanding (vaiśāradya), skill in verbal expression (vachana-śakti), recognition of ones merit (yaśas), elimination of doubts concerning what one has previously studied (pūrva-śrute sandehavatah), confirmation of the import of what one had already understood (bhuyo 'dhyavasāya). One would know, during such discussions, many things of which he was formerly ignorant; he would also be confided with many professional secrets. It is therefore that the wise recommend such discussions (*CS*, ibid., 15).

Medical discussions may fall into one of two categories: (1) friendly discussions among colleagues (sandhāya-saṁbhāshā), who are learned and competent; with abundant practical experience, and endowed with ready-wit; who are free from envy, anger, ill-will or desire to dominate and conquer; and whom it is possible to interrogate, argue and oppose without risking friendship; and discussion with whom one would learn how to explain clearly and to criticize frankly, all the while being polite (*CS*, ibid., 17); and (2) heated and hostile debates among opponents (superior to oneself, inferior, or equal to oneself) is the principal concern, techniques of correct and effective argumentation are learnt. The latter is necessary for medical learning, for it enables one to think clearly, present his views carefully, accept the valid arguments from the other side, and argue cautiously, for he is all the while exposed to criticism. But hostile debates should not turn into fights (kalaha), which are always condemned by the wise (*CS*, ibid., 18-24).

Medical Ethics: Medical profession, being motivated by compassion for the living beings (bhūta-dayā), has its codes of conduct which are elaborated in the classical texts (e.g. *CS*, vimāna, 8,8-13).

The medical student is expected to be calm, generous, noble-minded, virtuous, tolerant, persevering, modest, intelligent, rational, and compassionate. He must be good-looking, well proportioned in body, and free from defects and diseases. He must be interested in the science and art of healing and must be willing to help the people in distress even at the cost of his own comfort. His attention must be directed to discover facts about the disease, to understand the import of symptoms, to enrich his own knowledge and to provide himself with skill in practical management. He must be humble and loyal to his instructors. His love of study must be continuous. He should be free from addictions, irritability, greed, arrogance and intolerance. He must be enthusiastic in his profession, hard working and sincere (*CS*, ibid., 8).

Among the instructions that the medical student is given during admission, in a gathering of learned men and elderly physicians, are (*CS*, ibid., 13):

(1) "Your actions must be free from ego, vanity, worry, agitation of mind, or envy; your actions must be carefully planned, with concern for the patient, and in keeping with the instructor's advice

(2)Your efforts must be directed towards achieving professional success (karma-siddhi), earning wealth (artha-siddhi), attaining celebrity (yaśolābha), and also heaven after death (pretya svargaṁ)

(3) Your unceasing efforts must, at all costs (sarvātmanā), be directed towards giving health to the suffering patients (āturāṇām ārogyāya).

(4) You must never harbour feelings of ill-will towards your patient, whatever the provocation, even if it entails risk to your life ('jīvita-hetor api api cha āturebhyo nabhidrohavyam').

(5) Never should you entertain thoughts (manasāpi) of sexual misconduct, or thoughts of appropriating property that does not belong to you.

(6) Your appearance and dress must bespeak modesty.

(7) Take no liquor, commit no sin, nor keep company with the wicked.

(8) Your speech must be soft (ślakshṇa), pleasant (śarmya), virtuous (dhanya), truthful (satya), useful (hita) and moderate (mita).

(9) What you do must be appropriate to the place where you practice, and the time, and

you must be mindful in whatever you do (smṛti-mata).
(10) Your efforts must be unremitting (nityam yatnavatā cha) in enriching your knowledge (jñanotthāna) and promoting your health (upakaraṇa-saṁpat).
(11) Do not undertake to treat the criminals, traitors, other anti-social elements (mahājana-dveshi), excessively sophisticated folk (atyartha-vikṛta), wicked persons (dushṭa), and the moribund (mumūrshu).
(12) Do not undertake to treat a woman when her husband or any other relative of hers is not present (asannihita).
(13) Do not accept any gift presented by a woman-patient without ascertaining that it has been approved (anujñātam) by her husband or guardian.
(14) Never enter the house of your patient (ātura-kula) (unless you are invited) and take care to visit the patient only in the company of someone who knows (the patient and where he lives) (vidita), and who has obtained the patient's permission to enter the house (anumata-praveśi).
(15) When visiting your patient, take care that you are well-dressed (susaṁvita) and modest ('with head bent', avāk-śira), mindful (smṛtimān), and attentive (stimita); and your actions must be preceded by careful consideration of what must be done and what must not be done (avekshyāvekhya mānasa).
(16) When you have entered the patient's house, take care to confine your sense-organs, mind, awareness and speech on matters strictly relating to the patient's health and welfare; do not attend to anything other than the patient (anyatra āturāt), and what does not immediately relate to the well-being of the patient (āturopakārārthāt).
(17) Do not reveal to others what goes on in the patient's house-hold (ātura-kula-pravṛttayah).
(18) Even when you discover that the patient's life-span is severely limited (hrasitaṁ āyushah pramāṇaṁ, viz. that he is about to die soon), do not disclose this to the patient or to the near relatives of the patient, for such knowledge may cause a shock (upaghātāya saṁpadyate).
(19) Even when you are learned and proficient, do not show off (vikatthitavyaṁ), for people do not like such exhibition of one's own erudition and prowess".

"Difficult it is to master the entirety of medical science, therefore, one must be diligent (apramatta) in maintaining constant contact with this branch of learning. One must learn without ill-will even from his adversaries; for the wise folk, the entire world (viz. all human beings) is a teacher (kṛtsno hi loko buddhimatām āchāryah), while for the unwise it may turn out to be an adversary. Correct instructions which are conducive to celebrity (yaśa), health and longevity (āyushya), and personal growth and strength (paushṭika), and which have the merit of universal approbation (laukyam) must be received with gratitude, even when they come from an enemy" (*CS*, ibid., 14).

Medical Texts: Standard medical treatises are essential for a practising physician as well as a student. But the selection of suitable texts must be made considering one's own intellectual powers, place of residence, age, and time at his disposal for study. Several texts are available, but the desirable characteristics in a useful text are: it should have been used (āsevitaṁ), viz. relied upon by well-known, wise, and noble physicians; containing much import (artha-bahulaṁ) and being regarded highly by experts (āpta-jana-pūjitam); helping the mental development of the intelligent, average, and dull students alike (trividha-śishya-buddhi-hitam); free from defects of repetition (punarukti); compositions of ancient and enlightened sages (ārshaṁ); composed in good style (supraṇītaṁ,) viz. contents being properly arranged and ideas well elucidated; not containing vulgar or difficult expressions (anavapatita-kashta-śabdaṁ); directed towards the ascertainment of the subject-matter in an orderly manner (kramāgatārthaṁ, artha-tattva-niśchaya-pradhānaṁ); free from contradictions (saṁgatārtham); devoid of confusion regarding division of contents (asaṅkula-prakaraṇaṁ), enabling quick comprehension (āśu-prabodhakaṁ); and containing definitions, explanations and illustrations (lakshaṇavac-chodāharaṇa-vaccha). Such a text is like the Sun, which drives away darkness and lights up everything (*CS*,vimāna, 8,3).

Medical Treatment, Value of : *CS* (sūtra, 10) contains a discussion between Maitreya and ĀTREYA-PUNARVASU regarding the value of medical treatment or therapeutics (bheshaja). Maitreya argues that medical treatment is useless (akiñchitkaram), for some patients who are attended by the best of physicians, treated by the most effective medicines and nursed well, are seen to die (all the therapeutic help being little more than a drop of water thrown into a pond, or a handful of dust on a heap of dust), while others, with none of these advantages, survive and recover, nevertheless. Medical treatment is useless in the former case and unnecessary in the latter. The main thing is 'fate' (karma), which being strong will help the patient to survive, and being weak allows him to die, regardless of the presence of medical treatment or its absence.

ĀTREYA-PUNARVASU replies that this argument is incorrect and improper (mithyā). To say that patients were attended and treated properly by the best of physicians is not borne out by facts observed (anupapannam).In cases where diseases are curable (sādhya, *See* CURE), therapy is surely effective. Without prompt and correct therapy, the disease may get complicated and may become incurable. Where, however, the diseases are incurable, therapy may not be of much avail.

It is not that all patients who are treated are cured; some do die, despite the best of medical aid. In such cases, it is 'fate' (karma) that prevails. Like diseases being curable or incurable, 'fate' also is either strong or weak. When it is strong, a patient dies at the appointed time, despite all treatment. In cases where it is weak, treatment certainly helps [*See* KARMA]. Even when a patient is cured without any treatment, any given treatment would not be in vain. It is like helping a healthy man get up when he has slipped and fallen down; he could, of course, get up on his own, but help would make him get up quicker and more easily (*CS*, ibid., 10,5, cf. also CHKP on it).

The physician must (like a clever archer) examine each case and decide about the curability or incurability of the disease before he proceeds with the treatment (*CS*, ibid.,) [*See* DISEASE, PHYSICIAN].

Medical Wisdom: Medical wisdom is acquired by three methods (upāyāni): (1)study (adhyayana), earnest and continuous, involving intelligent recapitulation of the texts and intent contemplation on their import; (2)teaching (adhyāpana) after examining the student and ascertaining his character, ability, health and interest, and imparting lessons concerning life in general, medical profession, medical ethics and the science of medicine; and (3) academic discussions (tadvidyā-saṁbhāshā) with colleagues and fellow-students, in order to enrich ones own knowledge, to obtain clarity of knowledge and to get rid of doubts, to deepen ones understanding and to learn new methods and ideas, and to become skilled in expressing ones thoughts. (*CS*, vimāna, 8,6,16). [*See* TADVIDYĀ-SAMBHĀSHA].

Medicated oils and ghee: Extensively used in Āyurveda from very ancient times, the unctuous preparations made by boiling (sneha-pāka) oil or ghee in which selected drugs are put are prescribed for external use (usually oil) as well as internal (usually ghee) administration. There are decoctions of vegetable drugs made in an aqueous medium (menstruum); such as milk or water or juices from fresh drugs. This is added to oils (usually oil from sesame seeds, also called gingelly oil; sometimes cocoanut-oil, castor-oil or neem-oil is used); or ghee and paste (kalka) prepared by finely grinding some drugs together and the whole thing boiled down to one-fourth its volume. The usual proportions are: one part of paste, four parts of oil or ghee, and sixteen parts of the aqueous medium (*SaS*, II, 9, 1).

Boiling (pāka), which is the most important detail in these preparations, is continued till all the water evaporates, leaving only oil. Boiling is done in three degrees: (1) 'soft' (mṛdu), viz. underboiled, leaving the boiled paste soft because some water remains; (2)'medium' (madhyama), where all water has been lost, leaving the paste dry and just soft, so that pills may be made out of it using the fingers; and (3) 'hard' (khara) viz. overboiled, the dehydrated sediment being fried in oil till it becomes coarse in texture, turned hard and dry, entirely devoid of moisture. (*CS*, kalpa, 12, 105-107). Boiling beyond this point (dagdha-pāka) is useless.

The oil needs to be first purified by heating (to deprive it of its watery content) and then some drugs like mañjishṭhā *(Rubia cordifolia)*, haridrā *(Curcuma longa)*, lodhra and mustaka *(Cyperus rotundus)* are steeped in it; a small quantity of water is then added and the whole thing is laid aside for a day, before being boiled till all the water evaporates. Then after straining the oil and adding to it the herbal paste or decoction, boiling is again resorted to, for eliminating the watery portions. It is ready for use when cooled.

Ghee (clarified butter) is likewise initially purified by heating (to deprive it of its water content), and by adding a small quantity of turmeric juice. Then it is melted on a mild fire, before adding the herbal paste to it. The mixture is then boiled until the watery portion evaporates. The ghee then acquires the colour, taste and smell of the drugs introduced into it.

The three degrees of boiling as in the case of medicated oils, are resorted to here. The ghee that is 'soft'-boiled (mṛdu) is used for nasal inhalations (snuff), the 'medium'-boiled for internal administration, and the 'hard' boiled for external application.

The unctuous element (sneha) in the preparation is ascertained by indications such as freedom from froth in ghee and the presence of froth in oils, the paste in the oil or ghee becoming amenable to being rolled by the fingers, combustibility of this material without producing any sound when put on a fire etc. In case the unctuous element is deficient (āma-pāka), the medicinal value is little, and when taken it weakens the digestive process (*SaS*, II, 9, 17). [PREPARATIONS]

Mental Hygiene: Indian medicine believes that prevention of a disease is better than its cure, and prescribes measures for preserving health (both of body and mind). These measures are applicable to all human beings but takes note of the social group to which a person belongs and the place where he resides. These are collectively known as 'sadvṛtta' ('wholesome conduct'), which is especially a means of preserving mental health (*CS*, sūtra, 8, 17-35).

Mind (including sensory functions), when disturbed, would bring about diseases. It is important, therefore, that it should not be disturbed; one must strive to maintain its normal composure ('prakṛti-bhāve prayatitavyaṁ'). One must resort to actions only after carefully considering the wholesomeness or otherwise of those actions, keeping in mind the propriety of the transaction between the sensory functions and their respective objects (sātmyeṇdriyārtha-saṁoga), ones own constitutional peculiarities (ātma-guna), place of residence, and time of the year (deśa-kāla). Such conduct, done with mindfulness (smrti) becomes wholesome, for it accomplishes the welfare of the individual (ātma-hita).

The purpose of such conduct would be two-fold, maintenance of health (ārogya), and mastery over the sense-functions (indriya-vijaya). It involves performance of religious duties and details of personal hygiene:hair-cut, shave and nail-pairing thrice during a fortnight; wearing of neat and clean clothes; applying oil to the head, ears, nostrils and soles of feet; daily bath and frequent washing; cheerful countenance; helpful attitude, courteous manners; soft, clear and relevant speech; self-restraint; sense of duty; humility; tolerance; respectful attitude towards elders and teachers; calm and steady gait while walking; use of umbrella, footwear, and turban while travelling; avoidance of dirty, impure and dangerous places; friendliness and modesty; accommodating nature; calm bearing and avoidance of aversions as well as excessive attachments.

Avoidance is prescribed of falsehood, misappropriation of property, sinful conduct, wickedness, fault-finding, company of mean, cruel, degraded and treacherous folk, avoidance of dangerous vehicles, uncomfortable seats and beds, uneven ground for walking and places where fire abounds; avoidance of loud laughter, laughter without covering the mouth, expulsion of bodily wind with sound, yawning, sneezing, nail-biting, grinding of teeth, improper postures of the body, meaningless and nervous movements (like digging into the earth with the toe, fingering the parts of the body, chewing straw etc.), enmity with good folk and friendship of the wicked, solitary haunts and dangerous places, wild and vicious animals, easterly wind, snow and storm, and quarrels.

Food should be eaten only after taking a bath, wearing fresh clothes, offering ablutions and rinsing the mouth; eating good and clean food in pleasant and congenial company, in neat and clean surroundings and in clean vessels and plates; eating a variety of dishes but moderately, without making a sound; eating food while seated in an erect posture and with a pleasant frame of mind; avoidance of drinking water excessively during, immediately before or immediately after meals are recommended [*See* FOOD].

Avoidance of sneezing in a prone position, of attending to any work while the natural urges prevail (*See* SUPPRESSION OF URGES). of discharging urine, faeces or sputum on public roads, in water, near fire, when the wind is blowing or in the vicinity of sacred buildings and trees is a measure of health.

Care must be taken not to insult womenfolk, nor to trust them indiscriminately; avoidance of sexual misconduct (intercourse with a diseased, uncouth, unfriendly, or unexcited person; having affairs with persons already married to others;) sexual activity in any organ other than the genitalia; copulation in public buildings, cross-roads, sacred spots, hospitals, cemetery, garden, and water; sex activity during dawn, daytime or dusk; sex-indulgence without great desire for it and without erection, or when one is hungry or overfed, or when a natural urge prevails, when one is fasting or when he is physically fatigued.

Also prescribed are avoidance of studying in unfavourable periods; not breaking the common codes of conduct (for example, not walking in the open at night; not taking food or studying or indulging in sex during forbidden periods, like dawn and dusk; not making friends with persons much younger than oneself or with avaricious or ignorant people; not insulting anyone even under provocation; avoidance of arrogance, haughtiness, slander, violent or overmuch speech; trusting one's people and looking after the servants and dependents; not relying on others for all things; not being in the habit of procrastination; performance of actions only after examination and deliberation; not subjecting the sense organs to intense, unnatural or frequent stimulations; not discharging one's normal duties when excited or indignant; avoidance of conceit when successful, or despair when failure comes; constantly reflecting on one's own nature, aspirations, abilities and limitations; and having self-confidence at all times.

This prescription helps one to maintain his health, avoid ailments, curtail needless desires and actions, live for a hundred years and avoid untimely death. He will achieve dignity in society and salvation thereafter (*CS*, ibid. 30-33). (*See also* HEALTH, HYGIENE, PREVENTIVE MEDICINE].

Metabolism: The action of 'fire' (agni) in the body, which not only digests food but builds up the living tissues of the body from the nutritive portions of the assimilated food. Generally referred to as 'cooking' or 'maturation' (pāka), this process takes place in each of the seven body-constituents (chyle, blood, muscle, fat-tissue, bone, bone-marrow and semen)and hence called dhātvagni-pāka, as distinguished from digestion which is called jāṭharāgni-pāka. Digestion transforms the ingested food into an assimilable form; metabolism transforms the nutritive portions of the assimilated food into the constituent elements of the body structure. Involved in this process, is the separation of the nutritive portions (sāra) from the waste products (kiṭṭa) which are expelled from the body. (*See* DIGESTION, DHĀTU, MALA, FIRE].

Mind: Along with the ten organs (indriya), five of cognition, and five of action, [*See* SENSE-ORGANS], mind (manas, also called sattva) is a sense-organ, which, according to *SS* (Sarīra, 1, 4) is an evolute of the sattva-dominated egoity (vaikārika-ahaṁkāra), and shares the characteristics of cognition and action (ubhayātmaka), [*See* SĀṀKHYA], and which, according to *CS*, is a composite product of the five primary forms of matter (bhautika).

It is regarded as a substance (dravya) [*See* NYĀYA-VAIŚESHIKA] among the nine (viz. the five primary forms of matter, soul, mind, space and time), substratum of action and phenomenal properties (*CS*, sūtra, 1, 48 and 51). The mind is not physical and is independent of the five forms of matter. It is counted among the individual (adhyātmika, viz. non- physical but pertaining to the living, experiencing and behaving individual) collection of substances and properties: mind (manas), objects of mind (manortha, viz. thoughts), individualized consciousness (buddhi) and soul (ātmā) (*CS*, sūtra, 8, 13). As a substance, mind is 'atomic' and unitary (*CS*, śarīra, 1, 19).

While it is a sense-organ, for it shares the characteristics of cognition and action in common with the other sense-organs (*SK*, 27), it is a 'super-sense' (atīndriya) in that the objects of all the other senses are objects to it and no sense-organ can function independent of it (*AS*, śārīra, 5, 45). In fact, one of the functions of mind is to activate the sense-organs and regulate them ('indriyābhigrāha', *CS*, śarīra, 1, 21 cf. also 'sarvendriya-para', *BS*, 6, 1, 2).

"The mind, body and the soul are like the 'tripod' (tridaṇḍa) on which the individual rests and functions" (*CS*, śarīra, 1, 46); they are interrelated. The body is inert and cannot provide its own motivation; the soul is beyond the field of action but provides the motivation by its very presence (*CS*, ibid. 75). It is in association with the mind that the soul is able to do this ('yuktasya manasā tasya', *CS*, ibid). The soul, in fact, is defined as 'the body with mind' ('samanaskam śarīram', *KS*).

When the sense-organs are associated with the mind, they are able to prehend the sensory objects. but what the sense-organs prehend is only an indeterminate mass (nirvikalpa); the mind, however, continues its operation after sensory prehension (ūrddhvam) and provides meanings and resolves on the sensory data (*CS,* ibid., 22). The mind, thus, is not only the cause of sensory function, but the very source of the sensory abilities (*BS,* 6, 8, 4). It acts as a 'driving force' for the sensory processes ('cheshṭāpratyaya-bhūtam', *CS,* sūtra, 8, 4).

Other functions of the mind independent of the sensory processes include thinking (chintya), considering (vichārya), imagining (ūhya), attending (dhyeya), and deciding (saṁkalpya) (*CS,* śarīra, 1, 20). The expression 'buddhi' is used in the context of mind in the two senses: the higher mental process of determining (adhyavasāya, niśchaya) (for example, *CS,* śarīra, 1, 21), and the preliminary sensory apprehension (indriyabuddhi) (*CS,* ibid., 32). BHELA, for instance, distinguishes between the sensory or peripheral mind (manas), which is confined to the field of sensory data (and, therefore, located in the 'brain') and the higher mental processes or the central mind (chitta) which is located in the 'heart' (*BS,* 6, 8, 4).

In the course of the foetal development, mind (manas) is said to make its appearance in the fifth month and the organ for higher mental processes (buddhi) in the sixth month (*SS,* śarīra, 2, cf. acc. to *AHr*, śarīra, 1, the organs are unmanifest alongwith consciousness chetanā in the fifth month, and buddhi develops in the sixth). Among the views cited in *CS,* (śarīra, 6, 21) regarding the first organ to develop in the foetus, the view of KUMĀRAŚIRĀ-BHĀRADVĀJA was that the 'head' (śiras) appears first, for it is the seat of all the sense-functions, and the view of KAṄKĀYANA, the physician from Bāhlīka, was that heart (hṛdaya) develops first, for it is the seat of consciousness (chetanā). Accordingly, two views have prevailed in Indian medicine regarding the location of mind: the 'brain' (mastishka, the organ between the top of the head, śiras, and palate, tālu) and the heart. But the general trend is to assign mental functions to the heart. *BS,* however, makes brain responsible for mental processes which are associated with the sense-organs, and 'heart' for all higher mental processes (ibid, cf. also *CS.* chikitsā 9, 5, 'buddher nivāsaṁ hṛdayaṁ'). *KS* (1, 3, 6) holds that the sense-functions as well as mind emerge from the heart (cf. also *CS,* sūtra, 17, 12). *AHr* (7, 12, 13) holds that the sādhaka-pitta [*See* PITTA] located in the heart is responsible for the higher mental processes (buddhi, medhā, abhimāna, cf. also *SS,* sūtra, 21, 10 and CHKP on *CS,* 1, 12).

There is some discussion in recent years about the exact significance of the location of the mind in the 'heart' as found in the classical texts of Āyurveda (*SS,* śarīra, 4, 30). GAṆANĀTH SEN suggested that the 'heart' here actually signifies 'brain', (viz. the brāhma-heart in the ājñā-chakra) (*PS*): DHIRENDRANĀTH BANERJEA points out that there are six 'hearts', out of which the 'heart in the head' (śirogata-hṛdaya) is referred to as the seat of the mind. But the arguments are far-fetched and have little justification in the classical texts. The heart situated in the thoracic cavity (urogata-hṛdaya) is the heart that is referred to in the texts as the seat of the mind [*See* BRAIN]. Even in lay literature, hṛdaya, chitta and manas are expressions which are used synonymously in the sense of mind (e.g. Amara-kosha, Tattirīya-Upanishad, 1, 6 'manomaya-purusha' in hṛdayākāśa'). *CS* (sūtra, 30, 3-4 and vimāna 8, 7) mentions in clear terms that mental functions are located in the heart (in the thoracic region).

Mind is said to be tripartite in its nature ('trividhaṁ', *CS,* śarīra, 4, 30): 'pure' (śuddham), 'excessively active' (rājas) and 'extremely indolent' (tāmasa), in accordance with the three guṇas (*SK* 14). While the bodily disturbances are caused by all the three doshas (vāta, pitta and kapha), mind which is itself sattva is affected by rājas and tamas only, which are pathogenic so far as the mind is concerned (*CS,* ibid, 34).

Among the diseases, three types are recognized: (1) endogenous (nija), caused by the morbid doshas of the body; (2) exogenous (āgantu), caused by extraneous factors like poison, wind, fire, accident etc; and (3) mental (mānasa) caused by contact with undesirable objects and separation from the desirable objects (*CS*, sūtra, 11, 45) [*See* MENTAL DISEASES]. [*See also* BRAIN, DISEASES, GUṆA, MENTAL DISEASE, PRAJÑĀPARĀDHA, ERRORS OF JUDGEMENT, SATTVĀVAJAYA].

Mithyā-Yoga: Improper employment of the mind, speech and body by the individual is known as 'mithyā-yoga', for such employment leads to undesirable results (ahita), and it is distinguished from 'excessive employment' (ati-yoga) and 'non-employment' (ayoga) (*CS*, sūtra, 11, 40). Suppression of natural urges, preoccupation with unwholesome images or ideas, harsh speech, excessive inhalation of foul air, too much exposure to bright light, loud sound etc. are examples of improper employment. The opposite of it is sama-yoga (balanced employment), leading to health and happiness.

Modaka: A pill or bolus, usually larger than the guṭika. One part of powdered drugs are added to two parts of cold syrups or jaggery treacle (guḍa) and stirred well until a uniform mixture is obtained, and then made into a bolus. (*BP* 1, cf. 'yavāsa-śarkarā' *RN*). [*See* PILLS].

Muscle: [*See* MAMSA].

N

Nāḍī: Meaning a tubular stalk or flute (from nada, hollow reed which grows in the rainy season) the word is as old as the Vedic literature, (*RV*, 10, 135, 7; *AV*, 6, 138, 4) used in the sense of a conduit, duct, vein or artery in the human body. It is often used synonymously with dhamanī (*RV*, 2, 11, 8; *AV*, 1, 17, 3 and 4), sirā (or hirā, although a distinction is sometimes made, e.g. *AV* 7, 35, 2 'a hundred dhamanīs and a thousand hirās') and snāyu (tendons, *AV*, 9, 8, 11 and 12; 12, 5, 69. The diminutive form, nāḍikā, is also used (*AV*, 5, 18, 8) [*See* SIRĀ, DHAMANĪ, SNĀYU].

In the Vedic context, nādī means conduits in the sense of spermatic ducts and cords (*AV*, 6, 138, 4). One of the Upanishads (Katha, 6, 16) speaks of a hundred and one nādīs of the heart, and another (Praśna, 3, 6) of the hundred nādīs of the heart with their thousand branches.

However, the meaning of pulse, amenable to examination and helpful in diagnosis and prognosis, is absent in the Vedic literature. The concept of nādī-parīkshā (pulse-examination) is likewise absent in the classical texts of Indian medicine (*CS, SS, KS, BS, AS, AHṛ, MN*). Its first occurrence appears to be in *SaS* (pūrva-khaṇḍa, 3, 1-11), about the thirteenth century. It is also mentioned in *BP*, (1, 7, 11-22), *BYT, YR,* DHANVANTARI'S Sarva-roga-nidāna, and Gada-saṁjīvinī. There are about 50 works dealing exclusively with this topic (e.g. KANĀDA'S Nāḍī-vijñāna, RĀVANA'S Nāḍī-vijñāna, ŚAṄKARA-SENA'S Naādī-prakāśa, RAGHUNĀTHA-PRASĀDA'S Nāḍī-jñāna-tarangiṇi,, and several anonymous works like Nāḍī-jñāna-tantra and Nāḍī-Darpaṇa). In course of time, pulse-examination became very popular not only as a variety of examination by touch (sparśa-parīkshā), but as a valuable aid for discovering the errant condition of the doshas.

The examination of the pulse was introduced into Greek medicine as early as 320 B.C. by Praxagoras of Cos. Herophilus is said to have evolved a system of counting the pulse by a water-clock. Pneumatists evolved an elaborate pulse lore. And it entered the field of Arabic medicine, and thence into the Yunāni system. Chinese medicine had an ancient literature concerning pulse-examination. It cannot be ascertained with any degree of certainty when or how pulse-examination was introduced into Indian medicine. But its popularity during the middle ages and in the recent past is beyond doubt.

Pulse-examination is a difficult art, and presupposes not only long and assiduous practice but insight into the normal human constitution as well as pathogenesis. Its special value consists in helping diagnose the diseases of patients who cannot communicate, like dumb folk, patients with paralysed speech, patients who have lost consciousness, patients who are 'possessed' and talk irrelevantly. Amidst the welter of confusing symptoms, the pulse can provide an accurate picture of the diseased conditions of the body 'like objects being illumined by a lamp'. It tells the physician the condition of the three doshas (vāta, pitta and kapha), severally (vyasta), in pairs (dvandva or yugalīkrta) and collectively (samasta, or sannipāta). It also suggests to him the ease or difficulty with which treatment could be effected, or whether the disease is altogether incurable (śādhyā-sādhya-viveka').

There are said to be three crores and a half crore of nādīs, gross and subtle, in the human body, all rooted in the region of the umbilicus and spreading upward, downward and across. Among them 72,000 are gross, and carry the properties of the five sense-functions. The subtle ones (called sirā, in *SS*, sarīra, 7, 3) are 700 in number; and they carry uninterruptedly the food-juice' (anna-rasa) prompted by the body wind to all the parts and satiate the entire body, 'like a hundred rivers that flow into the sea'. They pervade the body from head to foot, and are covered by the skin even as the mṛdaṅga (a percussion instrument) is. Not all of them however, are visible; only 24 are. And among them one alone (which extends to hands and feet) can be examined (cf. *SKD,* Toḍala-tantra, 8). It is directly related to the heart, and therefore the condition of the entire body is reflected in it. In men, this nādī is to the right, and in women to the left. Its condition is perceptible on the wrist of the right hand of men, and of the left hand of women. It is also perceptible in the foot, but in practice the wrist is preferred.

The pulse for examination is to be found in the wrist immediately below the thumb. This pulse (nādī, dhamanī) is described as the 'witness of the life-process in the body' (jīva-sākshinī), and as the evidence of happiness or misery within the body. When the physician presses against this pulse with his three fingers of the right hand (the fore-finger, the middle finger and the ring-finger), he can feel by the first finger movement that is diagonal in the part of the pulse that resembles a barley-seed. This portion of the nāḍī indicates the condition of vāta. He can feel by the second finger the movement that is quick and constant but in one point. This portion of the pulse indicates the condition of pitta ('fire' in the body). He can feel by his third finger movement that is oblique (horizontal) but slow and almost non-existent. This indicates the condition of kapha. The physician must press the pulse three times with his three fingers and release it, before he begins to feel exactly the condition of the three doshas. During examination, however, he must first discern pitta (with his middle finger), then vāta (with his fore-finger) and finally kapha (with his ring-finger) (*GOML* Madras, vol. 23, no. 13086).

The three doshas are perceived in the pulse as transverse movement (vāta like the movement of the wind), unsteady (pitta, like the flames of the fire), and steady (kapha, like the settling water). When vata is aggravated, the pulse at the point appropriate to this dosha, is perceived like the moving serpent or a crawling leech. When pitta is aggravated, movement in the pulse appears like the flight of the crow or a sparrow, or like the hopping of a frog. When kapha is aggravated, movement in the pulse is similar to the measured strutting of a peacock or the slow floating of a swan on water. When two doshas are together aggravated, the movement in the pulse is sometimes slow, sometimes fast. When all three doshas are troubled (sannipata), the movement in the pulse is extremely erratic, sometimes very slow, sometimes very fast, resembling the flight of a quail (lava) or a partridge (tittirī). The physician will understand by pulse-examination whether the disease is hard to cure (kṛcchra-sādhya) or impossible to cure (sthana-vichyuta). The pulse that stops every now and then, the pulse that is extremely sluggish, and the pulse that is cold to touch indicate approaching death (Nadıprakasa, SKD) [*See* CLINICAL EXAMINATION].

Examination of pulse is to be resorted to early in the morning, when both the physician and the patient have finished their ablutions and bath, are in a calm frame of mind, and seated comfortably. The pulse is not to be examined immediately after a bath, or after eating a meal; nor after exercise or an oil-bath; nor when hungry or thirsty; nor while the patient is asleep. Very early in the morning, the pulse will be unctuous, in the afternoon warmth in the pulse will increase, and in the evening its pace is quickened. Therefore, these periods must be avoided for examination of the pulse.

Nidra: The word (derived from nidi, 'kutsayaṁ' 'to abuse' 'to throw away'), means sleep, which is a condition of tamas: 'When the heart, which is the seat of consciousness is overpowered by tamas, sleep results' (*SS,* śarīra, 4, 30). It is distinguished from the dream state, which is dominated by rajas ('rajoyuktena manasā' *SS,* ibid., 35), and wakeful state, where sattva (viz. mind and sense-organs) prevails.

When the mind is fatigued, the organs of cognition and action are also fatigued; and they are withdrawn from their respective functions and become inactive; it is then that one sleeps (*CS,* sutra, 21, 35). Mind, in this state, is located in a place beyond the realm of sensory functions ('nir-indriya-sthāne', CHKP). The sensory faculties are dependent upon the mind; but the mind can be independent of the senses. Dream is when the mind continues to be active, independent of association with the sense-organs. In sleep, however, the mind is also inactive (klānta). [*See* SLEEP].

Normal Pursuits: The normal pursuits (eshaṇā) of a healthy individual are threefold: to live long (prāṇaishanā), to earn wealth as means of fulfilment of passions and desires (dhanaishaṇā), and to have a pleassant existence beyond (paralokaishaṇā). The instinctual urge of survival is the first; equally instinctual inclinations to enjoy pleasures of life and obtain emotional satisfactions are included in the second; and the religious predispositions in the third. (*CS,* sūtra, 11, 3-6).

Āyurveda is the science of the first of these pursuits which also is the foundation for the other two. The person must possess a mind which is not diseased (anupahata-sattva), intellect (buddhi), strength (paurusha) and courage (parākrama) in order to fulfil these pursuits (*CS,* ibid.).

Nyāya: An ancient system of thought, which developed the art and science of reasoning, in order to understand aright the reality, and to provide a consistent and effective method of such understanding. It is technically defined as "examination of reals by means of valid knowledge" ('pramaṇair arthaparīkshaṇam') (VĀCHASPATI). The system also discusses the nature and value of the means of knowledge (pramaṇa); hence called 'pramāṇa-śāstra'

The background of this system can be traced in the examination of sentences by sentences, to arrive at conclusions (vakovākya) in the *Chhāndogya-Upanishad*, inferential knowledge (anumana) in *Taittirıya-aranyaka*, logic (tarka) in the *Katha-Upanishad*, reasoning (yukti) in *Aitareya-brahmana* and discussions (vada) in *Ramayana*. It was a well recognized system even prior to the days of Pāṇini (300 B.C.), for the system as a method of logical reasoning has been mentioned by him (Ashṭādhyāyi, 3, 3, 122).

The immediate precursor of Nyāya was the science of critical study or scrutiny known as 'anvıkshikı', which has been described by Kauṭilya (about 327 B.C.) as "the light which illumines all sciences and which is the means for all activity" (*Artha-śāstra*, 1,2). It was one of the four necessary disciplines for an administrator, the other three being the three-fold Scripture (*trayı*), commerce and agriculture (*vārttā*), and polity (*danda-nıti*). Included in 'anvıkshikı' were the Sāmkhya, the Yoga, and the Lokayata systems. The sage DATTA-ATREYA is said to have taught this subject to disciples like ALARKA and PRAHLĀDA (*Bhagavata-purāṇa*, 1,3,12 and *Markaṇḍeya-purana*, 16, 12).

MANU was acquainted with 'anvīkshikı' as the "science of the soul" ('ātma-vidya', *Manu-Saṁhita*, 7,43), although he employs the expression only in the sense of 'the art of reasoning' ('hetuvidyā) or in that of discussion ('vādavidyā') (*Manu-Saṁhita*, 6,50; 8,269 etc.). Manu's attitude towards this subject was ambivalent. While he praises it (12,106; 7,43), he also condemns it as atheistic and anti-Vedic, and prescribes that the person who takes up this branch of learning should be excommunicated ('sādhubhih bahishkāryo nāstiko vedanindakah', 2,11). The epics also take the same attitude (for example, *Ramayaṇa,* Ayodhya, 100,36-39; *Mahābharata*, Śanti, 180, 47-49, and Ādi. 1,67).

It is suggested that the 'anvīkshikī' in its logical aspects evolved as the Nyāya system (*Nyāya-bhāshya,* 1,1,1 and VĀCHASPATI'S *Tātparya-ṭıkā* on it). The expression 'anvīkshikī' (*anu* + *ikshā*) signifies scrutiny of a subject-matter after it has been known by observation or testimony. It is the technique of determining the right meaning of an experience, or of ascertaining the true nature of a thing.

The earliest systematic treatise on the subject is the *Nyāya-sutra* ascribed to GOTAMA (-AKSHAPĀDA), whose date has been variously given by scholars (about 600 B.C., Gopīnāth Kavirāj; pre-Buddhist, but sūtra post-Māhāyāna, about second century A.D., H.P. Sastri; after Nagarjuna in second century A.D., A.B.Keith; between 200 and 500 B.C. H.Jacobi; about 300 A.D. Suali; post-Christian era, Garbe; between the middle of fourth century and second century B.C., Kuppuswāmi Śāstrī). While the tradition holds that GOTAMA and AKSHAPĀDA were names of the same person, Satīś Chandra Vidyābhūshaṇa argues that while GOTAMA, who was the author of the earlier part of the Sutra, lived about 550 B.C., AKSHAPĀDA, to whom the latter part may be ascribed, is assigned to about 150 A.D. (JRAS , 1918). GOTAMA (-AKSHAPĀDA) is identified with the Vedic seer who was born blind, DIRGHATAMAS.

Vaiseshika-sūtra appears to have been redacted earlier than the *Nyaya-sūtra* [*see* VAIŚESHIKA]. VĀTSYĀYANA, whose commentary (*Bhāshya*) on the *Nyāya-sutra* is the earliest treatise expounding the Nyāya System, was very well acquainted with the Vaiśeshika system. He was perhaps the first Nyāya thinker who attempted to incorporate Vaiseshika ideas. VĀTSYĀYANA's date too has been variously given: about 200 B.C., Windisch; second or third century B.C., Gopīnāth Kavirāj; beginning of fourth century A.D., H. Jacobi; middle of fourth century, Keith, Randle; middle of fifth century, S.C. Vidyābhūshana. The most probable date, however, is about A.D. 375. He was a realist, who defined the real as something apprehended by a pramāna. He was also a pragmatist who made successful activity the critical test of reasoning, and made valid knowledge the precondition for successful activity.

UDDYOTAKARA (about 500 A.D.) wrote a critical annotation on VĀTSYĀYANA'S *Bhāshya* called *Nyāya-vārttika,* where he defended the Nyāya position from the attacks of the Buddhist logician DIGNĀGA. He was mainly responsible for the amalgamation of the Vaiśeshika system with the Nyāya. VĀCHASPATI-MIŚRA (about A.D. 899), whose *Tātparya-tīkā* on the above defended UDDYOTAKARA against the attacks of the Buddhist DHARMAKĪRTI, was a great Nyāya writer. UDAYANA'S *Pariśuddhi* is a gloss on VĀCHASPATI'S work which was prepared around A.D. 984.

During the twelfth century GANGEŚA-UPÁDHYÁYA'S *Tattva-chintāmani* inaugurated a new development in the Nyāya school. While the old school ('prāchīna-nyāya'), which relied heavily on the works of GOTAMA, VĀTSYĀYANA and UDDYOTAKARA, was interested in philosophical issues like the nature of the soul, the value of dispassion, and salvation, the new school ('navya-nyāya') was interested in developing talent in debate, and skill in exposition.

Nyāya technically means what is right, viz. right judgement by means of syllogistic reasoning consisting of five steps: proposition (pratijñā), reason (hetu), explanatory example (udāharana), application (upanaya), and conclusion (nigamana). Reasoning is said to work neither with regard to things that are not known at all, nor with regard to things that are well ascertained, but with things that are doubtful ('saṁśayite'rthe'). According to VĀTSYĀYANA the procedure involves three steps: enumeration (uddeśa), definition (lakshana) and examination (parīkshā). The earliest example of syllogistic reasoning, called sthāpanā, however, occurs in CHARAKA'S *Saṁhitā* ('vimāna', chap. 8). Nyāya came to mean the critique of five topics: method (pramāna), object of knowledge (prameya), the art of discussion (vāda), syllogistic members (avayava) and examination of the prevalent philosophical systems (anya-mata-parīkshā).

The five topics were accommodated in sixteen categories (padārthas), the correct knowledge of which would help dissipate the ignorance which is the root-cause of all suffering. The goal that was held out in Nyāya was salvation (apavarga), or the absolute elimination of twenty-one varieties of suffering (pertaining to the six sense-organs, to the six sense-objects, to the six sense-experiences, to the physical body, to the bodily experiences of pleasure and pain).

Of the sixteen categories enumerated, objects of knowledge (prameya) and means of valid knowledge (pramāna) constitute the core of the philosophical system that Nyāya represents. They constitute the real issues, but an inquiry is impossible without the aid of the other fourteen categories. The third category is doubt (samśaya) which is the source of, and reason for, inquiry. The fourth is the purpose of such inquiry (prayojana), viz. salvation, or elimination of suffering. The remaining topics pertain only to the art of reasoning, employed in debates and discussions, illustrative instances which occasion inference (drshtānta), tenets or the viewpoints accepted by both parties involved in debate (siddhānta), syllogistic sequence (avayava), hypothetical reasoning to help the pramāna (tarka), ascertainment of truth by any recognised method (nirnaya), discussion involving arguments and counter-arguments (vāda), wrangling in order to defeat the opponent (jalpa), destructive criticism aimed at silencing the opponent (vitaṇḍā), deliberate fallacious reasoning (hetvābhāsa), quibbling and unfair arguments (chhala), far-fetched analogy in order to refute an argument (jāti), and points of the opponent's defeat (nigraha-sthana).

The entire group of topics, beginning with illustrative instances and ending with clinches (or points of defeat), appear to be relevant only in the situation of debates and discussions. But the implied purpose is to formulate one's own arguments without flaw. The topics aid the construction of a valid viewpoint. Ayurveda has adopted many of these topics. In fact, they figure early and prominently only in the Nyaya system and in the Indian medical school as crystallized in *CS*. CHARAKA, for instance, attaches importance to meaningful discussion (vada); and within the field of medicinal debates, the method known as 'saṁbhasha-vidhi' (arguments to supplement to discourse) has been explained by him. Charaka includes wrangling (jalpa), cavil (vitaṇḍā), rejoinder by far-fetched analogy (jati) and non-reason (ahetu, viz. hetvābhāsa) in the discussion. He is acquainted with syllogistic reasoning (avayava) as 'demonstration' (sthapana).

In CHARAKA'S work, some of the topics enumerated in the traditional Nyāya have been given without much modification (for example dṛshṭanta, prayojana and vitaṇḍā), while some others have been formulated differently (for example jalpa, and Chhala); and nigraha-sthana has altogether been omitted. More importantly, however CHARAKA'S work contains numerous logical categories which are not found in the Nyaya-sutra, like the pratishṭhāpanā, jijnasa, vyavasaya, vākya-dosha, vākya-praśaṁsā, upalaṁbha, parihāra and abhyanujna. The significance of these categories lies in the attempt to make clinical discussions meaningful, and academic criticisms creative.

In the category of 'object of knowledge' (prameya), Nyāya enumerates twelve topics, which comprehend physical, psychological and spiritual details. The self as the experiencer, is involved in the existential transactions which are productive of suffering; it is also capable of eliminating the mass of suffering. The body (śarīra) constitutes the physical ground on which the soul's experiences are structured; the five sense-organs (indriyas) are the physiological tools that the soul employs for structure-specific experiencing; and mind (manas), as an internal and structure-free organ, is general in its function, and is the medium through which meaningful experiences take place. There are real objects outside the individual , which provide the data for the individual's experiences. The transaction between the individual and the objects in the world which materializes as 'experience' (bhoga) is the subjective cognitive principle (buddhi). Such is the psycho-physiological constitution that encounters the physical world.

The remaining six topics pertain to individual behaviour, bodily, vocal and mental (pravṛtti), the motivations for such behaviour (dosha, approach, avoidance, and ignorance), existential continuity in successive births (pretyabhāva), the resultant experiences of pleasure and pain (phala), the conviction that all is misery (duhkha) and the final elimination of this misery (apavarga, salvation). The arrangement of these topics assumes a clinical framework: 'to-be-eliminated' (heya, viz. existential continuity, resultant experiences, and misery); the reason for the occurrence of this 'to-be-eliminated' (heya-hetu, viz. individual behaviour, and motivations thereof); 'to-be-pursued' ('upādeya, viz. the final elimination of misery); and the means by which the 'to-be-pursued' is accomplished (hetu, viz. correct knowledge of reality, 'tattva-jnana').

CHARAKA recognizes the category of 'the objects of knowledge' (prameya), but does not enumerate the twelve topics as above (which is the account in *Nyāya-sūtra*). It appears, as Dāsgupta suggests (HIP, vol.I.,p.302), that CHARAKA was not acquainted with the *Nyāya-sūtra*; it is likely that when CHARAKA wrote his work, the *Nyāya-sūtra* had not been compiled, or redacted, as yet. It is also probable that both CHARAKA and the *Nyāya-sūtra* relied for their enumeration and description of categories on an earlier Nyaya text, which it is now difficult to identify. Dāsgupta also suggests that CHARAKA'S account is an earlier version than the *Nyāya-sūtra*. For CHARAKA, the theory of the soul is an aspect of the general issue of 'anvīkshikī'. The soul (which is the seat of desires, volitions, cognitions, and experiences of pleasure and pain) and the body (which is the locus of behaviour, sense-organs and mental processes) are alike substances that are inferred from their 'marks' (liṅgas).

The means of valid knowledge (pramāṇa) is an important issue in the Nyāya system. It is looked upon not only as the special source of the correct knowledge of a thing (arthopalabdhihetu), but as a precondition for successful activity (saphalapravrtti). Correct knowledge leading to the elimination of wrong knowledge, which in turn leads to the cessation of misery is discussed in detail in the Nyāya treatises, with regard to its nature, causation, and involvements. The Nyāya writers accept four instruments of correct knowledge: observation (pratyaksha, viz. employment of sense-organs and mind), inference (anumāna, based on observation), analogical reasoning (upamāna), and testimony of a reliable person (śabda).

In the last group is included not only the Veda, but testimony from any trustworthy person; a sage (rshi), a refined insider (ārya), or an alien person who is reliable (mléccha) (VĀTSYĀYANA). This forms the fundamental methodological position of Indian medicine. CHARAKA discusses this problem in his *Samhitā* (*CS*, sūtra 1,35-38). While he accepts the four-fold pramāna of the traditional Nyāya thought, he employs expressions like 'examination' (parīkshā), and 'rational inquiry into causation' (hetu-pramāna). And he provides testimony a wider context. It includes instructions of a well-meaning expert (āptopadeśa), word of authority (śabda), and traditionally communicated wisdom (aitihya). He does not appear to have known the subdivisions of inference that became popular in the Nyāya thought but ignored in the Vaiśeshika school (pūrva-vat, śesha-vat and sāmānyato-dṛshta). He uses a variant expression for analogical reasoning: aupamya, instead of the upamāna of the Nyāya-sūtra.

The philosophical position of the Nyāya is described as ontological realism and pragmatic pluralism. The categories it enumerates are taken directly from common human experience. In consonance with the general Indian outlook, empirical existence is looked upon as an invariable source of misery, and the living being as having an irrepressible urge for happiness. The desire for happiness, however, is rarely fulfilled, thus occasioning disappointment, frustration and misery. The mistaken notion (mithyā-jñāna) that the body-sense-mind complex is the soul which experiences pleasure and pain is postulated as the material cause for craving (trshnā) for survival, resulting in the succession of births. The break in this continuity, viz. the absence of rebirth, is salvation (apavarga). It also means the absolute and final cessation of all misery that is incidental to existence. The salvation that thus results from the elimination of mistaken notion (mithyā-jñāna) is a condition that is similar to deep sleep, where there is neither pleasure nor pain. [*See also* NYĀYA-VAIŚESHIKA, VAIŚESHIKA, PRAMĀNA, ĀTMAN]

Nyāya-Vaiśeshika: Nyāya and Vaiśeshika were originally two distinct systems, which developed independently till about the early centuries after Christ. While we cannot be certain when exactly the two systems coalesced or became syncretic, we find that the great Nyāya writer of the fourth century, VATSYAYANA minimized the gulf between them. UDDYOTAKARA (about A.D. 500) introduced the typically Vaiśeshika concepts into the Nyāya framework. By about the twelfth century, the Vaiśeshika treatises were employing extensively the Nyāya technicalities (for example, VARADA-RĀJA'S TARKIKA-RAKSHA, 1150, VALLABHA'S NYAYA LILAVATI, twelfth century, KEŚAVA-MIŚRA'S TARKA-BHASHA, 1275).

The two systems were greatly similar in form as well as content, and are therefore described as 'samana-tantra'; they could easily be amalgamated into a common approach. The integrated system came to be known as 'Tārkika-darsana', underlining the predominantly rational spirit of inquiry and analysis. 'Tarka' is reason (yukti), logic, inference (anumāna). However, the two systems are alike oriented towards salvation (moksha, interpreted as total cessation of bodily association and existential pain, called 'nihsreyasa' in Vaiśeshika and 'apavarga' in Nyaya). Right knowledge is held by both systems as the means for the achievement of this ideal. And the formulation of epistemological problems and the discussion of pramāṇa have been undertaken in the context of right knowledge; that ignorance is the root cause of existential pain is the basic assumption in the two systems.

The two systems agree on the essential framework, and on several issues, opposed to the Mımaṁsa views (such as the self-validity of the Scriptures, belief in God as creator, eternality of sound, and immediate perception of the Self in the ego). However, they differ among themselves in details, as for instance the number of pramāṇas (four according to Nyāya, and two according to Vaiśeshika) and the enumeration of categories (sixteen according to Nyāya, and seven according to Vaiśeshika) covering the whole of reality. The idea of pramāṇa, which figures prominently in the Nyāya system, is included in the Vaiśeshika category of 'quality' (guṇa).

While the two systems are thus closely allied, there is a difference in emphasis. The Nyāya system is concerned mainly with methodological and epistemological problems, and hence styled as 'pramāṇa-śāstra' (the science of how we know). The Vaiśeshika, on the other hand, is more concerned with the categories of reals, the contents of knowledge; hence called 'prameya-sastra' (the science of what we know). We find that the Nyaya system does not discuss the Vaiśeshika categories of substance, quality, activity, particularity and generality.

The Nyāya-Vaiśeshika approach takes a hard common-sense view of reality, and rejects both the Buddhist idea of evanescence and the Sāṁkhya theory of Cosmology. Unlike the Sāṁkhya, this approach accepted time as a real, substantial and meta-human dimension as also space in a relative context. It assumed the atomic doctrine of four primary elements (bhuta, earth, water, fire, and air) with eternal and all pervading akasa as the fifth substance. The soul (atma) too was looked upon as a substance, all pervading but distinct for each body. Mind (manas) is atomic in size, and is the vehicle of memory. Its function is to connect the soul with the senses.

The approach is thus pluralistic. And no attempt was made to reduce the multiplicity that is evident in experience to any hypothetical unitary principle. The syncretic viewpoint emphasized the role of reason in understanding reality, but reason was not allowed to interfere with the data gathered from direct experience. Abstractions of logical categories and coherence in arguments (made much of in the Nyāya) were not pressed towards the dismissal of the main categories of experience (enumerated in the Vaiśeshika).

There arose in due course points of difference between the two systems (such as the idea of number, application of atomic theory, qualitative changes in heat, the apprehension of non-existence, and the concept of salvation), but they appear to be mainly matters of interpretation. The two systems became inseparably linked, especially in the minds of the advocates of the other systems of thought in India.

Āyurveda relies heavily on the Nyaya methodology as well as the Vaiśeshika categories, although when the early treatises on Āyurveda came to be written, the two systems do not appear to have become as yet hyphenated. [*See also* NYĀYA, VAIŚESHIKA, PRAMĀNA].

O

Ojas: The essential product of all the seven body constituents (dhatu), especially of the seventh, viz semen (śukra), is called ojas (from vaj, 'bodily strength', 'ability', 'vital power'). It pervades the entire body, although its principal seat is the heart (hṛt): its flow starts from the heart and permeates every minute subdivision of the system.

Its function is to endow the physical system with warmth and help in all the activities. Efficient functioning of the sense-organs, formation and growth of flesh, physical strength and nourishment are all due to this factor. Its normal quantity in the human body is eight 'drops' (bindu). Decrease in ojas (due to such causes as physical injury, wasting diseases, emotional stresses like anxiety and fear, fatigue and hunger) leads to shortening of life and death (*SS*, śarıra, 15, 18-27).

It is white in colour, with a touch of red and yellow (because its nature comprises 'fire', agni and 'moon', soma). It is of the nature of kapha. Its prevailing properties are: soft, cool, tranquil and mobile. [*See also* VITALITY].

Ojas: The word means vigor, vitality or bodily strength (from vaj 'to increase', 'to be able'). It is the principal factor responsible for the effective functioning of the body and the sense-organs, and is described as the final emergent of the metabolic processes that occur in the seven body-constituents (dhātu). [*See* VITALITY].

Organs: Called indriyas, they are faculties or abilities which help in individual survival and transaction with the world outside. They are grouped into two types: organs of cognition (jñānendriya, sense-organs, five in number, meant for vision, audition, gustation, olfaction and touch) and organs of action (karmendriya, five in number for locomotion, prehension, speech, elimination of waste, and procreation). [*See* SENSE-ORGANS].

Oshadhi: Any medicinal herb, especially the soma-plant, in the Vedic literature; the later employment of this expression was with regard to the annual plants or herbs [*See* PLANTS].

P

Padartha: Literally anything that can be denoted by words (abhidhevatva), but more usually, object or thing that can be cognized, and also expressed in language. The constituent word 'artha' in the expression 'padā-artha' ("word-object") is explained as 'that object towards which the sense-organs move ('rechati indriyāṇi yaṁ prati'). Such an object may be concrete (viz. apprehended by the five external sense-organs), or abstract (viz. apprehended by the internal organ, mind). The other constituent word 'pada' means whatever could be predicated or represented in a symbol (saṅketa). In this sense, 'padārtha' is the object of valid knowledge ('pramitivishaya'). In a broader sense, it means the 'categories' of reality.

Most of the Indian schools of thought accept as an axiom the independent reality of such knowable and nameable categories. Vedānta accepts but two categories: ātman and non-ātman. Vaiśeshikas postulate six positive categories and a negative category [*See* VAIŚESHIKA] and the Nyāya school has sixteen categories in the sense of topics [*See* NYĀYA]. The Sāṁkhya school enumerates twenty-five categories [*See* SĀṀKHYA], physical, psychophysical and psychological; and the Yoga system adds iśvara to this list.

Āyurveda accepts the Vaiśeshika position with regard to categories in a general way, but adopts the categories to its own practical framework. While Suśruta does not refer to the Vaiśeshika background, CHARAKA begins his work with an enumeration of categories that obviously reminds us of the Vaiśeshika account; in fact, his commentator, CHAKRAPĀṆI, actually relates CHARAKAŚ ideas to the *Vaiśeshika-sūtra.*

The Vaiśeshika school is pluralistic, with no interest in any hypothetical unitary principle. It postulates that all things in the universe are ultimately reducible to atoms (paramāṇus), which are eternal (nitya), and irreducible (niravayava). These atoms, however, are discrete, and occur in several final categories (padārtha). Betwixt these atoms is a peculiar separating 'substance', called particularity (viśesha), the emphasis on which has given the school its name.

Substances (dravya) have a two-fold attribution (dharma), constant and fleeting. The constant attributes are called 'qualities' (guṇa) and the fleeting ones constitute 'action' (karma). Qualities are of 24 kinds, and actions of five varieties [*See* VAIŚESHIKA]. In actual life-experience, qualities and actions are perceived as different in nature; and therefore, they are taken as distinct categories. Things occur in the world in their generality (sāmānya), so that the concept of a class or species is justified; things appear to belong to different groups, and within each group, the members share common characteristics. Things are also distinct from each other, and despite generality, two things do not merge into each other. The particularity or individuality (viśesha) is also a fact of life. Finally, things and their qualities, or things and their classes, do not exist apart from each other; they are related in a constant, intimate and inseparable inherence (samavāya).

These are the six categories recognized in the Vaiśeshika school: substance, quality, action, generality, individuality and inseparable inherence. To these, a seventh category a negative one, viz. non-existence (abhāva), was added during the later history of the school [*See* VAIŚESHIKA]. CHARAKA'S enumeration of the categories begins with generality (samānya) and the particular (viśesha) qualities, and goes on to the substance (dravya), qualities (guṇa), action (karma), and inseparable inherence (samavāya). Neither the usual Vaiśeshika order of categories is followed, nor are the usual explanations for categories given in the Vaiśeshika texts reproduced in *CS* (sūtra, 1, 48 ff). CHARAKA'S account bears a distinct stamp of its own, although generally following the Vaiśeshika outlook. Relevance in the clinical context is never lost sight of.

The twin concepts of 'generality' (samānya) and 'particularity' (viśesha) constitute the rationale of dietetical prescriptions and the pharmacological action of the herbs. The need to reduce a pathogenic factor is fulfilled by appropriate articles of food or medicine, which increase or accentuate the contrary factor. The two expressions 'samānya' and 'viśesha' are not used in the usual Vaiśeshika sense of 'class concept' and 'specific differentiating properties'. A new interpretation has been given for them. The fact of generality among the characteristics or constituents of substances (food or drug and the body condition) tends to increase or accentuate (vṛddhi) those characteristics, at the cost of others. The underlying principle is that of 'common direction' (tulyārthaṭā), with an urge towards unification (ekatvakara). Particularity, on the other hand, has dissimilar characteristics, and therefore diminishes (hrāsa), weakens and separates (pṛthaktvakṛt). The physician's choice of a drug should naturally be guided by these considerations. [*See* PHARMACY].

Substances (dravya) are important inasmuch as they support qualities (guṇas); and qualities figure prominently in the Āyurvedic context. The five elements (khādīni, earth, water, fire, air and ākāśa), self (ātmā), mind (manas), time (kāla), and space (dik) are listed under the category of substance. The quality that is especially important to the physician is that of intimate and mutual association (saṁyoga) between mind (sattva), soul (ātmā) and body (śarīra): it is likened to a tripod, and the entire transactional world is said to be founded on it (*CS*, ibid., 46) [*See* MIND, ĀTMAN].

CHARAKAŚ account of qualities (guṇa) utilizes most of the details of the Vaiśeshika enumeration of 24 qualities [*See* VAIŚESHIKA], but follows an independent line of thinking with regard to their descriptions and grouping. He includes sensible qualities (sensory details), physical or objective qualities ('heaviness etc') without mentioning the other qualities in the group, intelligence (buddhi) without, however, explaining it, qualities beginning with para (explained in CHARAKA as referring to superiority, by virtue of the country, climate, age, time, measure, potency, taste, maturation etc) and ending with prayatna (effort). It is likely that CHARAKA had before him different accounts of the Vaiśeshika categories, for his enumeration does not tally with the standard Vaiśeshika list that has come down to us.

The explanations of the categories given by CHARAKA are also characteristically different. 'Effort' (prayatna) for instance, is defined by CHARAKA as that which, when occurring, would move the mind to activity. 'Reason' (yukti) is a new quality mentioned by CHARAKA, explained as the care with which a medicine is properly selected and prepared with reference to the disease ('doshādyapekshayā bheshajasya samīchīna-kalpanā') (cf. *CS*,sūtra,26, 27-29).

'Action' (karma) as a category is defined as the movement which is of the nature of deliberate effort ('prayatnādi cheshṭitam'; the commentary explains that the sense in which 'ādi' is used is 'of the nature of' 'adi-śabdhah prakāra-vāchī, 1,1,48). Inseparable inherence,(samavāya) is explained as permanent (as the Vaiśeshaka account explains), but dominant or recessive in specific instances (cf. *HIP*, vol II, pp.366-373).

Pañchabhūta Theory of: Basic to Indian medicine is the assumption of the fundamental unity of man and nature: "whatever occurs in the material world (loke) also occurs in man (purushe), and whatever is in man is also in the world. The wise would employ this attitude" (*CS*, 4, 4, 13). That matter in its five primary forms (pañchabhūta) is the stuff of which the world is made, is the Nyāya-Vaiśeshika doctrine, which Indian medicine has adopted. Man, who is the special frame of reference in Indian medicine, is but a special organization of matter. "In medicine, our inquiry does not go beyond matter" (*SS*, śarīra, 14). The human body (śarīra), causes of diseases (hetu), diseases themselves (vyādhi), and treatment of diseases (chikitsā) are all within the scope of matter in its five forms.

Indian medicine not only assumes that everything in the world (including man) is matter, but holds that the five primary forms of matter are related to each other (paras-parasamsarga), that they depend upon each other (p-anugrahana), and that they penetrate into each other (p-anupraveśa), (*SS*, sūtra,42, 3). This explains the infinite diversity as well as the dynamic character that we find in the world. This applies to diseases also, and to the treatment procedures.

The five primary forms of matter are: earth (prthvī), water (ap), fire (agni or tejas), air (vāyu) and space or emptiness (ākāśa). However, no form of matter occurs in its pure or isolated state: all things in the world contain all the five forms, but in varying proportions, relations, dependences, and combinations. The Nyāya-Vaiśeshika distinguishes between the unmanifest and isolate conditions of the primary forms (tanmātras) and the manifest and complex condition (mahābhūtas). But CHARAKA does not mention the former condition; and it is not relevant in the practical context. If a thing ('substance' dravya) contains the earth form predominantly, it is known as 'earthy' (pārthiva), if water, 'watery' (āpya), if fire, 'fiery' (taijasa or āgneya), if air, 'airy' (vāyavya), and if ākāśa, ākāśiya or nābhasa. Each of these is characterized by a dominant or special quality (guna): earthy by smell (gandha), watery by taste (rasa), fiery by colour or shape (rūpa), airy by touch (sparśa), and ākāśiya by sound (śabda).

In general, all solid and concrete things are described as earthy, all liquids as watery, all shapes and colours are fiery, all activities are airy, and all intervals and empty space as ākāśīya. In addition to the special qualities mentioned above, each of the five primary forms has characteristics or qualities that characterize it. The earthy substances are rough (khara), hard (kaṭhiṇa), slow (manda), stable (sthira), and clear (viśada). The watery substances are unctuous (snigdha), cold (śīta), slow, soft (mrdu) and slimy (picchila). The fiery substances are hot (ushṇa), acute (tīkshna), subtle (sūkshma), light (laghu), dry (rūksha), and clear. The airy substances are light, cold, dry, rough, clear and subtle. The ākāśīya substances are soft, subtle, light, smooth (slakshṇa), and separating (vivikta).

The five primary forms are also associated with the gunas that make them what they are. The earthy substances are dominated by tamas [*See* GUNA], the watery substances by sattva and tamas, the fiery by sattva and rajas, the airy by rajas, and the ākāśiya by sattva.

The human body is made up of the same five primary forms of matter, and is produced by the three gunas; the three gunas support the body like three pillars (*SS*, sūtra,21). The earthy element in the body is illustrated by whatever is solid, gross, rough, heavy, firm and hard (for example, bones, teeth, nails, flesh, skin, faeces, hair, and tendons). The watery element is illustrated by whatever is liquid, unctuous, mobile, slow, soft and viscid (blood, fat, mucus, bile, urine, sweat and vital sap, rasa). The fiery element is illustrated by whatever has warmth, lustre, radiance and colour (digestive process, bile, etc.). The airy element is illustrated by whatever is dry, clear and light, and whatever makes for mobility (inhalation, exhalation, batting the eyes, contraction, expansion, movement, prehension, impulsion). The ākāśīya element is illustrated by whatever is soft, porous, light and productive of sound; channels in the body also represent this element.

The sense-organs likewise are products of the combinations of the five primary forms of matter, and each organ of sense represents the predominance of one of the forms: the earth element makes for odour in the world, and the olfactory sense in body; the water element makes for taste and the gustatory sense; the fire element makes for colour and the visual sense; the air element makes for touch and the cutaneous sense; and the ākāśa element for sound and the auditory sense.

The concept of attributes specific to the five primary forms is important. Ākāśa, subtlest of the forms, is equipped only with sound. Air has two—sound and touch. Fire has three—sound, touch, and colour. Water has four—sound, touch, colour, and taste. Earth has five—sound, touch, colour, taste, and smell. The ultimate (viz. irreducible) form of matter called tanmātra (bare presence), has only these attributes, although in an unmanifested manner. The combinations, inter-penetrations, and relatedness of these primary forms result in the gross forms of matter that we call substances (dravya), ranging from the invisible sky to solid earth in the world outside, and from the pores in the body to the muscle-tissues in the human body. The objects of the world available to the organs of sense as well as the organs themselves are looked upon as substances, dominated by one or the other of the five forms.

The equipment of the organs of sense renders their possessor 'conscious'; and their absence is characteristic of inert matter ('sendriyam chetanam dravyam; nir-indriyam achetanam', *CS,* sūtra,1,48). Consciousness is thus material in its context as well as content; it is a physical substance (dravya), a category of matter. It needs to be mentioned that CHARAKA departs from the general Sāmkhyan position (which holds that the organs of sense emerge from egoity) by considering the organs as direct modifications of the five primary forms of matter.

The five primary forms, which are manifest, are the bricks out of which the bodily constituents as well as the propensities are built. Among the basic body tissues (dhātu), the earth element is in the muscle tissues (māṁsa); the water element in chyle (or plasma, rasa) lymph and other fluids, fat tissue (medas), bone marrow (majjā) and sperm-ovum (śukra-rajas); the fire element in red blood corpuscles (rakta); the air element in bone tissue (asthi); and ākāśa is present throughout the body, especially in the pores inside the body. Thus the peculiar modifications of the five primary forms of matter called 'dhātus' cooperate, mutually contribute and supplement the actions of each other, and thus sustain the body. When these conglomerations (samudāya) are in proper proportion, and effective in their beneficial interaction (samayogavāhi), health is the result. When, however, their normal measure is disturbed and their interaction becomes troublesome we call that condition 'disease'.

The tripartite categorization of propensities (dosha) also is in accordance with the five forms of matter: earth and water elements predominantly contribute the kapha, fire makes for pitta, air and ākāśa for vāta. The waste products of the body (mala), which are principally threefold (urine, faeces and sweat), and which need to be eliminated regularly are also composed of the five primary forms of matter. [*See* DHĀTU, DOSHA, MALA].

Thus the balance of these five forms as dhātu, dosha, and mala renders the body efficient, and sustains it against odds. We call this health. Any disturbance in this equillibrium is disease, which, if left uncorrected, would lead the body to decay and death. The correcting drug, food or regimen too must be composed of the five forms of matter. The selection of a drug, or prescription of a regimen, is made with a view to restore the balance of the five forms. The skill of the physician and the success of the treatment consists in understanding which of the five forms has gone errant, how, and why.

Drugs, therefore, are classified according to the preponderance of one or the other of the five primary forms. Drugs by their attributes and actions counteract the deficiency or excess of the attributes and actions of the five forms of matter present in the body. In order to facilitate the proper selection of the drug, drugs are also classified in terms of the tastes (rasa), characteristic of the five forms: sweet in substances which are predominantly composed of earth and water; sour in water and fire, saline in earth and fire; pungent in air and fire; bitter in air and ākāśa; and astringent in air and earth. [*See* TASTE]. Likewise, the attributes (guṇa), potency (vīrya), and the taste that results after digestion (vipāka) also determine the drug that is appropriate. Drug action should facilitate readjustment of the material constituents within the body [*See* DRUGS].

Food which produces and sustains the body is also composed of the five primary forms of matter. Digestion is the process by which the five forms present in the food are adequately transformed into their counterparts (viz. the dhātus) in the body. Even as the physical fire cooks the food, the digestive fire converts the consumed food into vital sap (rasa), which is essential for health and survival [*See* FOOD]. Each of the five constituents of the physical body (earth, water, etc.) is regarded as fire in its own right to cook the corresponding physical form in the food that is eaten (*CS*, 6,15,13).

Pāpmā: Literally disease, originating in sin or wickedness (pāpa). But the notion of sin here involves the transgression of the normal laws of health and hygiene, which interferes with the performance of prescribed duties and precludes effective assumption of the social role. Indian medical texts as well as religious manuals insist that preservation of health is a duty (dharma) of all citizens; and that to fall ill is a transgression, a sin (adharma). However, the expression is employed for disease in general [*See* DISEASE].

Parīkshā: [*See* EXAMINATION]

Paste: Called kalka (also prakshépa or avāpa; nugdha in Yunāni), it is a medicinal preparation made by soaking in water selected fresh or dried parts of plants and grinding them on a stone (dṛshadī) with a muller so that a thin paste, leviated powder or wet mass (piṇḍo rasa-pishṭānām) is got for administration. In this preparation, the active substances in the drug as well as the other parts of the plant (like stem) enter, and therefore this form of decoction is regarded as lighter than the expressed juice (sva-rasa), where only the active ingredients of the drug are involved.

In case honey, ghee or oil is added while being administered, the proportion should be two parts of this substance to one part of the paste; if sugar or jaggery is to be added, the proportion must be equal to that of the paste; and if any other fluid is to be added, it must be four times.

The dosage is one karsha (tola) if the drugs involved are mild in potency, half a karsha if the potency is medium, and one quarter of a karsha if the potency is intense. When during administration ghee, oil or honey is added, the dosage of the paste is to be doubled. [*See* PREPARATIONS]

Peśi: Peśī (from *piś*, 'to give form') are structures that provide form and contour to the muscles, that are responsible for all muscular activity (with their ability to contract and expand), and are the source of physical strength of the body. Although translated usually as muscle', the peśī is different from the body constituent known as 'māṁsa': it is brought into being by the latter and is a secondary body-constituent (upa-dhātu), it does not participate in the production of the 'muscle-fat' (medas).

The peśīs constitute half the weight of the

body. They number 500; 400 in the extremities, 66 (60 according to GAYADĀSA) in the trunk, and 34 (40 according to GAYADĀSA) in the region above the clavicle. Women have 20 extra peśīs, 10 in the two breasts (five in each), reaching their full growth during puberty, four along the parturient passage (two about the external orifice of the vagina, and two in the internal orifice), three about the region of the Os (garbha-chhidra), and three along the passages of sperm and ovum.

The peśī covers up and thus protects, supports, gives strength to the joints, ligaments (snāyu), and veins (sirā). It is kept soft, and is nourished by the lasika-secretion (called 'muscle-juice') from the network of veins (sirā) and arteries (dhamanī). On death, this secretion solidifies, and then the peśīs become rigid and get contracted (rigor mortis); and decomposition of the body begins.

The peśīs contain also the channels of awareness (saṁjñā-vaha-nāḍī); and as the muscles contract and expand the faculty of this sensation is stimulated. This is different from the faculty of touch-perception in the skin, inasmuch as the former provides the knowledge of such details as weight etc. [*See* BODY).

Pharmacology: Man's knowledge of the medicinal properties of substances, especially plants, is of hoary antiquity. In India, even the Vedic literature contains a fairly extensive pharmacopoeia. There is also a suggestion that man discovered the medicinal properties of plants by observing the behaviour of wild animals and birds in disease (*AV*,8,7,23-25). Even *CS* concedes the knowledge of pharmacognosy on the part of primitive hunters, cowherds and denizens of forests. But classification of drugs, identification of their properties, and preparation of medicines were achievements of Āyurveda as a scientific approach to man's health and ailments.

Even in the course of the Vedic literature, we find that many of the drugs unknown to the poets of *ṚV*, were known to the compilers of *AV*, like apāmārga (*Achyranthes aspera*), alābu (*Lageneria vulgaris*), jāṅgiḍa (*Terminalia arjuna?*), kāśa (*Saccharum spontaneum*), māsha (*Phaseolus mungo)*, rohiṇī (*Soymida febrifuga*), Śīrsha-parṇī or śirīsha (*Albizzia lebbeck*) and Yashṭi-madhu (*Glycyrrhiza glabra*). Many of the plants known to the *RV* poets had to wait for *AV* to discover their medicinal properties, like śamī *(Prosopis spicigera*), śigru (*Moringa pterygosperma*), trāyamāṇa (*Gentiana kurroo*) and ulapa (*Imperata arundinacea*).

Many of the substances (plants as well as natural objects) mentioned in the Vedic literature were later used as drugs, when their medicinal value was understood. Datūra (*Datura metel*), for instance, was known from early times as one of the organic poisons. But it has not been noticed in *CS* at all, and *SS* mentions it briefly, the oil extracted from its seeds being useful for external application as well as internal use (as alarka-visha). *AHṛ*, however, prescribes the expressed juice (svarasa) of the leaves of datūra, and *RRS* illustrates its extensive use in diverse disorders like fever, tuberculosis, sprue syndrome, and colic pain; RĀJA-MĀRTANDA prescribes it for snake-bite, and CHAKRADATTA for insanity. There is also an interesting use of this poison to counteract the toxic effects produced by the ingestion of the same poison. *DN, SN* and *RN* are acquainted with the excellent curative properties of datūra. Likewise tuvaraka (*Hydnocarpus wightiana*), which was unknown to *CS*, has been highly praised in *SS* as a specific for skin diseases and urinary troubles. *GN* gives pharmaceutical details of this drug.

When medicine developed not only as an art but more as a science, the number of drugs naturally increased, and their properties ascertained by empirical observation of drugs (like taste, rasa), clinical observation of their action on the constitution (like changes in the system, vipāka), inference (like potency, vīrya), and logical assumptions (like systematic effect, prabhāva). The nature of the drugs and the responses of the body to them were carefully correlated, and an elaborate materia medica was evolved early in the history of Indian medicine. Early compilations like *CS* and *SS* themselves suggest the existence of such lists of drugs.

The early materia medica was little more than pharmacopoeia of synonyms. It was only later that descriptive pharmacology emerged. Works belonging to this type not only listed the synonyms of drugs (like *PRM*) but produced information about the drug, drug-properties (guṇa) and drug-action (karma) (like *DN*). Classification of drugs on various bases became an important feature. The early *DN* has a simple classification of drugs into herbs, trees, fruits, flowers and metals. *SN*, however, grouped the drugs into 27 groups (including the previous groups, and adding drinks, milk and its products, oils, sugar-cane, honey, fermented liquor, cereals, preparations of food, meat, urine etc.). There were also pharmacological works (like *ŚM*) which classified drugs on the basis of the physiological principle of dosha.

India has been in contact with its neighbouring countries since the earliest periods of recorded history. India's association with Assyria, Babylon, Egypt, Persia, Central Asia, Africa and China made Indian pharmacopoeia rich and varied. Many drugs not indigenous to India have been in use in India for thousands of years; many of them were grown here, and some imported. During the middle ages, contact with Turkisthan, Afghanistan and Europe enlarged the Indian materia medica. Besides the drugs of plant origin, many metals and animal products came to be included. Historical pharmacology would reveal the fact that many of the drugs currently used extensively in Indian medicine were not all indigenous; they arrived on the Indian soil at ascertainable periods.

Madhu-yashṭi (*Glycyrrhiza glabra*), is among the drugs of foreign origin that were accepted by physicians in India even during the days of *CS* and *SS*. Native to South Europe, Asia Minor, Persia and Turkey, it was imported to India, and hence known as 'klītaka'. Vatsanābha (*Aconitum chasmanthum*), another drug not known in ancient India, is counted by DṚḌHABALA, the redactor of *CS*, among the plant poisons; *AS* prescribes it as an important drug to counteract poison; it was made much of in the tāntrik cults and alchemy. *RRS* has an elaborate section on poisonous drugs employed to fight poison. Vijayā (*Cannabis sativa*), known popularly as bhaṅga, was probably of Chinese origin. Even in *PRM*, the expression Vijayā has been used to signify harītakī (*Terminalia chebula*). It is in *SN* that we find bhaṅga being prescribed as a drug for the first time. Likewise, in *GN* of the same author (SOḌHALA) we find the earliest reference to opium (*Papaver somniferum*), which perhaps was native to China. It came to India via Arabia; the Indian word for it, ahiphena, is merely the Sanskritized form of the Arabic word aphyum; *DN* knows it as aphūka. Kumāri (*aloe*), which is not to be found in *CS* or *SS*, is mentioned for the first time in *AN*, and later in BHOJA'S *Rāja-mārtaṇḍa*. It was native to the African islands, especially near Kenya, and hence known as Kanāri, from which 'Kumāri' was coined. Its use in the two works mentioned is limited to external application. But *GN*, a later work, recommends its internal use as Kumāryāsava. Pārasika-yavānī (*Hyoscyamus niger*, called Khurāsānī-ajwān) entered the Indian materia medica during the ninth century owing to contact with Arab merchants. It was grown in Europe and Central Asia. *DN* calls it *yavānī-viśesha;* and *Vṛnda-mādhava* (which makes the first reference to it) prescribes it as a anthelmintic. Chopa-chīnī (*Smilax china*) which was native to China and Japan, came to India during the sixteenth century; known here as dvīpāntara-vachā, it was prescribed to fight syphilis (phiraṅgāmayanāśanī), which disease itself was brought to India by the Portuguese adventurers. Sindūri (*Bixa orellana*) was a plant native to America, but has been known to *MV, RN* and *BPN*. Isabgol (*Plantago ovata*) is a Persian plant, used extensively in Yunāni medicine; it has found its way into the Āyurveda materia medica as īshadgola (*SN*). Tamākhu (tobacco, *Nicotiana tabacum*), originally grown in Central and Southern America and later cultivated in France and Spain, was brought to India by the Portugese in the sixteenth century. Its first mention as a drug is to be found in *Yogaratnākara* (seventeenth century).

Many of the names of the indigenous drugs listed in the nighaṇṭus are of Vedic origin; quite a number of them are of folk origin. As new drugs were incorporated into our materia medica their native names were accepted in their Sanskritized forms (like ahiphena for aphyūm, tamākhu for tobacco, kumāri for Kanāri, Kuliṅjana for Khalaṅjan, pūga for poka, isabagola for aspagol); or new names given, like jayapāla for *Croton tiglium*, ākarakara (or ākarakarabha in *BP*) for *Anacyclus pyrethrum*, madhu-yashti *for Glycyrrhiza glabra*, Vatsa-nābha for *Aconitum chasmanthum*, rāmaṭha for *Ferula foetida* (hiṅg). The names of many drugs leave no doubt about their foreign origin, for example, pārasika-yavāni (*Hyoscyamus niger*), khurāsāni-yavānī (*Trachyspermum ammi*), dvīpāntara-vachā (*Smilax china*), turushka (*Styrax officinale*), Barbari (*Ocimum basilicum*) and revanda-chīnī (*Rheum emodi*).

Some drugs have been named after the animals and birds which suggested to man the medicinal properties of those plants, like vārāha (*Tacca aspera*), nākulī (*Aristolochia indica*), sarpa-gandha (*Rauwolfia serpentina*), kāka-māchī (*Solanum nigrum*) and aja-śṛṅgī (*Gynandropsis pentaphylla*). Some others have got their names owing to their appearance, like aṇu (*Panicum miliaceaum*), sahasra-chakshu or vishāṅka (*Saussurea*), punarnava (*Boerhaavia diffusa*) and nitatnī (*Solanum nigrum*, also called Kākamāchī). Some names are descriptive of the parts of the plant, like maṇḍūka-parṇī (*Centella asiatica*), mayūra-śikhā (*Elephantopus scaber*), śara-puṅkha (or tushṭa, *Tephrosia purpurea*), nāga-kesara (*Mesua ferrea*), Chitra-parṇī (*Uraria picta*) and uttāna-parṇa (*Cissampelos pariera*). Some again are named after their colour (like arjuna, *Terminalia arjuna*, pīta-dāru, *Berberis aristata*, and pāṭalī, *Schrebera swietenioides*), taste (like madhuka, *Glycyrrhiza glabra*, lavaṇī, *Cicca acida* and amlika, *Tamarindus indica*), and smell (like aśvagandhā, *Withania somnifera*, and sugandhikā, *Zanthoxylum alatum*). And many plants are named after the drug-action they are capable of, like atibalā (*Abutilon indicum*), kāraskara (*Strychnos nux vomica*), jīvantī (*Leptadenia reticulata*), rohiṇī (*Soymida febrifuga*), takma-nāśana (or kushṭha, *Saussurea lappa*), dhātrī (*Emblica officinalis*) and ugraushadhī (*Imperata cylindrica*, darbha).

Indian pharmacology deals with medicines prepared from three classes of substances: (1) of plant origin (audbhida), (2) of animal origin (jaṅgama), and (3) obtained from earth (that is, minerals and metals, prthivījanya). Medicines from plants constitute the major portion of any Indian materia medica [*See* DRUG]. The use of animal products is extremely limited in Āyurveda, although pharmacopoeia do contain numerous prescriptions. However, milk and urine are extensively used. Honey plays an important role in Āyurveda. [*See* HONEY, MILK, URINE.] The employment of minerals is likewise limited. The Siddha system of medicine as well as the Rasa-school of therapeutics are distinguished by a fairly extensive use of minerals (like mercury which is called rasa, and metallic ores or uparasas, for example, sulphur, mica, iron, pyrites, arsenic, orpiment, realgar, calamine and sulphate of copper) metals (dhātu, like silver, gold, copper, tin, iron, zinc and lead), salts of eight kinds (lavana, five of which are in common use), and nine varieties of precious stones (ratna, like diamond, pearls and corals). This group also includes mud, sand, and lime. [*See* MERCURY, METALS and PRECIOUS STONES.]

Poisons (visha) also figure in Indian pharmacopoeia. They are of two kinds: plant origin (sthāvara) and of animal origin (jaṅgama). There are about twenty plants which contain poison of therapeutic value like Vatsanābha *(Aconitum chasmanthem)*, Vishamushti (*Strychnos Nux vomica*), arka (*Calotropis gigantea),* Jaya-pāla (*Croton tiglium*), and karavīra (*Nerium odorum).* They are again grouped into virulent poisons (visha) and subsidiary or mild poisons (upa-visha). There are nine poisons listed, among which vatsa-nābha (*aconitum ferox)* is the best known. Ahiphena (opium), gunjā (*Abrus precatorius),* karavīra (*Nerium odorum*), vijayā (*Cannabis indica*) and seeds of datūra (*Datura alba*) are illustrations of subsidiary poisons. [*See* POISON].

In accordance with the basic theory that all substances are composed of five primary elements (earth, water, fire, air and ākāśa), the drugs included in the Indian materia medica are, like the human constitution itself, composites of all elements in essential nature, but each drug is distinguished by the preponderance of one or more of the elements. Drugs are, therefore, classified as belonging to one or the other of the elemental groups. Further, the drugs as substances are grounds for certain characteristic properties (guna), potency (vīrya), taste that emerges after digestion (vipāka), specific actions (prabhāva). Classification of drugs within these frames of reference has also been made.

More importantly, however, the grouping of drugs is made on the effect they have on the constitution in health or in distress (for example, *CS*,1,4):

(1) drugs which promote longevity (vitaliser, jīvanīya); (2) drugs which promote nutrition and corpulency of the body (bṛṁhanīya); (3) drugs which emaciate the body or reduce corpulency (lekhanīya or kshīnakara); (4) drugs which are laxative (by disintegrating the compactness of waste products (scybala-breaking, bhedanīya); (5) drugs which heal by helping union of fractured parts of the body (sandhānīya); (6) drugs which increase the appetite (stimulate the digestive fire, (dīpanīya); (7) drugs which increase bodily strength (tonics, balya); (8) drugs which improve complexion (varṇya); (9) drugs which are expectorants and which are beneficial to the throat and voice (by removing hoarseness, kanthya); (10) drugs which promote cheerfulness or relish (cardiac) hrdya; (11) drugs which remove the sense of satiety and reduce kapha (antisaturative) (trptighna), (12) drugs which cure piles (anti-haemorrhoidal, arśoghna), (13) drugs helpful in leprosy and other skin diseases (anti-dermatoses. kushthagna); (14) drugs which cure itching(anti-pruritic, kandūghna), (15) drugs which are anthelmintics (removing intestinal worms, krmighna); (16) drugs which are antidotes to poison (vishaghna); (17) drugs which help increase secretion of milk (Galactogogue or lactiferous, stanyajanana); (18) drugs which improve the quality of milk (galacto-depurant, stanyaśodhana); (19) drugs which increase the secretion of sperm in semen (śukra-janana); (20) drugs which eliminate the defects of semen (semen-depurant, śukra-śodhana) and which promote sexual vigour (vājīkara or vrshya); (21) drugs which promote smoothness and softness of skin (emollients), used as adjuncts to fat therapy (saboleative, snehopaga or snehopayogaa); (22) drugs which facilitate perspiration, used in sweat therapy (anti-diaphoretic, svedopaga or

svedopayoga); (23) drugs which are emetics, and useful in emetic therapy (subemetic, vamanopaga); (24) drugs which are purgatives and useful in cathartic therapy (subpurgative, virechanopaga); (25) drugs which are used as enemata in decoction, enema therapy (subcorrective enemata, āsthāpanopaga); (26) drugs which are used as oily or unctuous enemata (anuvāsanopaga); (27) drugs which are used in nasal insufflation (errhine, śirovirechana); (28) drugs which stop vomiting (anti-emetic, chhardi-nigrahaṇa or vami-nigrahaṇa); (29) drugs which relieve abnormal thirst (antidypsic, tṛshṇāghna or tṛt-praśamaṇa); (30) drugs which relieve hiccough (hikkāghna); (31) drugs which relieve looseness of the bowels and make the stools consistent (intestinal astringent, purīsha-saṅgrahaṇīya or saṁgrāhi); (32) drugs which correct the colour of stools (faecal depigmenter, purīsha-virajanīyam); (33) drugs which reduce urination (mūtra-sangrahanīya); (34) drugs which correct the colour of urine (mutra-virajanīya) and diuretics (mutra-virechanīya); (35) drugs which cure cough (anti-tussive, kāsa-hara); (36) drugs which cure asthma (dyspnoea) (anti-dyspnoeic, śvāsa-hara); (37) drugs which cure dropsical swellings (anasarca, anti phlogistic, śotha-hara or śvayathu-vilayana); (38) drugs which cure fever (febrifuge), antipyretic in action (jvara-hara); (39) drugs which relieve fatigue(sramahara); (40) drugs which relieve burning sensation in the body (refrigerant, dāha-praśamana or nirvāpa); (41) drugs which relieve the sense of coldness or shivering (calefacient, śīta-praśamana); (42) drugs which cure urticaria (anti-allergic, udarda praśamana); (43) drugs which relieve body-ache (anga-mardaprasamana); (44) drugs which relieve colic pain (intestinal antispasmodic, śūla-praśamana); (45) drugs which stop haemorrhage (styptic) or haemostatic (śonita-sthāpana); (46) drugs which relieve pain of wounds (analgesic, vedanā-stapana); (47) drugs which restore consciousness (resuscitative, samjñā-sthāpana); (48) drugs which cure sterility (anti-abortifacient, garbha or prajā-sthāpana); and (49) drugs which prevent ill effects of old age (gerontologic, Vayah-sthāpana or vayasya).

SS, however, divides drugs into two broad groups: (1) drugs which are correctives (saṁśodhana), like purgatives, emetics and errhines, and (2) drugs which pacify the excited dosha (saṁśamana). And it provides a long list of drugs in 37 groups (*SS*,1,38). Although the classification is made on the basis of the drug-action, the names of the groups are given according to the main drug in the group, like (1) vidāri-gandha, etc; (2) āragvadha, etc, (3) sāla-sāra and so on. [*See* SAṀŚAMANA, SAṀŚODHANA, DRUG-ACTION] Correspondence between the lists of drugs provided by *CS* and *SS* have been worked out, and there is a fair degree of unanimity with regard to the identification of drugs and their actions, as for example, the jīvanīya group of *CS* and the kākoli, etc group of *SS*, the bṛmhaṇīya-group of *CS*, and the vidāri-gandha group of *SS*, the lekhaṇīya-group of *CS*, and the musta etc. group of *SS* (cf. P.V.Sarma, *DGV*, part I, p. 80-81. [*See also* DRAVYA-GUṆA, DRUG, PHARMACY, RASA, VIRYA, VIPAKA, PRABHĀVA, KARMA].

The Physician: Physicians (bhishak or vaidya) as a professional group of healers are an ancient institution in India. References to them and their art are to be found even in the early Vedic corpus (*RV*,2,33,4 and 7; 5,42,11; 8,79,2; 10,97,6, etc.). Several Vedic gods (like Rudra, Soma, Indra, Varuna and the Maruts) were regarded as patrons of medicine and physicians. The Aśvins of course were the divine forerunners of all mortal physicians [*See* AŚVINS]. Charaka's wandering physicians may also have been contemporaneous with the early Vedic age. Among the Vedas, the *Atharva* was especially devoted to diseases and their cures by physicians and magicians. [*See* ATHARVA-VEDA]. There seems to have been a period when physicians were denied decent position in the class hierarchy; but the situation does not appear to have lasted long. The Buddhist texts reveal not only the prevalence of physicians, but their honoured place in the society.

It is natural that during the early days, the distinction between magicians who cured diseases by charms, spells, amulets and magical formulae (daiva-vyapāśraya), and the physicians who cured diseases by herbs, drugs, dietary regimen and other rational practices (yukti-vyapāśraya) was rather slender. The Kauśika-sūtra (supplement to Atharva-veda) presents an indiscriminate admixture of magic, witchcraft, herbal medicine, nature cure, and diet. But gradually the drug system of medicine was segregated from the mass of folk magico-religious practices. [*See* ATHARVAVEDA]. The physician was no longer obliged to rely on charms for effecting cures. He could ply his trade with a certain knowledge of the human body and the diseases that it get, and with a rational acquaintance with herbs and minerals.

The physicians, even when they took to rational therapeutics, continued their formal affiliation with the *Atharva-veda,* for the main objective of therapeutic as well as magico-religious prescriptions was 'to benefit life' (āyushah hitāya, *CS,* sūtra, 30,20-21). But even CHARAKA recognizes that the therapeutic practices in *Atharva-veda* are mainly gifts, pacificatory rites, benefit-invoking rituals, penances, fasts, and so on. He distinguishes this complex from the rational therapeutics, which are his main interest. And, in this context, he gives a rather elaborate description of what a physician should be like, and his training (*CS,* sūtra, 1, 9, 14-28; 1, 11, 53; 3, 8, 1-6 etc.) He has also comments to make on quacks and physician-pedlars (sūtra, 9, 15-17; 29, 7-8 etc.). SUŚRUTA also has interesting comments on the nature, qualifications and training of physicians and surgeons (sūtra, 2; 1,4; 9-10; 25,44; 34, 19-20, etc.).

The physician must be learned (śruta), not only in the medical lore but in several other disciplines. SUŚRUTA makes it clear that one who is acquainted with but one branch of learning will not be able to understand aright even that discipline; therefore, he advises, the physician must be learned in many branches of study ('tasmad bahuśrutah śāstram vijānāyīcchikatsakah'). CHARAKA prescribes expert acquaintance with the texts, and more importantly an understanding of the import thereof (tattvādhigata-śāstrārtha). The physician's knowledge of the medical texts must be profound and clear (paryavadāta).

His knowledge must comprehend causes of diseases (hetu), symptoms (linga), curing the diseases (praśamane rogānāṁ), and preventing the recurrence of diseases (apunarbhave) (*CS*, sūtra, 9,19). He must be knowledgeable so far as medicine is concerned (vidyā); he must be learned in other branches of study (vi-jñāna, according to commentary 'śāstrāntara-jñānaṁ'); he must be capable of reasoning (vitarka); his memory must be powerful (smṛti); he must be hardworking, and devoted to his calling (tatparatā) (ibid. 1,9,21).

He must have extensively watched his own teacher and other physicians diagnosing diseases and administering medicine (bahuśo'-dṛshṭa-karmatā); and he must have himself practised (svayaṁ-kṛtī). He must be capable of preparing the medicines himself, and administering them to the patient (sajjopaskāra-bheshaja). If he is merely learned but not acquainted with practice, he would be scared out of his wits when confronted by a patient, even as a coward would be at the battle-front. If, on the other hand, he sets out to practice without acquainting himself with the texts he will become the laughing-stock, and he deserves to be punished by the administration (*AS,* 1, 2, 10 and 11). Learning is like a light (jyoti or pradīpa); it will extend the horizon of one's vision and refine one's native talents.

He is the chief among the four props of medical practice: the physician, the drugs, the attendant, and the patient himself. It is the physician who knows about the drugs (vijñātā), who instructs the attendant (śāsitā), and treats the patient (yoktā). The other factors being dependent upon him, he should be competent in textual knowledge, in developing insights, and in therapeutics (*CS*, sutra, 9,10). Even when the other factors are wanting, he alone will be able to bring succour to the patient, even as a clever boatsman leads the raft across safely. (*SS*, sūtra, 34,18). [*See* FOUR PROPS IN MEDICAL PRACTICE].

The physician must conduct himself with dignity and decorum. "He should not visit a patient uninvited; and when he visits the patient's house, he should not indulge in any talk other than what relates to the patient's health. He dresses himself neatly, and examines the patient carefully, and without haste. He will not communicate to others what might embarrass the patient. He will never decide on the drug or treatment on an impulse, nor will he waste time on this account. His action will be timely and well-decided" (*AS*, 1,2,15-17).

The qualities that bring credit to the physician are friendliness (maitrī), kindness for the suffering (kāruṇyaṁ ārteshu), eagerness to do his best to alleviate the suffering (śakye prītih), and withdrawal of treatment from one whose condition is definitely moribund (upekshaṇam prakṛtistheshu). (*CS*, sūtra, 9,26). The physician acquires just renown when his instructions are clear and firm (ājñā), when he is ready to sacrifice for the sake of the patient's well-being (tyāga), when he is patient and forgiving (kshamā), when he is steadfast when confronted by different cases (dhairyaṁ), and when he is uncommonly courageous (vikrama) (*SS*, sūtra, 34, 10).

Charaka's humanistic ideal becomes evident in his advice to the physicians (*CS*, 6, 1,58-62): "He, who practices not for money nor for caprice but out of compassion for living beings (bhuta-daya) is the best among all physicians. The physicians who set out to sell their skill like merchandise only lose sight of the gold and attain but heaps of dirt. Hard it is to find a conferer of religious blessings comparable to the physician who snaps the snares of death for his patients and proffers renewed life to them. The physicians who regards compassion for living beings as his highest religion fulfils his mission (siddharthah) and obtains the highest happiness"

CHARAKA humorously classifies physicians into two types: those who remove diseases and give life, and those who give diseases and remove life itself (*CS*, sūtra, 29,5). The former hail from respectable families, are adequately educated, have served as apprentices under masters, are competent and sincere, have self-control, are well-equipped, and are themselves free from defects. They look upon every patient as their own mother, father, brother, or other relative; they are essentially kind-hearted,' and are solely interested in relieving the suffering of the patient.

The other type of physicians lack decorum as well as honesty. As soon as they hear of anyone being ill, they will rush to him proclaiming their own merits, and have their eyes on the fees. When they find that they are unable to cure, they lay the blame on the patient's non-coöperation and lack of restraint. When the case is hopeless, they promptly disappear. They flatter themselves before ignorant folk, but avoid knowledgeable people, as travellers avoid a dangerous forest (sūtra, 29, 7 and 9). Such are the quacks who masquerade as efficient physicians and roam about the country, as veritable thorns, owing to the negligence of the administrators (*CS*, sūtra, 29,8).

Three types of physicians are distinguished

(*CS*, sūtra, 11,50-53): quacks who are in fact not physicians at all (bhishak-chhad-macharāh); quasi-physicians who have acquired some celebrity owing to factors not really connected with medicine (siddha-sādhitāh); and genuine physicians who are knowledgeable, well trained, and whose only objective in life is to contribute to the well-being of people (prayoga-jñāna-vijñāna-siddhi-siddhāh).

CHARAKA is aware that the fame of some healers, who are neither learned nor trained, spreads because stray instances of diseases are cured. "The quack, who cures purely accidentally some patient who is destined to live longer, may soon kill many patients, whose longevity is not predetermined!" (sūtra 9,17). He comes down heavily on the physicians who take a casual attitude while treating patients (sūtra, 1, 126-133). One who wants to become a physician must previously become thoroughly knowledgeable, and cultivate virtues; he must work hard ('param prayatnam ātishṭhet'), for he is 'a saver of lives' (prāṇadah) of human beings. Medicine is whatever contributes to health; and therefore a good physician is one who frees human beings from ill-health (sūtra, 9, 134). The commentary adds: "It is only the serious-minded and knowledgeable physician that can restore health. Chance cures effectd by quacks cannot be called restoration of health. The cure here is due not to the medicine, but to patient's fortune" (*NS*, ed., p. 23).

The medical profession was considered to be lucrative even during the Vedic and Buddhist periods. Physicians were well rewarded. A Vedic hymn (*RV*,10,97) speaks of horses, cows, and clothes being given to the physician who cures diseases by herbs. JĪVAKA the personal physician of the Buddha, was a very wealthy man; but the texts require the physician to treat poor people, ascetics, and superiors without receiving any remuneration. A verse advises the physician not to sell his wish-fulfilling gem (chintāmaṇi) for a few glass-pieces (viz.money)!

The physician is a great benefactor inasmuch as he facilitates people to attend to the three main objectives in life, viz. virtue, wealth and enjoyment, as all three depend upon health. He is to be looked upon as a generous donor (dātā), for he gifts bodily well-being and life. (*CS*, sūtra, 17, 38) [*See* also FOUR PROPS OF MEDICAL PRACTICE, MEDICAL ETHICS, VAIDYA].

Pills: Pillulae, pills or bolus (vaṭi, vaṭika, guṭika, guḍa, piṇḍa, modaka) are solid or semi-solid globular masses, meant to be swallowed as such (without being masticated in the mouth).

Medicinal substances are well-dried, finely powdered, ground on a mortar with juices or decoctions, and made into a paste which is rolled between fingers (slightly smeared with ghee), and made into pills. The wet pills are then dried in shade so as to assume hardness and solidity. Presence or persistence of moisture interferes with the preservation of pills. Pills are also prepared by adding the powdered drugs to water, milk or a herbal decoction which is boiled down to a thick consistency, so as to give a mass which may be rolled into pills. The proportion of the fluid is two parts to one of powdered drugs.

Rolling the powder into the pill form is facilitated by adding powders to a treacle of jaggery, sugar or honey, or to an adhesive (gum-resin) substance like guggulu (Balsamodendron mukul). The proportions of sugar, jaggery and guggulu or honey to the powders are respectively 4:1, 2:1, 1:1.

Pills are advantageous inasmuch as they are easily portable, easily administered, and contain the exact dosage of the drugs. [*See* PREPARATIONS].

Pitta: One of the three doshas involved in the constitution of the living organisms, it corresponds to 'fire' as the elemental principle, and with rajas as the essential functional mode [*See* DOSHA]. The word 'pitta' is derived from the root 'tap' which means 'to burn' (dāhe), 'to agitate' (santāpe). It is so called because it is responsible for the generation of heat in the system ('tapati', ushmāṇam utpādayati), and it burns up (viz. digests) the food that is ingested ('tapayati dahati bhuktaṁ āhārajātaṁ'). It is thus described figuratively as the 'fire' in the body (*CS,* sūtra, 12, 11): for though not occurring in the form of the physical fire, it discharges the functions of fire, viz. combustion (dahana, burning) and cooking (pachana, chemical actions) (*CS,* sūtra, 21, 9). There is no 'fire' in the body apart from pitta (*SS,* ibid.). It is called 'internal fire' (antarāgni) the presence of which is suggested by pitta and body warmth (ushmā) (CHKP on *CS,* sūtra, 12, 11).

The concept of pitta is a broad-based one: it comprehends many anatomical structures and physiological functions which are vital, such as combustion or oxidation (burning the nutrient substances, dahana), generation of heat in the body (tapana), digestion of food involving conversion of external, heterogeneous substances into internal, homogeneous and assimilable substance (pariṇamana), transmutation of the nutrients in the body (prāvṛtti), and separation (saṁghāta-bheda) of the nutrient portions of the food (sāra-bhāga) from the waste-products (kiṭṭa). In short, it is described as pāchaka-pitta (pitta that is responsible for digestion and metabolism). [*See* AGNI].

Besides this major involvement, the pitta, which is present all over the body, is responsible for many other functions. Even in the days prior to *CS,* the importance of pitta was recognized. The sage Marīchi, for instance, held that this principle was directly responsible for normal functions such as promotion of digestion (pakti), visual perception (darśana), production of normal heat in the body (mātraushma), normal colour or body complexion (prakṛti-varṇa), courageous disposition (śaurya), cheerfulness (harsha), and lucidity of mind (prasāda), and also for the morbid manifestations of all the above (*CS,* sūtra, 12, 11). *AHṛ* (sūtra, 11, 2-3) adds to the list: hunger (kshut), thirst (tṛṭ), relish for food (ruchi), suppleness of the body (tanu-mārdava), understanding (buddhi), retentive memory (medhā) and intelligence (dhī).

Located in different regions of the body, pitta has different functions. Located in the region between the stomach (āmāśaya) and large intestine (pakvāśaya) it digests food; and is therefore called 'pāchaka-pitta' (digestive). Located in the region including stomach, duodenum, liver, spleen and pancreas, it imparts pigment to the chyle (rasa) which is thus transformed into blood (rasa-rañjanāt), and is hence called rañjaka-pitta (pigment-giving). Located in the heart (hṛt), it enables one to accomplish his objectives by intelligence, memory, understanding, self-confidence and so on ('buddhi-medhā-bhimānādyair abhipretārtha-sādhanaṁ'), and is hence called sādhaka-pitta (accomplishing). Located in the optical structure (dṛk), it enables one to perceive clearly and meaningfully the form of objects (rupālochanatah), and is hence called ālochaka-pitta (perceiving or image-forming). Located in the skin (tvak), it imparts lustre to the skin (bhrājanatvāt tvachah), and is hence called bhrājaka-pitta (lustre-endowing) (cf. *AHṛ,* sūtra, 12, 13; *SS,*sūtra, 21, 10).

Physical properties of the pitta are thus enumerated. According to *CS* (sūtra, 20, 15) and *SS* (sūtra, 21, 11), the inherent, natural qualities are heat, sharpness, liquidity, slight unctuousness, all colours except white and red (according to *SS,* it is either blue when immature, or yellow, when mature), fishy smell, acrid (normally) or sour (in improper digestion) in taste, and fluidity. Natural actions of pitta are production of burning sensation, heat in the body, suppuration, sweat, putrefaction, itching, discharge, redness, and manifestation of its smell, taste and colour (*CS,* ibid.). These characteristics are aids in diagnosis.

Among the symptoms due to the abnormalities of pitta are burning sensations in body, cracking pain in the body, acid eructation, pyrosis, high temperature, excessive sweating, foetid odour of the body, cracking of skin, tendency to bleed, red spots on the skin, blue moles, herpes, bitter taste in the mouth, smell of blood in the mouth, abnormal thirst, inflammation of the penis, fainting spells, conjuctivitis, jaundice, urticaria, and stomatitis. [*See* DISEASES OF PITTA].

The aggravation is caused by excessive intake of sour and pungent articles of food which are hot, burning or sharp, incompatible and irregular food habits, eating dry vegetables, drinking of alcoholic preparations, exposure to fire and sun, anger, fear, fatigue, etc. Treatment consists in diet and drinks which are bitter, sweet, or astringent in taste, exposure to cold wind and moonlight, residence in shaded places and underground, frequent sprinkling with water, purgation therapy, blood-letting and anointments.

There is an aspect of pitta which is regarded as a byproduct (mala) of blood-liver-bile. Pitta is intimately related with blood, in its location (both being located in the liver, yakṛit, and spleen, plīha), as well as in its physical properties (both having identical colour and smell). It has among its powers the capacity to vitiate blood (*CS,* chikitsā 14, 9-10 and *AHṛ,* nidāna, 3, 3-4). However, as a waste product it needs to be eliminated from the system [*See* MALA]. It is looked upon as corresponding to hepatic bile, especially in the context of the symptomatology of abnormal increase of pitta (pitta-vṛddhi) for example, yellowish urine, yellow colour of faeces, eyes and skin, excessive hunger and thirst, burning sensations in body etc). [*See also* DOSHA, AGNI, DIGESTION, KALĀ].

Plants: Substances used for treating are classified into three groups: animal products (jaṅgama, like honey, milk, musk, gorochana, blood, fat, urine, horn, skin, etc.), minerals and metals (pārthiva, like gold, silver, iron, rust of metals, mercury, mud, salts, sand, lime, etc.), and plants (audbhida). Plants are extensively used in Indian medicine since very early times. Their use was prevalent even during the Vedic times, and it continues to prevail today. Although it is believed that there is no plant without a medicinal use, the nighantus describe the physical appearances, properties, uses and preparations of as many as two thousand plants.

Plants are described as composed of the five primary forms of matter and possessed of internal consciousness (antahsaṁjñā), as distinguished from animals which although similarly constituted possess consciousness both internally and externally (bhair-antaschetanā). They are dominated by tamas, and therefore they do not move about, nor do they actively cognize the external world. "They are stationary (sthāvara), for they are covered by great ignorance" (mahāmoha) (*Garuda-purāṇa*). But being internally conscious, they are capable of experiencing pleasure and pain: having hidden consciousness (avyakta-chetanā), they are sensitive to pressure or touch which is felt inward (antahsparśa). They drink water from the earth, and their sap moves up (ūrdhva-retas).

Therefore, they are organic in nature (viz. possessed of sense-faculty, sendriya, and have much in common with the human constitution. They are easily assimilated in the human organism, either as food or as drug. Unlike mineral drugs, the plant-drugs require no prior or elaborate treatment (like incineration, purification) before they can be used. And the preparations of plant drugs, (decoctions, infusions, pastes, powders) are comparatively easy, simple and quick. Further, the patient's life or health is not endangered by an excessive dosage of the plant-drugs, and therefore are safer to use.

Above all, the raw-materials for plant drugs are easily available in the country. These are some of the reasons why Indian medicine employs plant-drugs almost exclusively.

The constitution of plants was likened in an old text to the constitution of the human body. Chyle (rasa) in the human body corresponds with the sap in the plant, blood with latex, muscle with mesoderm, bone with heartwood, bone-marrow with pith, sinews with endoderm, skin with epiderm, and body-hair with leaves. (*Bṛhadāranyaka-upanishad,* 3, 9, 1-6). The parts of the plant have been carefully enumerated and described by the Indian poets, philosophers and even grammarians (Pāṇini, Ashtādhyāyī, 4, 1, 64, Vārttika, 4, 3, 166 and PATAÑJALI, *Mahābhāshya* 1, 2, 45; 1, 4, 21; 5, 2, 94) (cf. *DGV,* IV). The medical texts have found use for all parts of the plant; root, stalk, bark, leaves, seeds, berries, fruits, flowers, latex, sprouts, gum, oil bulb, expressed juice, etc.

Plants are broadly classified into four groups: (1) tall trees, which generally grow in forests and are distinguished by fruits but no visible flowers (vanaspati, for example, the ficus group); (2) medium-sized trees, which are distinguished by fruits as well as flowers (vānaspatya, mango, etc); (3) shrubs and weak plants, which have a tendency to grow in clusters, spread on the ground, or climb on trees (vīrudha), like grass; (4) herbs, which are annuals or periodicals (viz. die as soon as they yield fruit or mature), (oshadhi like *hordeum vulgare,* yava etc (*CS,* sūtra, 1, 70)

Plants are further grouped into two main types from the point of view of their effect on the human organism: (1) medicinal (bheshaja) plants, which are again classified as (a) those that help maintain health (svastha-hita), usually included as food or diet or prescribed for post-prandial drink etc, and (b) those that cure the disorders (asvastha-hita), viz. drugs; and (2) non-medicinal (abheshaja) plants, which are deleterious and dangerous to the human organism, for example, poisonous plants which are dangerous, or fatal (bādhana), and plants having magical properties and thus used in witchcraft and sorcery (sānubādhana).

Plants were regarded as organisms in their own right. They too could fall prey to diseases; and these diseases could also be treated and cured. The management and care of plants, horticultural details, diseases of plants and their cure form the subject-matter of the branch of Indian medicine known as Vṛkshāyurveda. There are references to several texts on plant pathology in Sanskrit; but few of them have survived. A well-known text in this field is PARĀŚARA'S *Vṛkshāyurveda.* Ascribed to first century B.C. the Manuscript of this work was discovered by Jogendranath Bhishagratna of Navadvīpa (Bengal), and published by his son, N.N. Sircar, in 1950. It consists of six chapters (kāṇḍas) dealing with the culturing of plants, varieties, diseases and cures. VARĀHAMIHIRA'S *Brhajjātaka* contains references to the plant-horoscopes (vrksha-jātaka).

Plexus: Known as jāla (network), the plexuses are four in kind; muscular (māṁsa), vascular (sirā), ligamentous (snāyu), and bony (asthi). They are closely interconnected, and interwoven in the form of a network. The entire body is a chain-work (gavākshita) of these plexuses (*SS,* śārīra, 5, 11). [*See* BODY (HUMAN)].

Poison: Poison (visha) is so-called in Sanskrit because it causes concern to all beings ('jagad vishannam tena'), by making the organism grieviously ill and leading it to certain death. It is the exact opposite of vitality (ojas), which promotes health and preserves life. [*See* VITALITY]. Poison is defined as that which destroys vitality.

Poison is further defined as the substance which possesses all of the following ten qualities, and is thus capable of ten consequent actions (*CS*, Chikitsā, 123; *SS*, kalpa. 16): (1) light (laghu); and; therefore, spreads all over the body, making it difficult to control or cure, baffling the efficacy of drugs (duratikrama *CS*, duśchikitsya, *SS*); (2) rough or parching (rūksha); and, therefore, aggravates vāta (*CS*, *SS*); (3) quick-acting (āśu); pervades the bodily organs swiftly (*CS*), takes away life fast (*SS*); (4) pellucid (viśada); excites the locations of the doshas (*CS*, spreads in the body arresting the functions of the organs (*SS*); (5) capable of afflicting the entire system (vyavāyi); enters into the fluids of the body, and is quick in its deranging function (*CS*), enters into the very core of the constitution (prakṛti) (*SS*); (6) sharp (tīkshṇa); destroys the vital organs (marma), which are by nature soft (*CS*), and also causes loss of consciousness, and disintegrates muscles and limbs (*SS*); (7) capable of drying the bodily humours or disintegrating (vikāśi); takes away life (*CS*), wastes away the doshas, the dhātus and the mala (*SS*); (8) subtle or minute (sūkshma); and aggravates blood (which flows in subtle pathways) (*CS*), enters even the minutest capillaries of the body (*SS*); (9) hot (ushṇa); aggravates pitta (*CS*) and also blood (*SS*); and (10) unidentified taste (anirdeśya-rasa) (*CS*); pollutes kapha (*CS*); indigestible (avipāki) (*SS*), (only in artificial poison gara, *CS*,) because of unassimilability, proves troublesome for a long time and baffles cure. (cf. also *AHṛ*, uttara, 5).

All the above ten properties are also present in alcoholic liquor (madya), excepting that instead of the unidentified taste and the unassimilability of poisons, liquors have sour taste (amla) and are assimilable. Both alike are opposed to vitality, but liquors are slow and gradual in their life-destroying function, while poisons are quick and sudden.

The grave character of poisons is due to their ability to vitiate all three doshas. As they are light, quick-acting, widely spreading, deranging and subtle, vāta is aggravated; because of their unidentified taste and pellucid character, kapha is aggravated; and because they are sharp and hot, pitta is aggravated. They deprive the organism of life by first vitiating blood (as soon as they enter the body), then vitiating the three doshas as well as their respective receptacles (āśayas), and finally obtaining a lodgement in the heart causing total disintegration of the system.

Poisons are generally classified into 'natural' (akṛtrima) and 'artificial' (kṛtrima, also called gara). The former is again in two groups: (1) of vegetable origin (sthāvara), including, however, poisons of minerals and metals (dhātu), as they are also found on the earth, and (2) of animal origin (jaṅgama). Poisons of the first group are derived from different parts of the plant, roots (mūla), leaves (patra), flowers (pushpa), fruits (phala), bark (tvak), milky exudations (kshīra), pith (sāra), gum (niryāsa), and tubers or bulbs (kanda). The most effective poisons are those derived from tubers or bulbs. The nighaṇṭus give a list of eighteen poisonous plants, eight of which are to be employed for therapeutic ends (saktuka, mustaka, śṛṅgi, baluka, sarshapa, vatsanābha, kūrma and śveta-śṛṅgi) and others (like kālakūṭa, hālāhala, haridrā and pradīpaka, which are all terrible poisons) to be avoided. However, vatsanābha (Aconitum ferox) is probably the only poison-drug in common use.

The poisons of plant extract aggravate all the three doshas and especially produce fever, hiccough, froth in the mouth, difficulty in breathing (which are symptomatic of the disorders of kapha), irritating sensation in teeth, swelling of neck and throat (which are disorders of vāta), nausea and loss of consciousness (which are disorders of pitta). The last symptom which is also the final is systemic (sārvadehika), while the others are regional ailments (sthānika).

Poisons of animal origin are of sixteen

kinds: communicated by eye-sight (dragons), breath (some snakes), teeth (all snakes), nails (cats, dogs, monkeys), urine, excreta (some insects), semen (mice), saliva (spiders), mense-blood (some spiders), sting (scorpions), expelled air at the rectum, rectum (wasp), bone, bile (some fish), bristle (centipede), and carcass (insects, snakes). Of the animal poisons pressed for curative ends, the snake poison is well-known. There are 68 varieties of snakes in four groups, known to be poisonous. Poison extracted from a strong, youthful black-serpent (cobra) is said to have great healing properties: it pacifies instantaneously all three doshas, increases digestive power as soon as it is taken internally, antidotes diseases due to the aggravation of the three doshas together (sannipāta) and cures cholera (vishūchika).

While not all snakes are poisonous, the bites of even the most poisonous snakes are not necessarily dangerous. The bite may merely exude the saliva without the involvement of fangs (tuṇḍāhata); or it may only make a mark of two teeth on the skin, without rupturing the skin (vyālīḍha). These two conditions need not cause any anxiety. But when, as a result of bite, the skin gets ruptured and blood begins to flow out (vyālupta), or when three teeth tear into the muscles and the flow of blood is copious, continuous (daṁshṭraka), or when four teeth are involved (dashṭa-nipīḍita), the situation is serious and calls for immediate action. Psychological factors such as fear which aggravates vāta (sarpāṅgāhata), and suspicion (śaṅkā-visha) of a snake-bite which can bring about all the symptoms of an actual snake-bite are recognized (*AHṛ* Uttara, 36). There are twelve varieties of snakes whose bite is not at all poisonous (nirvisha). But the person who is bitten is easily scared, and the fright itself may cause not only troubles characteristic of poisonous bite, but even death. Instructive is the case of the python (ajagara) which does not bite, but kills the victim by its very grasp.

Most of the snake-bites, however, are easily remedied, especially soon after the bite. The poison after the bite will not enter the bloodstream until after 100 mātrās (time taken to count 1 to 100); it will be during this time limited to the actual part of the body that is bitten. Treatment given at this stage is the easiest and most effective. But once the poison has entered the blood-stream, the case becomes difficult and needs to be handled with great care. There are symptoms appearing at once (hiccough, difficulty in breathing, cough, and pain in the heart) which indicate certain death. Frothy vomit, loss of consciousness, inability to rouse the man even with an intense errhine (nasya), blackening of face, hands and feet, twisting of the nose, non-flow of blood from a cut on the body, are other symptoms of the approaching end.

Judicious blood-letting by puncturing appropriate veins (sirā-vyadha) is among the remedies suggested for snake-bite. To make the patient vomit is another. Drinking of plentiful ghee (clarified butter) and honey with some medicines mixed is also recommended; this would cover the heart with kapha so that the disorganization of vital functions is arrested (hṛdayāvarana). Numerous herbal preparations like the kernel of the jayapāla (*Croton tiglium*) seed, which is itself a powerful poison, macerated with lemon juice twenty-one times, to antidote snake poison are in use, as also incantations, charms and spells.

Among the disturbances of organic poison in the human body are coma, drowsiness, fatigue, inflammation, froth in the mouth, hair standing on end, swelling, and diarrhoea.

Snake poisons used for curative purposes must be initially purified and rendered powerful by mixing cow's urine with them and drying in the sun, or by mixing mustard oil with them, or by subjecting them to maceration (bhāvanā) with juice of tulasī (*Ocimum sanctum*) leaves or decoction of kushṭha (*Saussurea lappa*) thrice. Human saliva is also considered effective in controlling the spread of poison.

Artificial poison (gara) is composed of the toxins created mainly by medicines that contain inimical substances, by medicines that are improperly prepared or administered, and by medicines that involve powerful substances like mercury and mineral poisons. It may also be caused by eating articles of food which do not agree with each other (like milk and sour things) or with the person's constitution, or eating when the body does not need food. Unlike the natural poisons, the artificial poisons act more on the body constituents (dhātus) than on the doshas. Consequently, disorders like dyspepsia, anemia, emaciation, cough, hiccough, fever, drowsiness, depression, enlargement of liver and spleen, body-swelling, and dryness of feet and hands result.

Interesting is the account of dreams which are usual with the patients afflicted by artificial poison. Their dreams abound in wild animals (like jackal, wild cat, tiger, mongoose and monkey), dried lakes and withered plants. The person, if fair, would see himself as dark in complexion, and if dark, would see himself as fair; he would have a feeling that his nose and eyes are lacerated or absent altogether.

The effect of strong poison (vega) is said to have seven or eight stages. In the first stage, the body constituent, rasa, gets vitiated; the tongue turns black and rigid; there will be abnormal thirst, irritation of teeth, excessive flow of saliva, nausea, fatigue, unrest, and spells of fainting. This is followed by the vitiation of blood in the second stage; the body changes colour, there is sweating, trembling, burning sensation in the throat, giddiness, frequent yawning, difficulty in breathing, piercing pains all over the body, and pain in the heart. The poison at this stage would have entered the stomach (āmāśaya). The case is easily handled (sādhya) at this stage, as the poison can be thrown out by emetics.

The third stage is when the poison enters the large intestines (pakvāśaya); treatment becomes difficult (kashtasādhya) at this stage, for the vitiation of muscles would have begun here. Along with emetics, purgatives also are indicated. Severe pain in the stomach, rumblings in the intestines, cough, hiccough, dryness of palate, swelling of body, weakness, the discolouration of eyes and loss of clear vision result.

The fourth stage is characterized by heaviness of the head, burning sensations, nausea, fainting spells, and body-pain. The fifth stage finds the person suffering from frequent black-outs (tamasah darśanam), patches of blue and yellow before the eyes, excessive flow of saliva, tearing pain in the joints and in the intestines. In this stage, all the three doshas would be vitiated. The next stage (sixth) is marked by loss of consciousness (samjñā-nāśa), excessive purging, and unabated hiccough. The last stage (seventh) finds the person having lacerating pain in the shoulders and back. This is followed by death (*SS*, and *AHṛ*), which is counted as the eighth stage by *CS* (chikītsā, 27).

If the first of the above stages is marked by disturbances in the seat of kapha (viz. stomach), the second stage is predominantly a disturbance of pitta; the third and the subsequent stages, of vāta. The last stage is really incurable (asādhya), but the physician should try if he can manage the case by a conjoint administration of emetics (vamana), purgatives (virechana), enemata (basti), opthalmic ointments (añjana), purification of the system (śodhana), and errhines (nasya).

There is another account which identifies the seven stages preceding death by single prominent symptoms when poison enters into the system suddenly; (1) discolouration of skin (tvag-vikāra), (2) trembling (vepathu), (3) inflammation and burning sensation (dāha), (4) disfigurement and debility of body (deha-vaiklavya), (5) froth in the mouth (phenodgati), (6) lacerating pain in the shoulders (skandhayor bhangitā), and (7) loss of movement of limbs (jāḍya) (RJN).

Treatment of disorders by poisonous drugs is the subject-matter of many manuals, which described in detail the methods of purifying or neutralizing the poison in such drugs before administration (śodhana, māraṇa, etc). There are also details about the patient to whom poisonous drugs may be administered. These drugs act effectively when taken with a lot of ghee and milk, and when the patient observes the rules prescribed for the rasāyana treatment. Persons who are irritable in temperament, bilious in nature, impotent, worn out by hunger or thirst and fatigued by physical work, or by travel are not fit for these drugs. Patients whose skin is rough and devoid of natural oil, women in pregnancy, children and old people are likewise unsuited for this treatment. Administration of poisonous drugs is not advisable when the patient is quarrelling with the physician.

The patient who is under treatment with poisonous drugs must avoid sexual activity, and must be on diet; he must preserve his calm while taking the drugs, for anger also is a poison and will vitiate the drug-poison. He must prepare his body by taking a decoction of aśvagandha, triphala, and go-jihvā mixed with mercury (either incinerated, or in a state of compound with sulphur), and start taking the poison-drug from next day. The drug must be taken every day, early in the morning after drinking some ghee and taking some light repast. The patient's diet should consist of cow's milk, ghee, paddy-rice and articles of food that are cold in property (like sugar, milk, honey, goat's blood, madgura fish, and flesh of jāṅgala animals); he must drink cold water.

Winter and spring are suitable seasons for treatment with poisonous drugs; if it cannot be avoided, summer may also be alright, but the treatment must never be taken in the rainy season. The dosage must be gradually increased from the quantity equivalent to a sarshapa or mustard seed on the first day until one guñjā (equivalent of 36 mustard seeds), (two sarshapas on the second, third and fourth days, three for the next four days, four on the ninth day, and so on). The healthy man also may use these drugs for preventing senile decay, but his dosage must be limited to a yava (equivalent of six mustard seeds) a day. The patients suffering from leprosy, leucoderma and other serious skin ailments may take as much as one guñjā a day with advantage.

Those who are under this treatment must avoid things which are pungent, sour, saline and oily; they must also avoid the fierce rays of the sun. Cold weather, cold things, cold country, black pepper, rock-salt, sugar, honey, wheat, rice from boiled paddy are recommended. Poisonous drugs must be discontinued when one suffers from indigestion for they may even cause death. One who does not take plenty of ghee while under this treatment will fall prey to various illnesses like loss of eye-sight, deafness and diseases of vāta.

There is a classification of therapeutic poisons into virulent (visha) and mild (upavisha). The former group has nine vegetable drugs listed in the nighaṇṭus. But all of them, excepting vatsanābha (*Aconitum ferox*), are at present unidentified (haridrā, sakthuka, pradīpana, saurāshṭraka, śṛṅgi, kālakūṭa, hālāhala and brahma-putra). The latter group of drugs, having the same action as the virulent poisons, but much milder, owing to an imponderable specific property (prabhāva), is in extensive use: ahiphena (*Papaver somniferum,* opium), gūñjā (seeds of *Abrus precatorius*), dhattūra (*datura fastuosa* fruits), kara-vīra (roots of *Nerium odorum*), lāṅgalikā (*Gloriosa superba*), arka (milky exudation of *Calotropis gigantea*), and snuhi (exudation of *Euphorbia nerifolia*). Arsenic and orpiment are classed among mineral poisons.

There is another classification of poisons, according to the 'castes' (jāti) imputed to them. The 'brāhmana' class of poisons are white or tawny in colour, sweet or saltish to taste, and have hair-like structures over the surface. They are employed chiefly to prevent old age and to cure senile decay (rasāyana). The 'kshattriya' class of poisons are red in colour, and are used mainly in mercurial preparations (rasa-karma); they are administered to antidote other poisons. The 'vaiśya' class of poisons are yellow or grey in colour and are employed to cure skin-diseases, especially leprosy. The 'śūdra', class of poisons are dark in colour, and are fatal if ingested by a healthy person. But they are extremely useful in curing one bitten by poisonous snakes. The 'caste' of the poison is said to be ascertained by putting the poison into a pot filled with milk and watching the colour into which the milk turns (*RJN*).

Even mild poisons may kill a person when taken in excess. Its powerful action may be understood when we learn that when mercury is rubbed with a milk-poison, mercury will 'lose its wings', and grow 'hungry'; it is only then that mercury will be able to 'swallow' and 'digest' metals. All mild poisons which are used for therapeutic purposes need to be purified by subjecting them to maceration with the five products of the cow (pañcha-gavya, viz. milk, curd, ghee, urine and dung) by boiling them with milk in a dola-yantra.

Poisons that have found lodgement in the patient's body could be weakened and their action made mild and slow by conditions such as weather, nature of the place of residence, food, and persistent habits (like sleeping during daytime) which tend to aggravate kapha. They nevertheless vitiate the bodily constituents, and lead to the accumulation of toxins and waste products within the body. Hence they are called 'vitiating poisons' (dūshī-visha). Such poisons may also be weakened because of the action of drugs or by their own nature; or the body may get used to them, owing to their long residence in the body. Being covered over by kapha, they cease to be fatal in their effect, but need to be eliminated all the same. [*See* DŪSHĪ-VISHA]. [*See also* TOXICOLOGY].

Potency: The expression vīrya is taken in the sense of potency by which the drug acts; the presence of this potency renders the drug effective, while its absence renders it ineffective. The term 'potency' refers to the active principle in the drug which makes it act. It is distinct from property (guṇa), taste (rasa), and the post-digestive taste-transformation (vipāka); and it resides in substances. It is known by its action.

There are different views regarding the nature of potency. Some hold that it is another term for 'power of action' (śakti), and define it as that by which action is accomplished (*CS*, 1, 26, 'yena kurvanti tad vīryam'). Some others argue that the especially powerful properties (guna) of substances are known as potencies (*SS; AS*, 1, 17 'guru-ādyā vīryam uchyante śaktimantonyathā guṇāh,): eight among the twenty classical properties of substances [*See* GUṆA] are regarded as potencies, for they are supremely competent (para-sāmarthya), while the other twelve are mere properties. There is a third view that potency signifies the most essential aspect (or the most active principle) of the five primary forms of matter (dravya).

The tastes of drugs (rasa), of substances are apprehended directly, and the final transformation of taste after digestion (vipāka) can only be inferred. The potency of a drug, however, is sometimes directly apprehended (viz. by the contact of the drug with the tongue or skin, nipāta), sometimes referred by the action in the body (adhivāsa, after the contact of the drug with the tongue or skin, and before the final transformation of the taste consequent on digestion; the expression adhivāsa is explained as 'sahāvasthānam, yāvaccharīra-nivāsāt' , viz. as long as the drug is present in the body), and sometimes both directly apprehended and inferred. When the potencies are taken as identical with the properties, soft, cold and warm are apprehended by touch, slimy and pellucid are perceived by the eye as well as by touch, sticky and dry are perceived by the eye, and sharp by the trouble it causes in the mouth (*SS,* 1, 41).

The number of potencies is also a matter of some controversy. *RVS,* which argues for the independent reality of potencies on the ground that they are apprehended as such (upalabdheh) by the actions they perform, holds that there can be no fixed number of potencies; they can be unlimited in accordance with the infinite possibilities of action.

Nimi lists fifteen potencies in terms of the drug-actions like expulsion of waste-products, pacification, appetising, digestion, life-promotion, piercing, wound-healing, intoxication, etc. Better known, however, is the list of eight potencies given in *SS*. Out of the twenty properties of substances, the following are selected to merit the name of potency (vīrya-saṁjñakāh) (*SS,* 1, 42; cf. also *CS,* 1, 26). Their effect on the doshas as well as on the general body condition are also indicated (*SS,* ibid.):

(1) cold (śīta): composed predominantly of 'earth' and 'water' elements, pacifies pitta but aggravates kapha and vāta; heavy, exhilarating, cooling, moistening, arresting the flow of secretions, cleansing, life-promoting, and acting like a tonic;

(2) hot (ushṇa) composed predominantly of 'fire'; pacifies kapha and vāta, but aggravates pitta; light, heating, digestive, causing loss of consciousness, producing thirst, causing vertigo and depression, decreasing semen, helping purgation, diaphoresis, and emesis;

(3) sticky or greasy (snigdha): composed predominantly of 'water'; pacifies vāta; oleation, bulk-increasing; promoting sexual vigour, preventing old age, and providing satiation;

(4) dry or parched up (rūksha): composed predominantly of 'air'; pacifies kapha and aggravates vāta; astringent, roughening, and healing;

(5) heavy (guru): composed predominantly of 'earth' and water'; pacifies vāta; anointing, bulk-increasing, filling, promoting union, increasing sexual vigour and production of semen;

(6) light (laghu): composed predominantly of 'fire', 'air' and ākāśa; pacifies kapha; roughening, fluid-absorbing, healing, emaciating (reducing fat and body-weight);

(7) soft (mṛdu): composed predominantly of 'water' and ākāśa; pacifies pitta; saturates and clears blood and muscle; softening; and

(8) sharp (tīkshṇa): composed predominantly of 'fire'; pacifies kapha; constipates, promotes secretions, tearing.

SS is found to mention slimy (picchila) and clear or pellucid (viśada), instead of heavy (guru) and light (laghu); and this reading is regarded as better by CHKP, *NiS* and HEMĀDRI. Slimy is composed predominantly of 'water'; it pacifies kapha; it dries up, roughens and heals wounds. Pellucid is composed predominantly of 'earth' and 'air'; it is anointing, filling, joining, and is an aphrodisiac.

The view that there are only two potencies, hot (ushṇa) and cold (śīta) (*AS,* 1.17 and *AHṛ,* 1, 9) is very popular. Derived from the basic outlook that the entire world is mainly constituted by the twin principles of fire (or sun) and moon (agnī-shomīya), all the material things in the world are accommodated in dichotomous classifications like the sun and moon, pitta and kapha (vāta being only a yoga-vāhī, because of its vikshepa quality);

[*See* DOSHA], menstrual blood and semen, etc. Basically, there are only two prevailing properties of substances: hot (ushṇa) and cold (śīta), the former being principally composed of 'fire', and the latter of 'earth' and 'water'; the former representing the pitta group of entities and activities in the body and the latter the kapha group. Accordingly the potencies are generally either hot or cold.

The drugs of cold potency (śīta-vīrya) are sweet in taste (rasa) and sweet in the final transformation of taste after digestion (vipāka), like madhu-yashti (*Glycyrrhiza glabra*). On the other hand, the drugs of hot potency (ushṇa-vīrya) are sour and pungent in taste as well the final transformation of taste after digestion, like haridrā (*Curcuma longa*). However, there are some exceptions to this general law.

Potency is an important consideration in Indian pharmacology. It is considered a more significant detail than either the property of the drug, or the taste, for it is said to suppress the other details and accomplish its end (*SS,* 1, 40). In fact the drugs are prescribed and taken only because of their potency; a drug that has no potency (nirvīrya) is utterly useless (*RVS,* 1, 131). The earliest texts of Indian medicine have recognized the importance of potency in the drugs (ibid., 1, 140).

There is a view which recognizes two varieties in potency: (1) which can be rationally explained on the basis of properties, tastes etc. of substances, and in accordance with the principle of cause-effect relation (chintya); and (2) which can only be empirically recognized and not explained rationally (achintya). The latter is also called 'specific effect' (prabhāva) (*SS, RVS*) [*See* PRABHĀVA]. [*See also* GUṆA,VIPĀKA].

Powder: Called chūrṇa (also rajas or kshoda; safūf in Yunāni), it is a pulver or powder of crude drugs, meant to be administered internally. It is the dry variety of paste (śushka-kalka). Dry substances with active ingredients are reduced to a fine powder by pounding them well in a mortar with a pestle, and then the powder is sieved in a piece of fine cloth. It may be a single drug that is involved, or several of them. When several drugs are to be mixed, each drug must be powdered separatcly, but finally mixed altogether so that a perfectly homogenous and amorphous mass is got. In powders, the method of mixing is an important detail. And no active principle of any of the drugs used must be lost (cf. *SaS* II,6,1).

Because powders are bulky preparations and of rather complex nature, they take considerable time to act. Therefore, only those drugs whose active principles are easily soluble are selected. The substances that enter into the powder must be freshly procured and well cleansed; they must also be in a perfectly dry state. Substances which are old, stored for a long time, which have lost their original colour, taste or scent, and which are infested with insects are to be avoided. However, there are some substances which gain in merit as they are stored for long periods, provided they are preserved well (for example, embelia, long-pepper, coriander seeds, jaggery, honey, ghee).

In order to enhance the action of the active principles of the drugs in the powder, it is usual to add sugar, jaggery, common salt, rock-salt etc; the powder is also made more palatable thereby. When jaggery is added, its proportion must be the same as that of the powder, but if sugar is added, the proportion of sugar to powder should be 2:1. If hingu (*Ferula foetida*)) is to be added, it must first be fried slightly in ghee (*SaS,* ibid.)

It is important to select the proper vehicle (anupāna) to go with the powder, for it will enhance the action of the drug by quickly pervading all over the system. (cf. *SaS,* II,6,4 and 5), (*See* ANUPĀNA]. Water, milk, honey and ghee are the usual vehicles. Lemon juice and juice of pomegranate are also recommended in some cases, to enhance the action of the powder. When honey or ghee is used as the vehicle, it must be double the quantity of the powder; and when the powder is administered in a fluid (water, milk, or fruit-juice), the fluid must be four times the quantity.

If the powder is preserved well, its potency will remain unabated for two months, and thereafter it will gradually diminish until about a year; after a year, the powders become ineffective. [*See* PREPARATIONS]

Prabhāva: That by which a drug becomes specifically effective, in quite a different manner from other drugs which have the same pharmacological details (like property, taste, potency, final transformation of taste after digestion) as this one (*CS,* 1,26; and *AHṛ,* 1,9 'rasādisāmye yat karma viśishṭam'; Viśishta is explained as an overriding power in the substance, 'sarvātiśāyinī dravya-śaktih', also *AS,* 1,17). The example given is the differential action of dantī (*Beliospermum montanum*) and chitraka (*Plumbago zeylanica*), both of which are alike pungent in taste (rasa) as well as in final transformation after digestion (vipāka), and hot in potency (vīrya); but the former is purgative in action, while the latter is not.

The peculiar factor present in one drug and absent in other drugs of similar pharmacological description, and producing an unexpected effect is regarded as 'inexplicable' or 'imponderable' (achintya or anavadhāraṇīya), for its presence or action cannot be ascertained by any rational processes (like direct observation, inference on the basis of cause-effect relationship, invariable concomitance of properties, physical constitution, or chemical composition of the drug). Nevertheless, its presence or action can empirically be established.

The drug's power to act (śakti) is two-fold: (1) that which can rationally be understood (chintya); and (2) that which cannot be so understood (achintya). The former is known as 'potency' (vīrya), while the latter 'specific power' (prabhāva). The specificity in the latter is something which cannot be inquired into (amīmāmsya), which cannot be thought about (achintya), but something that is well-known as the very nature of the thing: its effect is available for observation, and its operation is evident. Therefore, this factor must be understood by the physician, and utilized by him only by traditional wisdom (scriptural authority, āgama) or oral instruction by competent authority, (āptopadeśa) (*SS,* 1,140).

Sometimes, this inexplicable factor is classified under potency (vīrya), but as an unascertainable factor (anavadhāraṇīya) inherent in the collocation of tastes and properties but producing an unusual potency (*RVS,* 4,24). Among drug actions, many are directly derived from the known potency (vīrya-janya) (like facilitation of digestion, increasing bulk, etc.), but others are due to some potency that is unusual and uncanny (like pacification, intoxication, elimination of poison etc.) It is more usual, however, to regard this inexplicable factor as the very nature of a drug (dravya-svabhāva) (*CS, AS,* etc.).

Drugs are grouped into two types: (1) the drugs the pharmacological actions of which are due to evident physical or chemical constitution, and are in accord with well-defined rules (samāna-pratyayārabdha); and (2) the drugs the pharmacological actions of which cannot readily be explained and are in the nature of exceptions to the general rule (vichitra-pratyaya). Some drugs act by their tastes, some by their digestive transformations, some by their properties, and some by their potencies. But there are some drugs that act by none of these, and in such cases the suggestion is that it is the prabhāva that is active (*AHr,* 1,9).

In Indian therapeutics, there are several cures which defy rational explanation. For instance, how poison antidotes poison (organic poison counteracting inorganic poison, and inorganic poison organic) is not readily explained; but that it does, is not doubted. Two drugs of similar pharmacological properties, madhu-yashṭi (*Glycyrrhiza glabra*) and mrdvīka (*Vitis vinifera*) are mysteriously divergent in action: the latter is a laxative, while the former is not. There are some drugs that cause vomiting or/and purgation, but the exact factor responsible for this action cannot be ascertained. Garlic (which is pungent in taste and in final transformation after digestion, unctuous, and heavy in potency) curiously does not aggravate kapha and vāta, but on the contrary pacifies them. And well known are the cures effected by precious stones (mani), sacred formulae (mantra), and wearing of certain herbs (like the root of apāmārga, *Achyranthes aspera*) in warding off evil influences and malefic stellar impact, removing poison from the system, eliminating burning sensations, and colic etc. All such cases are included in the category of inexplicable but specific potencies (*CS*,1,26; also cf. *RVS*, 1,132-140).

An attempt has recently been made to classify the action of this kind of specific potency: physical (like the extraction of foreign matter from the body by magnet, etc.), pharmacological (like emetics, purgatives, etc.), toxicological (anti-poison), bactericidal and vermicidal (anthelmintic), and spiritual (rituals, precious stones, etc.).

Prajñāparādha: Any action done (eating, exercise, sexual indulgence, conduct), bereft of intelligence, perseverance and mindfulness ('dhī-dhṛti-smrti-vibhrashtah karma', *CS*, śarīra, 1, 102 ff). It is to be avoided, because it will aggravate all the three doshas (vāta, pitta and kapha). An action done after the time it should have been done, or much sooner than it should be, or when it is not to be done at all, or executed in an improper manner (excessive, deficient or incorrect) is included in this category, as it is likely to become injurious (ahita) to the individual's body, mind, or both.

Examples given in *CS* (ibid., 102-108) include: suppression of natural urges, forcing the evacuations that are not ready, unnecessary show of strength, over-indulgence in sex, immodesty, enjoyment of unwholesome things, conduct improper for age, time, place or situation, company of wicked folk, neglect of regimen for health, undesirable emotions like greed, anger, jealousy, vanity and fear, intoxication and confusion. In all these cases, the defects of the mind (viz. rajas and tamas) are allowed to become dominant; and, thereby, the individual's intelligence (dhī), endurance (dhṛti) and memory (smṛti) get impaired. This, in turn, leads to unwholesome contact with the sense objects (asātmyārthasamyoga) which is the source of ailments and misery (*CS*, ibid., 98). [*See* ERRORS OF JUDGEMENT].

Prakṛti: The idea of original (pra) but inert nature, which is responsible for the effective (pra) production (kṛti) of all the details of the phenomenal world (pra karoti iti), as distinguished from the inactive but conscious spirit (purusha) [*See* PURUSHA] has been borrowed from the Sāṁkhya system [*See* SAMKHYA]. (*SS*, śarīra, 1,6). It is also called pradhāna ('important', 'chief') in the sense of being the main cause behind the world of evolution.

It is composed of three guṇas, sattva (white, knowledge, happiness, pra), rajas (red, activity, pain, kr), and tamas (dark, resistance or inertia, confusion, ti). Thus it is endowed with all the necessary and sufficient powers of production, preservation and dissolution of the phenomenal world. Mainly, it is the material cause of multiplicity (tattvāntaropādāṇa).

Usually it is regarded as eight-fold: (1) the original unmanifest condition (avyakta), when the three constituent guṇas are in a state of perfect balance (sāmyāvasthā); (2) the subsequent stage of the evolving principle (mahat, buddhi) which disturbs the balance and sets up activity by a preliminary and undifferentiated awareness (adhyavasāya) which however does not upset the unity of the unmanifest; (3) the subsequent stage of self-identified awareness (ahamkāra), which owns up the evolutionary direction, and brings about plurality (anekatva) and distinction between individual details of production (pṛthaktva), and which in the next stage would undergo a tripartite division into sattva-dominated (vaikārika), rajas-dominated (taijasa), and tamas-dominated (bhūtādi); (4-8) the five subtle, unmixed, discrete and primary forms of matter (tanmātra), represented by audition, touch, form, taste and smell (*CS,* śarīra, 1, 17, cf also CHKP on it).

There are sixteen modifications thereof (tanmātra): 10 organs (indriyāṇi), five of cognition, (viz. visual, auditory, tactile, olfactory and gustatory), five of action (viz. speech, hands, feet, organ of elimination and organ of procreation), objects of the five organs of cognition (vishaya, viz, form, sound, touch, smell and taste), and mind (which partakes of the nature of cognition as well as of action).

Thus are enumerated the twenty-four categories involved in prakṛti (*SS,* ibid., 6), which are all inert (achetana), and which are enlivened only by their conjunction of purusha, the twenty-fifth category (*SS,* ibid, 8). It is to be noted that according to Pañchaśikha, the purusha is included in the category of the unmanifest (avyakta) (cf. *HIP,* vol. I, p. 216, also cf. *CS,* śarīra, 1, 17).

The expression is also used in the sense of 'natural', 'innate', 'inherent' (svabhāva), as distinguished from 'deviant' 'disturbed', 'perverted' (vikṛti) (as for instance, in *CS,* vimāna, 5, 'the three doshas in their natural state help the body, while disturbed they bring about many diseases and torment the body' ; also ibid. 21, 1), 'tatra prakrtir uchyate svabhāvah', in the sense of 'untreated', 'original' or 'unprocessed' nature of drugs ('samskārādyakrtah', CHKP on it).

The expression has an extended use in the sense of constitution of individuals, dominated by one or the other of the three guṇas (sattva, rajas and tamas) or the three guṇas in a balanced state [*See* CONSTITUTION].

Prakṛti in the sense of natural disposition of the human being is classified into six groups : (1) according to the species (jātiprasakta) viz. natural to all human beings; (2) according to the family background (kula-prasakta), viz. natural to the social group one belongs to; (3) according to the place of one's birth and residence (deśānupātinī), that is, natural to territorial groups and climatic conditions prevailing in that territory; (4) according to the time (kālānupātinī), natural to seasonal changes; (5) according to the individual's age (vayonupātinī), for instance natural to boyhood, adolescence, youth and old age; and (6) according to one's own peculiar constitution (pratyātma-niyata), as for example, natural to the constitutional type one belongs to, innate tendencies, congenital disposition etc. [*See also* SĀMKHYA, PURUSHA, MIND, ORGANS].

Pramāṇa : The consideration of the means of correct apprehension or valid knowledge, occupies a significant position in all systems of Indian thought, philosophical, epistemological and medical. The topic has been especially discussed in the Nyāya school; and Āyurveda follows the discussions closely.

Valid knowledge (pramā) which has been referred to even in *RV* ('kāsīt pramā pratimā kim?', 10, 130, 3) has been defined as the apprehension of an object as it really is (Vātsyāyana). The Nyāya school is realistic and pragmatic in its general orientation, and credits the world outside human imagination with evident reality. To know the objects of the world as they are, is therefore an important involvement in this school. Cognitive experience must be definite, perfectly corresponding with objective details (unerring), and capable of resulting in successful activity in the practical world. Utility (pravṛtti-sāmarthya) as the test of truth is an assumption in the Nyāya school that is of great import. Validity of knowledge is determined or inferred only on the basis of how successfully we can act on it.

Valid knowledge is distinguished from invalid knowledge (apramā), viz. doubt, memory, error (illusion) and conjecture (hypothetical argument). Invalid knowledge presupposes the presence or operation of some limiting or distorting factor (dosha), like jaundice when things are seen as yellowish in colour, or distance which makes an object appear much smaller than it really is. Likewise, valid knowledge presupposes the operation of some facilitating factor (guṇa 'merit'). The presence of the facilitating factor is to be inferred. For each of the means of valid knowledge, there is a unique factor that is capable of generating knowledge that is not only veridical but practically valid *(Bhāshā-pariccheda)*.

Correct and useful knowledge of a thing depends upon the means that are employed to obtain such knowledge; what is measured depends upon the measure ('ṃānādhīnā meyasiddhih'). The means of valid knowledge is technically called 'pramāṇa' (pramā-karaṇam, 'instrument of pramā'). The means (or instrument) here is explained as 'unique cause' (asādhāraṇa-kāraṇa), that is, the special source of a particular valid knowledge. For a 'cause' to become an 'instrument', it should be unique (asādhāraṇa), and should have an active function (vyāpāra).

In the Nyāya school of thought, apprehension is an 'effect' like any other effect in the material world; and its production, like the production of any other object, is contingent upon the collocation (sāmagrī) of conscious and unconscious causes, which brings about an experience that is at once definite (asandigdha) and uncontradicted (avyabhichāri) (*Nyaya-mañjarī*). This particular collocation is called pramāṇa. It is in this sense that it is described as the cause of cognition ('upalabdhi-hetu'), or the evidence, or proof of the reality of an object.

There are ten possible instruments of valid knowledge: perception (pratyaksha), inference (anumāna), comparison (upamāna), verbal testimony (śabda), presumption (arthāpatti), non-perception (anupalabdhi), implication or equivalence (saṁbhava), legendary or traditional account (aitihya), gesture (cheshṭā) and elimination (pariśesha). The acceptance of these pramāṇas by different schools of thought in India depends on their particular philosophical orientations. The materialists (the Chārvākas) recognize only perception. The Vaiśeshika school recognizes inference in addition to perception; the Sāṁkhya system adds 'verbal testimony' to these two. The Nyāya thinkers recognize four pramāṇas, adding 'analogical reasoning' to the three accepted by the Sāṁkhya. Mīmāmsakas owing allegiance to the Prābhākara faction accept 'presumption' as the fifth, while Mīmāmsakas of the Kumārila faction accept, like the Vedāntins, six pramāṇas, adding 'non-perception' to the above. The followers of the legendary lore (paurāṇikas), naturally enough, accept 'legendary accounts' and 'implication' as additional sources to the above six.

The Nyāya school accepts four pramāṇas (viz. perception, inference, analogical reasoning and verbal testimony) as necessary, sufficient, and non-overlapping. Each of them has a peculiar causal collocation (sāmagrī), generating a specific species of knowledge, which manifests itself in a unique manner ('sāmagrī-bhedāc cha phala-bhedāc cha pramāna-bhedah', (*Nyāya-mañjarī*).

(1) Perception is knowledge brought about by the contact of sense-organs with their objects. Such knowledge is not only definite and unerring, but has a sense of immediacy or directness (sākshāt-pratīti).

The Nyāya system (like the Vaiśeshika and Jaina systems) recognizes six sense-organs, five of them external (visual, auditory, tactile, gustatory and olfactory), and one internal (mind). Accordingly, perceptual knowledge can be of six varieties;five external(sensory), and one internal (mental). While the sense-organs apprehend the appropriate details of external objects, the mind apprehends its own states (like desire, aversion, effort, pleasure, pain, cognition). The mind, called an 'internal organ', is not constituted (like the sense organs) by the material elements (earth, water, fire and air); nor is it limited (like again the sense-organs) to the cognitions of specific types (like visual, auditory etc). Its function is general, central, and integrative. [*See* MIND].

Perceptions are also classified into two types, depending on how the sense-organs function. Ordinary (laukika) perceptions entail the usual transaction between the sense-organ and the object present before it. They are of six types, as mentioned above, five sensory and one mental. Extraordinary (alaukika) perceptions, however, do not necessarily depend upon the confrontation of the objective detail in immediate time and space. They are of three types: universal apprehension (sāmānya-lakshaṇa), viz. knowledge of truths like 'all men are mortal'; apprehension by 'complication' (jñāna-lakshaṇa) like 'seeing' the fragrance of a flower, or like 'seeing' a snake in the rope; and intuitive apprehension (yoga-ja), viz. directly cognizing things which have been past, or which will come about in future, which are concealed, or of exceedingly minute size.

Perception is further grouped into (i) 'indeterminate' (nirvikalpaka) or primary and general cognition of the presence of an object, without however differentiating its details, (ii) determinate (savikalpaka), or cognition of an object as distinguished by details; and (iii) recognition (pratyabhijñā).

Perception is regarded as the most important of the pramāṇas, and as the ground on which other pramāṇas are based. Vātsyāyana argues that it is also superior to the other pramānas. [*See* NYĀYA]. Perception does not need the help of previous knowledge, or inference, or any manner of projection, or conjecture.

(2) Inference is apprehension of an object following (anu) some other knowledge, usually obtained by perception. This involves the process of reasoning on the basis of a 'middle term' (liṅga, also called hetu or sādhana). It involves relating a subject under consideration (paksha, minor term) with something that is sought to be established (sādhya, major term), through the relation of invariable concomitance (vyāpti). Inference usually takes the form of syllogistic reasoning in five steps: proposition (pratijñā), ascription of reason (hetu), an illustrative instance to represent a universal proposition (udāharaṇa), application to the issue on hand (upanaya), and conclusion (nigamana). It is important to note that in Indian logic, the dichotomy between induction and deduction is not recognized, and that the two reasoning processes are integrated in the formally valid syllogism.

Inferences are classified as those that are meant for one's own edification (svārtha), and those that are meant to be communicated to others (parārtha). The former group of inferences is informal, spontaneous, and pragmatic, while the latter assumes a formal syllogistic form. Three further subdivisions are made in the latter: reasoning from cause to effect (pūrva-vat) reasoning from effect to cause (śesha-vat), and reasoning based on common characteristics that are observed (sāmānyato-dṛshta).

(3) Comparison or analogical reasoning involves the obtainment of knowledge of a thing on the basis of its similarity with another thing already known. While most of the other systems of thought reject the independent validity of this means of knowledge,

the Nyāya thinkers have held fast to its value as a pramāṇa. The materialist Chārvākas are not inclined to concede analogy as a pramāṇa at all; the Buddhists, however, concede that it is a pramāna, but argue that it is little more than the conjoint operation of perception and verbal testimony. Vaiśeshikas and Sāṁkhya thinkers dispute its distinct character or its independent status; according to them, it is but a variety of inference. The Jaina logicians regard it as mere 'recognition'. The Mīmāmsakas and the Vedāntins, however, accept its independent status, but explain that the real process here is the recognition of likeness (sādṛśya-jñāna).

(4) Verbal testimony involves the employment of verbal knowledge as a means of correctly knowing an object. It is the knowledge derived from significant words and their organization in a sentence. The words (containing significative potency, śakti), in this case, must be in the form of instruction from a reliable authority (āptopadeśa). The idea of reliability proceeds on the assumption that the person who has direct and correct knowledge about the thing in question has also the desire and competence to communicate this knowledge to another. He may be, according to VĀTSYĀYANA, a sage (ṛshi) with direct intuitive understanding, a cultured and learned man (ārya), or an outsider (mléccha) who has knowledge of things in his own province. The three conditions necessary to make him a reliable authority are: knowledge of truth, communication that is truthful, and the desire to guide others *(Tārkika-rakshā)*.

Verbal authority is generally grouped into two types: secular (laukika) and scriptural (vaidika). The latter is perfect and infallible, while the former is not always valid. Again, what is communicated has been divided into ordinary things which may be verified immediately (dṛshṭārtha) and extraordinary prescriptions, predictions and promises (adṛshṭārtha).

Verbal knowledge is communicated through words whose meanings are defined by grammar, lexicons and popular usage (according to the Nyāya view), combined meaningfully in a sentence. The construction of a sentence becomes effective inasmuch as it satisfies four conditions (cf. *Bhāshā-pariccheda*): expectancy or mutual dependence of words in order to express the meaning of the sentence as a whole (ākāṅkshā), capacity of the words to accord with the sense of the sentence, and not contradict the total import (yogyatā), favourable proximity of constituent words (saṁnidhi), and the intended meaning (tātparya).

CHARAKA, following probably an older Nyāya tradition, postulates four pramāṇas, which he designates 'four-fold examination' ('chaturvidha-parīkshā', *CS*, sūtra, 11, 17): (1) instruction from a reliable authority (āptopadeśa); (2) perceptual knowledge (pratyaksha); (3) inference (anumāna); and (4) reasoning (yukti). While the first three are evidently the pramāṇas accepted by the Nyāya school (although in a different order), the fourth one is a new feature in Āyurveda. Further, the explanations given by CHARAKA for the first three pramāṇas are different from the usual explanations to be found in the Nyāya texts.

(1) Instruction from a reliable person is almost the same as the Nyāya 'verbal testimony' (śabda), to which a reference is made by the commentator, CHAKRAPĀṆI. The reliable person (āpta) is defined by CHARAKA as one who has completely rid himself of passion (rajas) and ignorance (tamas), by the power of penance and wisdom, who has developed unobstructed insight into the things in all the three segments of time (past, present and future), who is in conduct respectable (śishṭa, viz. who is in a position to guide mankind in the proper conduct, according to the commentary), and exceedingly knowledgeable (vibuddhah). His words are wholly trustworthy, for he always speaks truth. He cannot utter untruth, because he is

neither ignorant, nor prompted by passions (like desire and aversion). (*CS*, ibid., 18-19).

CHARAKA elsewhere in his work (vimāna, 4, 4,) refers to this pramāṇa. Āpta there is described as the person who is versatile and discerning, but free from prejudices and passions. It is therefore, that his words become authoritative. Contrarily, the words of the inebriated, the mentally unsound, the foolish or the wicked persons are not trustworthy. At another place (3, 8, 6) he includes legendary accounts (āitihya) under 'āptopadeśa'.

It is obvious that CHARAKA has in his mind trustworthy and competent human beings when he speaks of the āptas. He is concerned here with ordinary verbal testimony (laukika), and not scriptural authority (alaukika), although he refers to it (ibid., 27).

(2) Perception arises from direct association (saṁnikarsha) of the soul, sense-organs, mind, and the objects outside. The condition of four-fold ingredients in perception precludes experiences like pleasure and pain which are felt by the individual (commentary). Association (relation', saṁbandha, according to commentary of five kinds) is further explained as being definite (vyakta) and immediate (tadātva). Perceptual knowledge is thus distinguished from recollection and inference (*CS*, ibid, 20). Perceptual knowledge could either be sensory (visual etc) or mental (pleasures, pain, etc.) (*CS*, vimāna, 4, 4).

(3) Inference proceeds on the basis of perceptual knowledge, for the inferential process presupposes the apprehension of the middle term (hetu), whose invariable concomitance (vyāpti) is recognized only by perception. Three-fold is inference, contingent upon the time segment: (i) from the present effect to a past cause (for example, deducing sexual congress from the fact of pregnancy); (ii) from the present cause to a future effect (for example, deducing from the seed with facilitating factors the fruit which is yet to appear); and from a seen effect to the unseen cause, both in the present (like deducing from smoke the concealed fire). The order of the three types given here follows the commentary but CHARAKA'S own order would place the third here first. This bears some correspondence with the three-fold inference given in the standard Nyāya-texts: pūrva-vat, śesha-vat and sāmānyato-drshṭa (*CS*, ibid., 21-22).

(4) Reasoning is illustrated by the prediction of harvest on the basis of the conjoint operation of a ploughed field, water facility, seeds and the season, or the knowledge of the possibility of conception by the conjoint operation of the six constituents (viz. the five physical elements or primary forms of matter and the soul), or the knowledge of the production of fire by the conjoint operation of the stick, the contraption and the rubbing of the stick. The examples are directed towards clinical prognosis based on the conjoint operation of the four ingredients in medical practice (physician, patient, drug, and nurse) (*CS*, ibid., 23-24).

CHARAKA goes on to define 'reasoning' after these illustrations (verse 25). It is the intelligence (buddhi) that perceives a number of factors involved in a complex phenomenon; and reasoning functions in the three segments of time (past, present and future), and helps the individual attain the three goals of life (wealth, pleasures and spiritual welfare). The commentator calls it speculation or 'conjecture' (ūhā), based on the perception of relevant factors (causes, symptoms etc), and the consideration of their relationship. This has an obvious clinical context, and its refers to prognosis.

The commentater discusses the problem of how justified is the counting of 'yukti' among the pramāṇas. He concludes that it cannot truly be described as a pramāṇa (for it is only an inference of an effect from the causes), but argues that it facilitates the acquisition of valid knowledge, and that it is employed by all people in the form of practical and intelligent guesses and conjectures in daily life. According to him, the deduction of effect from the causes is not the relevant issue here, but the formulation of a conclusion on the basis of present conditions, by the employment of reasoning.

CHARAKA, later in his work (vimāna, 4, 3-4), refers to three pramāṇas as especially useful in understanding the diseased condition: (i) instruction from reliable authority (āptopadeśa) called aitihya (vimāna, 8, 41); (ii) perception (pratyaksha) got directly with the aid of the sense-organs; and (iii) inference (anumāna). And not only does he not enumerate 'reasoning' (yukti) as a separate pramāna, but he includes 'reasoning' along with logic (tarka) in the import of inference. The commentary explains 'logic' as non-perceptual knowledge, or apprehension of things not available for perception ('apratyaksham jñānam'), and 'reasoning' as the apprehension of invariant relationship ('saṁbandho avinābhāvah'). Elsewhere (vimāna, 8, 40), he states that inference relies on yukti.

While enumerating 'yukti' among the 'guṇas' (*CS,* sūtra, 26, 27-29), CHARAKA means by the term proper selection of medicines with reference to diseases ('doshādyapekshayā bheshajasya samīcīnakalpanā') [*See* YUKTI].

CHARAKA prescribes that the disease must be examined first by the total knowledge that arises from the employment of these three methods, and thereby, the disease must be faultlessly identified. He also gives the sequence by which the three methods must be employed: knowledge obtained by reliable persons (viz. medical treatises and experts), then knowledge obtained by actual observation, and finally inference. He also discusses the value of other factors and methods: doubts (samśaya), analogical reasoning (aupamya), purpose in view (prayojana), inquiry (jijñāsā), determination (vyavasāya), presumption (arthapatti), and hypothetical reasoning (saṁbhava) (cf. vimāna, 8, 39-49).

Prāṇa : Usually translated as 'vital air', 'life', 'body wind', 'respiration', 'breath' etc., it is in no sense identical with, or an evolutionary product of air (vāyu), as it came to mean in later Indian thought. In the Sāṁkhya school, on which the basic ideas of Indian medicine are based, it is a biomotor force, principally the action of the sense-organs (cf. Vijñānāmṛta-bhāshya, 2, 4, 10): "it is neither air (na vāyuh) nor the upward or downward air-current (ūrdhvādho-lakshana-vāyukriyā") (ibid., 9).

In Sāṁkhya, prāṇa is an evolute of prakṛti [*See* PRAKṚTI], and is identical with the mahat category. In its cognitive and assimilative aspects, it is called buddhi, while in its aspect of activity it is known as prāna: it is the power to initiate movements. It is referred to as vāyu, only because it shares with air the power of initiating movement. The so-called five vāyus ('winds in the body', prāṇa, apāna, udāna, samāna and vyāna) are many functions of the mahat in this aspect. The other categories, viz. buddhi (individualized consciousness occurring as resolve, intention), ahamkāra (ego), and manas (mind) are energies, each functioning in its own way, but all cooperating with each other; and this joint operation of the three categories is tantamount to the five-fold prāṇa which upholds the body (cf. GAUDAPĀDA on *SK,* 29).

The three categories (together called antah-karana, 'inner instrument') build up and maintain the bodily systems in the presence of the purusha, through the five activities, called prāṇas: (1) prāṇa as 'forward or exhaling air', pervading the whole organism from the tip of big toe through the navel and heart to the tip of the nose; (2) apāna as the 'downward or inhaling air', prevailing in the heart, back, ribs, intestinal canal, sex-organs and legs; (3) samāna as the 'equalizing air'' prevailing in the heart, navel and the joints and helping digestion and assimilation; (4) udāna as the 'ascending air', prevailing in the heart, throat, palate, skull and between the eye-brows; and (5) vyāna as the 'pervading breath', diffused throughout the organism and effective in circulation and distribution of vital substances in the body.

The prāṇa is regarded as a collective expression for 'fire' (pitta-agni), 'moon' (kapha, soma), 'wind' (vāta, vāyu), sattva, rajas, tamas, the five sense-organs (indriya) and the empirical soul (bhūtātmā) (*SS*, śarīra, 4, 2). [*See* SAṀKHYA].

Prapāka: Name given to digestion in the gastro-intestinal tracts (*CS*, 6, 15, 9-11). The prefix 'pra' in the expression signifies 'first' or preliminary (prathama, adikarmaṇi, CHKP on above). This is as distinguished from vipāka (or nishṭhā-pāka), or assimilation of food after the digestive process is completed. [*See* VIPĀKA, DIGESTION). This is more familiarly known as avasthā-pāka (CHKP on *CS*), for the six tastes of the food eaten are 'settled' into three digestive tastes, sweet, sour and pungent in three successive stages, [*See* AVASTHĀPĀKA].

Pratyaksha: Observational data derived by the individual as a result of actual contact of the sense-organs with their respective objects. They are of two types: (1) made available directly to the individual self (ātma-pratyaksha, viz. without the medium of the senses, purely mental), like happiness, misery, desires etc; and (2) made available through the sensory pathways (indriya-pratyaksha), viz. sounds, forms etc. (*CS*, vimāna, 8, 39). [*See* PRAMĀṆA).

Prayojana : Purpose or intended object of any undertaking like medical treatment. The patient, while taking medicines, deliberates: "Although untimely death is possible, I shall get better and prolong my life by taking these medicines" (*CS*, vimāna, 8, 44).

Precious stones: The employment of precious stones (maṇi or ratna) for religious, occult, and therapeutic purposes is ancient (cf. *Bṛhat-saṁhitā* of VARĀHAMIHIRA, *Vishṇu-dharmottara-purāṇa, Agni-purāṇa, Garuda-purāṇa, Ratna-śāstra* of AGASTYA, Yukti-kalpa-taru of BHOJA etc.). The precious stones are also used in the preparation of mercury and mercurial medicines. The preparations are meant to cure and prevent diseases and senile decay (rasāyana).

Of the numerous precious stones known and used, the well-known are:(1) diamond (vajra), which prolongs life, increases digestive power, pacifies all three doshas and enhances vitality (vṛshya); (2) emerald (marakata), which when properly incinerated cures fever, nausea, asthma, abnormal excess of the three doshas (sannipāta), swelling of the body, loss of digestive power, piles, poison and anemia; (3) ruby (māṇikya), padma-rāga being its best variety, which when purified and incinerated increases digestive power, removes the excess of kapha and vāta, cures the wasting diseases, eliminates the occult evil influences (bhūta, vetala), and antidotes all diseases caused by the previous inimical karma; (4) pearl (muktā), with several varieties such as 'elephant', 'hog', 'serpent', 'fish', 'frog', conch, oyster, etc, is generally cool and beneficial to the eye-sight; it pacifies the excess of vāta and pitta, removes inflammation, cures all digestive troubles (especially pearls of aquatic origin, viz. 'fish', conch and oyster), acts as a laxative, increases vitality, promotes longevity and antidotes poison; (5) garnets (vaikrānta) of different colours, angles and facets, which promote longevity, pacify all the three doshas, increase digestive power, cure many diseases, especially leprosy and phthisis, and strengthen the body; (6) quartz (sphatika), in several varieties, which, being balanced in potency (sama-vīrya, viz. neither too cold nor too hot) cures pitta, inflammation, impurities of blood, and wasting diseases (water kept in a quartz container pacifies pitta); (7) coral (pravāla), also in many varieties, which cures phthisis, haemorrhage, cough, eye- diseases, poison and indigestion; (8) topaz (pushyarāga), which cures nausea, indigestion, inflammation, haemorrhage, leprosy, and antidotes poison and excess of kapha and vāta; (9) lapis lazuli (rājāvarta), which prevents senile decay; (10) Zercon (gomeda), which is beneficial in wasting diseases, anemia, excess of kapha and pitta, skin troubles, loss of appetite, indigestion, and brain fatigue; (11) oriental cat's eye (vaiḍūrya), in three varieties, 'yellowish-black' (like the green bamboo leaf), 'reddish blue' (like the peacock's neck), and 'whitish black' (like the cat's eye), which cures haemorrhage, diseases principally caused by pitta, and difficulties in elimination of waste products from the body; and which promotes intelligence, strength and longevity.

Among the precious stones, five (pañcha-ratna) are regarded as therapeutically superior: diamond, emerald, ruby (the padmarāga variety), sapphire, and topaz. Nine of the stones (nava-ratna) are associated with the nine planets (nava-graha), whose movements are said to influence the health of people: ruby-Sun; pearl-Moon; coral-Mars; emerald-Mercury;topaz-Jupiter; diamond-Venus; sapphire-Saturn; zercon-Rāhu; and cat's-eye-Ketu.

Preventive Medicine: Indian medicine attaches great importance to the conduct, methods, and devices by means of which sound health is maintained, promoted, and corrected before it is greatly impaired. The context in which this subject is treated is 'preventive medicine' (rogānutpādanīya) (*CS*, sūtra, 1, 7; *AHṛ*. 1, 4 and *SS*, Uttara, 55). The assumption is that prevention (anutpatti) is better than cure (śānti) (*AHr*. 1, 4, 34); treating the disease in its early stages is better than grappling with it when it has advanced.

It is usual for Indian medical texts to contain sections entitled 'rogānutpādaṇīya' (e.g. *AHr*, 1, 4), which means 'non-occurrence of diseases'. *CS*, however, does not contain a separate section on this subject, but deals with the problem under the heading 'non-suppression of natural physiological tendencies' ('na-vegāṁ-dhāraṇīya', sūtra, 1, 7,). One who is given to suppression of natural tendencies of the body cannot possibly attend to the right conduct to Health (svastha-vrtta); and hence he would be unable to prevent diseases (*SsA* on *AHr*, 1, 4, introduction). *CS* makes it clear that medicine should concern itself not only with eliminating the diseases when they actually occur, but more importantly with prescriptions for the non-occurrence of diseases.

Prevention of diseases is considered under five heads: (1) suppression of natural bodily impulses (vega-dhāranā); (2) excessive and forced discharge of these impulses (vega-udīranā); (3) periodical cleansing of the system (śodhana) by throwing out the errant doshas that have got into the body constitutents and circulatory systems; (4) promoting health and energy (brmhana), depending on the digestive power (agnibala) of the person; and (5) non-contact with injurious influences (bhūtādyasparśana) such as evil spirits, poison, fire, accidents etc. Of the five, (1) and (2) are to be avoided (hāna), and the others resorted to (upādāna). By the avoidance of total suppression and excessive discharge of the natural tendencies, the causes for diseases are prevented from appearing (prāgabhāva); by cleansing the system often and taking tonics for enhancement of health and efficiency, the existent causes of diseases are eliminated in their early stages (pradhvamsa) and other causes are prevented from occurring (prāgabhāva) (*Ad* on *AHṛ* 1, 4, prefatory sentence, *NS* ed., p. 52). The fifth kind of prevention is by prayer, propitiation, rituals, etc.

There is thus an employment of prophylactic and curative measures in 'preventive medicine' as envisaged by Indian medical authorities. But these drugs and methods are not considered as specific to diseases which are dealt with in sections on the medicine proper (bheshaja). They are considered as pertaining to the causation of diseases in general (hetu). And they are dealt with alongside prescriptions of proper food, exercise, conduct etc. (cf. *Ad,* op. cit.).

Preventive medicine in the West has a history of not more than two hundred years, and is largely a matter of the preventive needle (vaccination and inoculation) against infective diseases like small pox, diphtheria, measles, whooping cough, tetanus, and prevention of deficiency diseases. Its foundation is the detection and identification of potential causes of diseases together with the knowledge of nutrition and diet. Indian medicine, on the other hand, has an ancient reliance on preventive aspects of medicine, but its concern has not been so much with the prevention of specific diseases as with positive and general health. Its foundation is the understanding of natural health, and its prescriptions are not drugs but right conduct.

Among the measures for preventing ill-health, four have general relevance (1) cleansing and evacuative processes (saṁśodhana); (2) measures to pacify and correct the doshas and dhātus (saṁśamana); (3) diet, and drugs taken as food (āhāra) and (4) correct conduct and regimen (āchāra). In addition to these, prayers, propitiations, expiations and spiritual practices are also recommended to be employed alongside the above, to ward off evil influences that may bring about diseases. [*See also* HYGIENE. HEALTH. SUPPRESSION OF URGES. DAILY ROUTINE. FOOD].

Pulse:[*See* NĀḌĪ].

Purusha: The inactive but conscious principle (chetanā) as the necessary factor in the production, preservation, growth and dissolution of the phenomenal world is distinguished from the active but inert principle of prakṛti which is the material out of which the phenomenal world is constituted [*See* PRAKṚTI]. While the older Sāṁkhya (represented by Pañchaśikha and adopted in *CS*) includes both the original state of prakṛti and the purusha in the same category of 'the unmanifest' (avyakta) and thus recognizes only twenty-four categories [*See* SĀṀKHYA], later Sāṁkhya (represented by *SK,* adopted in *SS*) recognizes purusha as the twenty-fifth category (for example, *SS,* śarīra, 1, 8).

The assumption of purusha (from puri śete, 'lies in the body') was necessitated because the assemblage of material objects, presupposes the fulfilment of the purpose of an intelligent being (who also guides and superintends the assemblage) which is two-fold: 'enjoyment' (bhoga) and 'isolation' (kaivalya). (*SK,* cf. GAUDAPĀDA on it). Purusha is also called 'kshetrajña' ('one who is aware of the field of action and cognition, viz. the body'), where the 'kshetra' (the field) is in a state of conglomeration.

In Āyurveda, the term purusha is employed both in the sense of the transcendental spirit (uncaused, eternal, unevolving and untainted), as in Sāṁkhya philosophy, and also in the sense of the empirical individual (rāśi-purusha) as the upholder of the sense organs and the experiencer of pleasures and pains. *SS* (śarīra,1 1, 22) defines purusha as a conglomeration of the five primary forms of matter (earth, water, fire, air and ākāśa) and the spirit that possesses the body (viz. ātman, 'pañcha-mahābhūta-śarīri-samavāyah purushah'). *CS* (śarīra, 1, 16) describes purusha in general as comprising of the above five primary forms of matter together with consciousness as the sixth constituent (dhātu), and specifies that this factor alone can be construed as consciousness. It is the unmanifest aspect (avyakta) of prakṛti, which coordinates (as nothing else can do 'yoga-dharam param') the faculty of individuated but undifferentiated consciousness (buddhi), sense-organs (indriya), mind (manas) and objects of sensory experience (artha) (ibid., 35) These constitute the twenty-four categories, the dynamic organization of which is the purusha ('chaturvimśatiko hy esha rāśih purusha-saṁjñakah'). This organization endures as long as rajas (activity) and tamas (resistance) last; and it is sattva (knowledge) that frees the purusha from the hold of rajas and tamas (ibid., 36).

In this organizational construct called purusha are founded the phenomenal processes such as life, knowledge, ignorance, activity, the results of activity, happiness, misery, appropriation of objects etc. (ibid. 37). Purusha is the real cause of all activities, equipped with instruments such as the sense-organs (ibid. 49) and its existence is empirically relevant, as it is the conglomerate that is engendered by ignorance, intentions and aversions unlike the Soul that is beyond (ibid. 53). [*See also* ĀTMAN, PRAKṚTI, SĀṀKHYA].

R

Rajas: Derived from rañj 'to colour' (and hence rāga, 'red'), the word denotes passion, impurity (dust, or dry mud floating in the air and clouding the sky as well as vision), and obscuration. More specifically, however, it signifies activity and change at the phenomenal level: it is a matter of 'becoming' (contrary to sattva, which is 'being'), constant mutation of things which obscures their real nature (distinguished from sattva, which reveals and shines forth). The word is frequently used for vapour, mist, and clouded atmosphere, as well as for passion, emotion, affection,

One of the three guṇas of prakṛti (other two being sattva and tamas), it is responsible for the variety of things and events in the world and for the manifold structure and function of the human constitution. It also determines personality types by its dominance, and the energetics in life.

In the sense of 'red' and 'impurity', the word is employed to signify the menstrual discharge in women (hence rajah-srāva, rajo-darśana, rajo-nivrtti). [*See* SĀṀKHYA, GUṆA, CONSTITUTION, PRAKṚTI].

Rakta: One of the seven body constituents (dhātu), the red fluid (or blood) is the most important among them, after chyle (rasa). It is regarded as the very basis of life (jīvanaṁ). Imbalance in the nature or normal quantity of blood in the body (which, according to *CS*, is eight añjali) has an impact on the nature or quantity of the other constituents (including chyle). Loss of blood would necessarily lead to the degeneration of other constituents.

Blood is formed when the subtle aspect of the cool (saumya) chyle (transparent extract of extreme fineness) reaches the liver (yakṛt) and spleen (pliha) during its course of circulation all over the body. There, it becomes subjected to the heating action of pitta (ranjaka-pitta), and acquires a red colour. The normal colour of blood is likened to that of ruby, cochineal (indragopa insect), lac-dye or guñjā-seed (*Abrus precatorius*). It is unctuous, warm, heavy, fluid, saline, and sweet in taste (*SaS*, 1, 6). Its principal seat is the liver-and-spleen, which is also the seat of pitta. Like the other constituents, blood is made up of all five primary forms of matter, although it is predominantly 'fire' (tejas). Accordingly, its properties are: raw (fleshy smell; owing to the earth ingredient), fluid (water), red (fire), light (air) and mobile (ākāśá).

Its main function is to nourish other constituents, provide physical strength, vitalize, and maintain the normal activities of life; it also endows on the body the natural glow of complexion. Its specific action is to reinforce (pushti) the immediately succeeding constituent, viz. flesh (māmsa), during the course of being cooked in its own 'fire' (rasāgni) [*See* DHĀTU]. Blood has two aspects: the concrete aspect that is blood itself, and the subtle aspect which inclines towards flesh. The secondary constituents (upadhātu) that are caused by blood are blood-tendons (kandara) and blood-vessels (sirā). Blood reaches all parts of the body through the blood-carrying channels [*See* SROTAS].

Blood may be spoiled by one, two, or all three of the doshas. If it is spoiled by vāta, blood becomes frothy, pink,tending towards black in colour, devoid of its natural unctuous property, thin like water, quick-flowing, and hard to congeal. If pitta is the spoiling agent, blood would turn yellowish, bluish or dark greenish, become thin, emit foul smell, and become hard to congeal; ants and flies would be expelled from it. If kapha is responsible for the spoiling, blood would be thick, glossy, unctuous, cold, and sluggish. If all three doshas together are the spoiling agents, blood would appear like water in which rice has been washed (sour gruel); and it may have many of the characteristics mentioned above.

Spoilt blood leads to a variety of diseases; inflammation of the mouth, eyes and nose, pimples, stomatitis, swelling of body, jaundice, erysipelas, abscess, leprosy, indigestion, irritability, insanity, skin diseases, enlargement of spleen, phantom tumour, ring worm, scabies, rashes, black and blue moles, freckles, haemorrhage through different channels in the body, red circular patches etc. If blood is in excess, flushing of the face, redness of the eyes, filling of the blood-vessels to their fullest capacity etc. are symptoms; if, on the other hand, there is decrease in the quantity of blood, loss of consciousness may result. [*See also* BLOOD, DHĀTU].

Rasa: Translated variously, but often misleadingly, as lymph ('sap', used since 1830), chyle ('juice', used since 1841), and plasma ('colourless liquid part of blood', used since 1845), rasa (from root ras, 'to move', 'gatau') refers to the food-essence and body-sap. It is regarded as the first and most important among the seven body constituents (dhātu, *See* DHĀTU). This is held to be the very source of all vital functions of the organism.

It is defined as 'the substantial but extremely fine aspect of the food that is properly digested, which partakes of the nature of fire (tejas): (*SS,* sūtra, 14, 3).

It is derived from the food that we eat. As the food is digested by the 'stomachic fire' (jātharāgni), the substantial portion (sāra), being separated from the waste-products (mala, urine and faecal matter), reaches the heart (which is the main centre of rasa) as 'the sustaining fluid'. From there it is circulated to all parts of the body through twenty-four channels (dhamanī, 10 going upward, 10 downward and 4 across), prompted by the forms of the wind in the body (vāta).

Its general purpose is to nourish the body, more especially the other body constituents (dhātus, blood, flesh, fat-tissue, bone-tissue, marrow and sperm). Circulating throughout the body, it has a soothing effect on the entire system and causes a systemic feeling of well-being (prīnana) and absence of tension (tushti). (*SS,* ibid, 7). Being itself the food-essence, it provides nutrition to all the cells of the body.

Its specific function is to feed the blood by its own subtle aspect. Each of the body constituents has a gross aspect and a subtle aspect. The gross aspect is the nature of the constituent itself, while the subtle aspect is contributory to the succeeding constituent. Blood (rakta) is the constituent that comes after rasa. The gross aspect of rasa is the fluid itself (chyle, lymph, plasma). But as it is 'cooked' in its 'fire' (dhātu-agri, *See* DHATU, AGNI) it is tranformed into its subtle aspect, viz. blood, at the end of five days (or 3015 kalā), and successively into other constituents until it is transformed into sperm (śukra, in men and ovum in women) at the end of one month (18, 090 kalā). When the watery rasa enters the liver and spleen, it turns red, and that is what we call blood.

SS (sūtra, 14, 12) holds that the entire constitution is ultimately derived from this transparent and extremely subtle fluid, which is the unseen cause (adṛshṭa-hetukena karmaṇā) of all physiological and psychological functions. Its movement in the body is likened to the horizontal spread of sound, the upward rising of the flame of fire, and the descending flow of water (ibid, 15, 17).

The obesity of the body and emaciation are alike due to this factor (ibid., 15, 38). One who habitually eats food which increases kapha, eats when the previously eaten food has not been digested, sleeps during daytime, or does not exercise his limbs sufficiently gets the food inside the stomach ill-digested; the food-extract is therefore transformed into a serum of sweet taste. When this fluid circulates in the body, because of its unctuous quality, it increases the fat-tissues beyond normal proportions, leading to obesity. The obese person is weak and incapable of much work, owing to excessive accumulation of kapha and fat-tissue. Therefore, the condition hinders the proper transformation into other successive constituents. Likewise emaciation of body is due to food which aggravates vāta, excessive manual labour, loss of sleep at night, insufficient intake of food, anxiety, grief etc. The food-extract is therefore parched up and robbed of nutritive elements. Bodily strength gradually diminishes (ibid., 15, 37).

It is this chyle that nourishes not only the immediately next constituent, viz. blood, but all the other constituents. There are two views in this context. One view is that the chyle nourishes blood, blood nourishes flesh, and so on, successively. The other view is that the main nourishing factor is the chyle alone, although the succession of constituents is not affected. The former view, acceptable to *CS*, offers the illustration of milk getting transformed into curds, curds into butter, butter into ghee etc., (kshīra-dadhi-nyāya). The latter view offers the illustration of the one water-canal being utilized to irrigate the entire stretch of a field (kedārī-kulya-nyāya); the areas near the source are watered first, and the more distant areas, in due course. This view appears acceptable to *SS*. However, both views emphasize the primary role of chyle, and concede the successive formation of the seven constituents.

An increase or decrease in the quantity of chyle would lead to metabolic disturbances. Increase of chyle manifests itself in excessive salivation and nausea, and decrease of chyle in cardiac pain, palpitation, tremor, weakness, abnormal thirst, and a feeling of emptiness.

Other ailments directly related to abnormalities of chyle include anorexia, distaste for food, bad taste in the mouth, inability to taste (agnosia), nausea, heaviness of limbs, drowsiness, body-ache, fever, fainting, pallor, obstruction of channels (śroto-rodha), impotence, wasting of body, loss of digestive power, premature formation of wrinkles, premature greying of hair.

In old age, the chyle (because of the aging of the physiological mechanisms) helps only to support the body and does not nourish the other constituents. (*SS*, sūtra, 14, 19). [*See also* DHĀTU].

Rasaliṅga: The mercurial icon to be installed and worshipped in the metallurgical and alchemical laboratories (rasa-śālās) on their eastern side. Pure gold lead, one and a half kola (one kola = half a tola, or about 63 grains) in weight, mixed with mercury, three times its weight, are rubbed for a yāma (about three hours) with some vegetable juice, sour in taste. The kneaded mass is fashioned into the form of a liṅga and put inside a lemon fruit, which is then boiled in gruel in a dolā-yantra for twenty-four hours. It is then taken out and installed for worship as the fiery goddess (Āgneyī) who brings prosperity (Śrīh).

The icon thus prepared is regarded as a composite symbol of the male (Śiva, white in colour, five-headed; three-eyed and with eighteen arms, seated on a corpse) and the female (golden-hued devī, clad in yellow garments, single-headed; with four-arms; holding rosary, goad and noose in three hands and suggesting protection by the fourth hand, seated on Śiva's lap) as parents of the universe and as the progenitor and patron-deity of the science of alchemy. The female aspect of this icon is known as Rasānkuśī (cf. *RJN*).

Rasāyana: [*See* REJUVENATION]

Rational Medicine : Cures effected in Indian medicine are broadly grouped into the two varieties: cures by invoking supernatural intervention (daiva-vyapāśraya), and cures by the employment of rational methods such as proper food and suitable drugs (yukti-vyapāśraya). This classification is ascribed to Atri-putra (*CS*, sūtra, 11, 54). The main stream of Indian therapeutics, however, belongs to the latter variety. Great importance is attached to the utilization of his rational faculties by the physician, both for understanding the causes and the nature of diseases, and for deciding upon the proper course of treatment. The theory of causality plays a significant role in Indian medicine, especially in the branch of pathology (nidāna).

Utilization of rational faculties is known as yukti, and has been accorded a special place in the medical consideration of means of valid knowledge (pramāna). Besides the usual objective sources of information (viz. observation, inference and analogy), yukti, (rational application) is regarded as having an independent value by CHARAKA. While his commentator is not prepared to accept that it is an independent means of knowledge, he explains that it is more than inference: it is not merely ascertaining the effect from the examination of the cause, but the formation of a judgement, or the arrival at a conclusion on the basis of numerous related reasonings (*CS*, sūtra, 11, 25). [*See* PRAMĀNA, YUKTI].

In this sense it is more than inference; in fact, inference is dependent upon 'rational application' (ibid., 3, 4, 6). When the physician's intelligence perceives a fact after careful consideration of numerous antecedent conditions, cause-effect sequences and related factors, he may then be able to make valid and effective judgements in order to facilitate the fulfilment of the three-fold purposes of life (viz. spiritual well-being, wealth, and satisfaction of mundane desires). This is described by CHARAKA as 'rational application' (yukti) (1, 11, 25). It is not just a species of empirical reasoning but an organized intellectual endeavour, a methodical device for discovering hidden relationships among several factors and for explaining how an effect is conjointly brought into being (ibid., 23 and 24).

It is also a careful and purposeful employment of a drug, or of a method of treatment. CHARAKA points out that the names and curative values of many herbs may be known to hunters, cowherds, shepherds, forest-dwellers and lay-folk, but that this can hardly match, or render unnecessary, the pharmacological wisdom of physicians. The physician's knowledge of the natural substances (dravyas) should be more valuable inasmuch as it comprehends not only an acquaintance with the precise properties of the natural substances (herbs, etc.), but also how, in what manner, when (kāla, time of day, season etc.), and in what measure (dosage, mātrā) they ought to be administered.

The physician's approach is guided by individual examination of the patient, and by judgements concerning the disease and drug (*CS*, sūtra, 1, 120-3). Rational application is thus the foundation for therapeutic success ('yuktih siddhau pratishthā').

The value of rational application is frequently brought out in medical discussions. Even necessary and naturally favourable things and practices may turn out to be evils, when the 'rational application' is ignored. Food, for example, or exercise, may be actually harmful if irrationally resorted to (ayukti-yukta), or in excess. Alcohol, taken rationally, would contribute to health; otherwise, it may spell ruin (ibid., 6, 24, 59). Even poison which in its natural state may be fatal, would prove beneficial if taken 'rationally' (yukti-yukta). On the other hand, even good drugs, irrationally administered, would work like poison. (ibid. 1; 1, 126).

The rational approach in medicine is cultivated when the physician participates in 'medical discussions and debates' (called saṁbhāshā or tadvidya-saṁbhāshā or parishad). This would supplement his own learning and apprenticeship under an expert, by exposing him to other points of view, to the experience of other medical men, and to fresh light on diseases, drugs and dosage. (cf. ibid., 3, 8, 15), [*See* MEDICAL DISCUSSION]. Medical wisdom should at no time be closed; and no judgement can be absolute. It is regarded as essential that the physician must be able to relate properly different factors; and this act of relating is referred to as yukti or yoga (ibid., 1, 1, 126).

AV (cf. Kauśika-sūtra, 4, 25 with gloss of KEŚAVA) distinguishes between ordinary diseases (caused by food etc.), and ailments brought about by sin etc. The glossator explains that the therapeutics of CHARAKA, SUSRUTA and VĀGBHATA deal with the former class of diseases. The rites prescribed in *AV* (austerity, penance, sacrifices, pacificatory rites, gifts etc.) acquire relevance in the context of the latter kind of ailments. *Kāśyapa-saṁhitā* describes 'medicine' (aushadha) as the proper utilization and application of natural substances (dravya-saṁyoga), while 'treatment' (bheshaja) consists of pacificatory rites (śānti-karma). However, a physician (bhishak) was expected to be acquainted with both types of curative methods, although his reliance would be on the former.

SUŚRUTA speaks of the collection of substances that have originated from the five physical root-elements (bhūta-grāma), and he holds that we cannot go beyond the physical elements in the field of medicine (śarīra, 14). [*See* PANCHA-BHŪTA THEORY]. For him, the body, the cause of disease, the nature of disease, and the treatment are all physical in nature, and are not outside the scope of bhūta-grāma. Therefore, the only valid system of medicine is that which employs the 'rational approach'. Diseases (vyādhi) are recognized as normal, physical occurrences with physical causes (nidāna); and also as curable by suitable methods (siddhi-upāya) involving physical substances like drugs and proper food (*CS*, vimāna, 8, 37). Admission of the possibility of supernatural agencies at work is more in the nature of a concession to popular beliefs than in that of a medical doctrine. The early works (*CS*, *SS*, and *AS*), in fact, seek to provide medical aid for all possible human ailments (e.g. *CS*, 6, 30, 288 'sarva-vikārāṇām chikitsitam'), and leave little scope for supernatural intervention.

CHARAKA is confident that the physician who knows his field well enough and who begins his treatment in time, aware of the gravity of the illness, is bound to succeed (sūtra, 10, 7); nothing else is mentioned as contributing to his success . Further, both CHARAKA and SUŚRUTA describe as sufficient and necessary the four props of successful medical practice, viz. the physician, medicine, the nursing attendant, and the patient himself (*CS*, sūtra, 10, 3; *SS*, sūtra, 34, 15 and 17). [*See* FOUR PROPS OF MEDICAL

PRACTICE]. It is important to realize that ideas like karma and divine intervention do not figure in this account of props of medical practice. CHARAKA pointedly mentions in this context that medical practice (bheshajam) is rational in approach (yukti-yuktam), and quite sufficient to restore health (alam arogyāya) (*N.S.* ed. p. 64). He also says: 'Any cures effected by the physician who does not employ reasoning are only chance cures (yadrcchā-siddhi) (8, 2, 28).

It is therefore that Indian medicine relies heavily on the Nyāya-Vaiśeshika system, which prescribes a thoroughly rational approach to reality, and on the Sāṁkhya system which outlines a rigorously realistic natural philosophy. Neither of these systems has a place for divine caprice or supernatural intervention in the scheme of things it formulates. [*See* NYĀYA-VAISESHIKA *and* SĀṀKHYA].

Rejuvenation Therapy: Literally "the way or movement (ayana) of the sap of life (rasa)", Rasāyana represents not rejuvenation therapy, or use of medicines that only cure all (even normally intractable) ailments, but also prevent old age and prolong life. Rasa stands for the fundamental fluid of the body [*See* DHATU RASA], and also for all the tissues that are nourished by this fluid.

Later, rasa came to signify mercury, probably because of the semi-fluid character and almost miraculous curative powers of mercury. Rejuvenation therapy made such an extensive use of mercury (along with other metals and mineral salts) that the term rasāyana was taken to mean exclusively mercurial preparations. The 'art' (kalā) of combining mercury (and metals) with herbal preparations is mentioned even in the *Kāmasūtra* of Vātsyāyana ('dhātu-aushadhīnām saṁyoga-kriyā').

Rejuvenation is essentially regeneration of vitality so that the individual, although old and worn out, would get a fresh lease of life, full of energy and stamina. *CS* enumerates the causes of premature senile degeneration: eating habitually raw, non-nourishing, heavy, dry or decayed food, excessively sour, salty or pungent in taste, or food that one is not accustomed to; irregular food habits; indifference to the condition of the digestive organs; sleep during day-time; excessive drinking of alcoholic beverages; over-indulgence in sex activities; fatiguing physical exercise; frequent episodes of anger, violence, fright, sorrow, dejection, and greed; and suppression of (or delay in) the natural urges (calls of nature).

These factors bring about serious disturbances of metabolism . They corrupt the seven body constituents [*See* DHATU], and hence the body becomes a victim to several ailments. The basic fluid (rasa) becomes impure, and the blood becomes putrefied and acidic; muscles and joints become lax and loose; the fats increase and turn into liquids; bone marrow diminishes in quantity; and the secretion of semen is lowered or ceases altogether. Vitality (ojas), which is the product of the combined and normal functioning of the seven body constituents, decreases. The three doshas are thrown into severe imbalance. As a result, various diseases manifest themselves; for example, anxiety, loss of inclination to work, sloth, depression, tensions and exhaustion.

The assumption is that senility is not an inescapable condition of old age, and that premature degeneration can be corrected. Conditions like degeneration of body tissues, loss of the efficient functioning of sense-organs, diminution in mental vigour (intelligence, memory and so on) can not only be prevented but can also be reversed. This outlook is shared alike by BHELA, SUŚRUTA and CHARAKA

Rejuvenation therapy aims in particular at restoring the normal balance of the three doshas, establishing the most effective interaction between the seven body constituents, recovering the vitality, invigorating the sense-organs, correcting the physical disorders stimulating the internal gastric fire, and removing mental conditions like fear, anxiety, depression and aversion to work. Youth is reestablished inasmuch as the body metabolism is once again rendered efficient, flabbiness of flesh is removed, zeal for life is enhanced, capacity for work is heightened, and complexion becomes lustrous.

There are two methods of this therapy in vogue: construction of a special kind of cottage in which the patient is confined for treatment over a length of time; he is altogether isolated from human contact as well as from the physical surroundings (including sun and fresh air); and the treatment is intense. This is known as kuṭī-praveśika. The other method, known as vātātapīya, permits the patient's exposure to sun and fresh air while under treatment, and allows him to pursue his normal avocations. The former, however, is preferable for good results.

Prior to the actual treatment by rejuvenation therapy, the patient is carefully cleansed and prepared by lubrication (snehana), perspiration (svedana), and a herbal preparation (harītakī, amla, guda, vachā, vāyu-vidaṅga, haridrā, maricha and śuṇṭhi, all powdered and strained, taken with hot water at bedtime). Care is taken to purge the intestines of all faecal accumulations, by administering a rehabilitating diet of barley-gruel mixed with ghee for several days. On the bowels being cleansed, therapy for revitalization starts, and its description varies according to individual needs and capacities.

While this treatment is on, it is important that the patient should strictly regulate his diet (like avoiding pungent, bitter, sour or salty dishes, and taking milk, honey, butter, buttermilk, sweet tastes), and his conduct (like avoiding fatiguing labour, sexual activity, sleep during daytime, aimless wandering, irrelevant preoccupations, emotional outbursts, etc. and cultivating qualities like patience, piety, tranquillity, generosity, etc.).

The diet should in particular exclude foodstuffs that are vidāhī in character (those that cause inflammation, burning sensation, thirst, acidity, and simultaneous aggravation of vāta and pitta). Sour things must be especially avoided; and too much of salt is contra-indicated. When salt is used, rock-salt is to be preferred. Milk is recommended, but for those whose digestion is weak, and those who suffer from flatulence, colic, phantom tumour (gulma), recent fever, diabetes, chronic diarrhoea, spermatorrhea and disorders of vāta need to avoid milk. However, there is one preparation known as parpaṭi in which milk plays a predominant role; and when this is being administered, milk proves beneficial. Likewise, ghee (cow's ghee) is recommended for its capacity to increase strength, enhance mental powers, pacify all the three doshas, and vitalize generally. But it should be avoided in conditions like diabetes, enlargement of the liver and spleen, intestinal obstruction, fever, loss of digestive power, diseases due solely to kapha or to pitta, disturbances resulting from excessive intake of alcoholic drinks, etc. Ghee is also not indicated when patients are quite young or very old. Using ghee at night in winter or during daytime in summer has bad effects.

The aim of the therapy is to reorient the individual's inclinations and reorganize his constitution (both physical and mental). But persons who are already virtuous, cool and collected, patient, moderate in their habits, tranquil and truthful, benefit more by this therapy. Those who are not given to drinking liquor, or indulging in sex activity, or engaging themselves in excessive manual labour, and those who habitually take milk and ghee in good measure will also profit. Considerations in deciding on the therapy include the patient's age, constitution (prakṛti), digestion (agni), adaptability (sātmya), habits (āchāra), and general physical condition. Therapeutic methods as well as the drugs selected would vary according to these factors.

Rejuvenation therapy utilizes several plant products, metals, alloys, metallic compounds, salts, poisons, and sulphur. The alternative action of the drugs administered is calculated to (1) raise the nutritional value of rasa, thus providing immunity to pathogenic agents and conditions; (2) improve the digestive power (agni) of the patient by correcting and invigorating the metabolic processes; and (3) cleanse and tone up the circulatory systems (srotas).

The drugs commonly used include āmalakī (*Emblica officinalis*), harītakī (*Terminalia chebula*), vibhītaka (*Terminalia belerica),* brāhmī (*Herpestis monniera*), punarnavā (Boerhaavia diffusa), mandūkaparṇī (*Hydrocotyle asiatica*), viḍaṅga (*Embelia ribes*), yashti-madhu *(Glycyrrhiza glabra*), śaṅkha-pushpī *(Evolvulus alsinonides);* poisonous products like bhallātaka *(Semicarpus anacardium)* and vatsanābha *(Aconitum heterophyllum)*); mercury, sulphur and gold made nontoxic and assimilable; and mineral products like gairika (ochre), manah-śilā (realgar), girisindūra (lead peroxide) and śilājitu (bitumen).

These drugs are normally more effective in correcting disorders on empty stomachs rather than immediately after food (vīryādhikam bhavati bheshajam annahīnam). But persons who are weak, old or very young as well as women, should avoid taking these drugs on empty stomach, for weakness and exhaustion may ensue. Drugs, in these cases taken along with food are better assimilated in the system. Further, these drugs are not to be taken when the patient is thirsty, or is weakened after prolonged fasting. Medicines containing poisonous ingredients should not be administered to children under nine years of age or to old men above 80 (*RJN*). [*See also* CHYAVANA-PRĀŚA.]).

Roga: Disease, sickness or distress in general. The word highlights the presence of bodily pain as well as mental torment (rujā) in diseases. [*See* DISEASE].

Rtu-Charyā: [*See* SEASONAL CONDUCT].

S

Śabda : Word (or verbal knowledge), regarded as one of the valid means of knowledge, is explained as four-fold: (1) 'pertaining to observed facts' (drshtārtha) (like the three-fold reasons for the aggravation of the doshas, six-fold therapeutic measures to bring the doshas to normalcy, and the fact that sensations like sounds can be apprehended only when the auditory apparatus like the ear are present and operative); (2) 'not pertaining to observed facts' (adrshtārtha) (like the possibility and nature of life after death, and the possibility of emancipation from mundane bonds); (3) 'pertaining to things as they are (satya)' (or factual, like the instructions of Āyurveda, the fact that curable diseases can be cured by standard medical treatments, and that medical treatments do have their effects); and (4) 'not pertaining to things as they are (anṛta) (or false, viz. contrary to the nature of things). (*CS*, vimāna, 8,38).

The word in this context comprehends both scriptural authority derived from a divine source and the authoritative works composed by the enlightened sages of yore who were human beings (CHKP. on the above). [*See* PRAMĀNA].

Śālākya : Described as minor surgery (from 'śalākā', 'surgical instrument'), this branch of

Indian medicine deals with the diseases of the region above the clavicle (ūrdhva-jatru viz. ears, eyes, nose, mouth etc), and their treatments principally with surgical instruments (*SS*, sūtra, 1,2).

Salts : Salts (lavana) are used extensively in Indian medicine both as drugs and as adjuncts to drugs. Some of the salts in use are naturally obtained, while others are prepared artificially. Of the several varieties of salts known, six are in frequent use:

(1) Rock-salt or sodium chloride (saindhava), named after the Indus region where it is found, is regarded as the best among salts, being the only one which is cold in potency (śīta-vīrya). There are three kinds, of which the pure white and crystalline kind is preferred. Saltish-sweet in taste, it is light and soft; it is an appetiser, and it increases the digestive power. It adds to the taste, and cools the system. It is especially indicated for alimentary purposes, constipation, etc. It is beneficial to the eyesight, and it increases semen. It can enter even into the minutest parts of the body (sūkshma). It cures boils. Its action is on all three doshas [*See* ROCK-SALT]

(2) Marine (sāmudra), or common salt (sodium chloride), is sun-dried sea-salt, produced by evaporating sea-water. It is digestive, acrid, light, an appetiser, and a laxative (sara). It aggravates kapha and pitta, but pacifies vāta. It is hot in potency [*See* COMMON SALT].

(3) Black salt (bida, vit) is artificially prepared, mostly in the upper parts of the country, especially in Bhevāni (Hissar district). It consists chiefly of sodium chloride with traces of sodium sulphate, alumina, magnesia, ferric oxide, and sulphide of iron. Reddish brown in colour, granular in shape and shining, it is saline in taste but also slightly nauseating. Its medicinal uses are many, and, therefore, it is also called "physician's salt" (vaidyaka-lavana). It pacifies kapha and vāta, while aggravating pitta. It is useful in colic, constipation, flatulence, indigestion, heaviness in heart, dyspepsia, intestinal tumour, enlargement of spleen and liver, and spermatorrhoea. It is a laxative, an aspirant, and a stomachic.

Two methods of preparing this salt are in vogue in our country. One of them is to take 82 parts of sea-salt and one part each of harītakī (*Terminalia chebula*), āmalakī (*Emblica officinalis*) and sarji (refined natron), all powdered well, and to heat the whole in an earthern vessel till they are intimately combined into a lump. The other method is to take eight parts of sea-salt and one part of powdered āmalakī, and to heat them on a strong fire until they are mixed together intimately. When the mass is cooled, it becomes 'black-salt'.

(4) Salt-petre (sauvarchala, audbhida or ūshara-kshāra) is both an alkali and a salt. Dark coloured, aromatic and agreeable, it is made by dissolving common salt in a solution of crude soda, and evaporating it. It contains chloride of sodium and sulphide of soda; but it is devoid of the carbonate of soda. It is digestive, stomachic, purgative, demulcent; it is indicated in abdominal tumour, dysentery and intestinal worms [*See* SALT-PETRE, ALKALI].

(5) Sambar-salt (romaka) is obtained by evaporating salt-water from the now extinct river Romavatī which flowed from Sambar lake in Rājāsthān. It is obtained as clear rhomboidal crystals in shape (like alum), and is regarded as the purest among evaporated salts. It is pungent in taste, also slightly bitter, hot, acrid, light, and saline. It increases digestive power, and acts as a laxative and a diuretic. It pacifies vāta, and helps emission of kapha through eyes and nostrils (abhishyandi). It aggravates pitta, and causes inflammation.

These five salts administered in combination (one part of rock-salt, two of marine salt, three of sambar-salt, four of salt-petre and five of black salt) is known as 'pañcha-lavaṇa', which is prescribed for its carminative, stomachic, laxative and tonic actions. It is widely used in colic, indigestion, and enlargement of spleen and liver. Groups of two (rock-salt and marine salt), or three (marine-salt, black-salt and salt-petre) are also employed. While it is usual to enumerate five varieties of salts (as above and as given in *Amara-kosha*), the lexicons provide lists of six (with the addition of challikā or navasāra, sal ammoniac; and nine salts (adding three more, viz., gādha, drauneya and ūshara). (cf. *RN* 20, *SKD*).

Salts in general have the following properties: purifier, appetiser, digestive, softening of body, slackening the organs and joints, impairment of strength and sexual vigour, causing inflammation in the cheek and neck, and inducing watering in the mouth. It aggravates kapha and pitta, but pacifies vāta. Taken in excess, salts tend to cause thirst, eye-troubles (opthalmia), intestinal ulcer, loosening of teeth and falling of hair, skin diseases, and erysipelas.

Samāgni : Meaning 'equalized fire', it refers to the digestive condition being balanced and normal, being influenced by all the three doshas (vāta, pitta and kapha) equally (viz. with none prevailing over the others; vāta prevailing would lead to vishamāgni, pitta to atyagni and kapha to mandāgni). Food, taken at regular intervals and in proper measure, is easily digested, without causing any irregularities or disturbances. [*See* AGNI, ATYAGNI, DIGESTION, DOSHA, VISHA MARGA].

Samāna-Vāyu : One of the five kinds of winds in the body, it is said to function chiefly in the stomach (āmāśaya) and intestines (pakvāśaya). Its function is to 'equalize'; being associated with 'fire', [*See* JĀṬHARĀGNI] it digests the food that has been taken in and separates the essential nutrient parts (rasa) from the waste-products. Disturbances in this wind may lead to dysentery, impaired digestion, gulma, etc. [*See* DOSHA, PRĀṆA and VĀTA]

Sāṁkhya : An ancient system of thought (tantra), which has left a deep impression on all the other systems of thought in the country, including Indian medicine. Both CHARAKA and SUŚRUTA (the latter almost exclusively) rely on the Sāṁkhya ideology for providing a philosophical foundation for medical prescriptions and practices.

However, much of the original literature on this system has been lost. There appears to have been frequent breaks in the continuity of the tradition of this school. It is also probable that there were variant viewpoints within this school. The Chinese tradition mentions as many as eighteen schools of Sāṁkhya (Johnston). There have been attempts to trace the historical development of the Sāṁkhya thought (Garbe, Keith, Edgerton, Dasgupta, Frauwallner, van Buitenen, Chattopadhyaya, Johnston and others), but the problem continues to be enigmatic and unsettled. The traditional Indian view has always been that the Sāṁkhya system as a full-fledged and complete philosophy was the contribution of an ancient sage, KAPILA, even as the Nyāya system was the work of GOTAMA, and the Vaiśeshika system the work of KANĀDA. Sāṁkhya provides the theoretical background and counterpart to the Yoga system formulated by PATAÑJALI. The two systems have been linked together since ancient times, as gnosis and askesis.

While Sāṁkhya is in its intent a method of emancipation, it constructed a system of thought, enumerating the principles (tattvas), and analyzing them with a view to aid discrimination (viveka). The expression 'Sāṁkhya' (from saṁkhyā) suggests this import. The seeds of this thought are to be found in some of the Upanishads (like *Katha* and *Śvetāśvatara*), and the first formulation in the 'Moksha-dharma' section of the epic *Mahābhārata* (12, 187, 239-240) (cf. Johnston, van Buitenen, Frauwallner). An early account of the Sāṁkhya system is also to be found in *Charaka-saṁhitā* and AŚVAGHOSHA'S *Buddha-charita*. In fact, Dasgupta refers to the account in *CS,* as almost an authentic version of early Sāṁkhya. The thought was crystallized by ĪŚVARA-KṚISHṆA (about the fourth century A. D.) in his *Sāṁkhya-kārikā,* and this has been referred to as "Classical Sāṁkhya"

Sāmkhya as a thought-system, appears to have receded into relative oblivion till about the fourteenth century mainly because of the growing popularity of the rival thought-systems, Vedānta, Mīmāmsā, and Nyāya. The commentaries on *Sāṁkhya-pravachana-sūtra* by VIJÑĀNA-BHIKSHU. MAHĀDEVA. ANIRUDDHA and others (about the fourteenth century) revived the academic interest in Sāṁkhya; but the Sāṁkhya as expounded by them involved an unmistakable accommodation to Vedānta ideas.

Among the major texts dealing with this school of thought, if we exclude the epic accounts (such as 'Moksha-dharma' in *Mahābhārata*), are included *Shashṭi-tantra*(a work of doubtful authenticity, whose contents are incorporated in the Pāñcharātra text, *Ahirbudhnya-saṁhitā,* and which is said to reflect the viewpoint of VĀRSHNAGAṆYA), *Sāṁkhya-kārikā* (a work in verses, ascribed to ĪŚVARA-KṚSHṆA. and on which there are several commentaries like the *Bhāshyas* of VYĀSA and GAUḌAPĀDA) *Tattva-kaumudī* of VĀCHASPATI-MIŚRA. *Yukti-dīpikā* and *Jayamaṅgalā, Sāṁkhya-pravachana-sūtra* (an aphoristic work ascribed to KAPILA. and, on which ANIRUDDHA. wrote his *Vṛtti* about A.D.. 1500 andVIJÑĀNA-BHIKSHUhis *Bhāshya* in the sixteenth century) and also *Tattva-samāsa* (a late work despite its deceptive aphoristic style). The traditional list of Sāṁkhya teachers includes after KAPILA. ĀSURI and PAÑCHAŚIKHA (*Mahābhārata,* Śanti-parvan, 219). PAÑCHAŚIKHA has been described as an important link between the Upanishadic ideas and the classical Sāṁkhya viewpoint.

As a system of thought, its approach is characterized by the recognition of the primary material cause (pradhāna-kāraṇa) in contradistinction to the spiritual Absolute (Brahma) of the Vedānta. It made a distinction of far-reaching significance between the 'male', non-material, passive purusha (the conscious subject) and the 'feminine', material and active prakṛti (primordial nature). It has been interpreted as the differentiation between matter and spirit (Richard Garbe), 'Being' and 'Becoming' (Paul Oltramare), permanence and change, teleology and ontology. And it emphasized the material aspect of nature (macrocosmic as well as microcosmic), and employed a perfectly rational theory (sat-kārya-vāda).

It enumerated in its early phase as many as 24 principles (tattvas), to which was added another (purusha) in the classical Sāṁkhya. The enumeration is justified by observation (pratyaksha) as well as reason (yukti). The principles were psychical and material; they included the elements out of which the stuff of the universe is constituted as well as the organs and objects that emerged during the course of evolutionary change (pariṇāma). The system subscribed to a theory of evolution, both 'horizontal' (involving the sequence of incorporated awareness or buddhi, mind, sense-organs and the elements) and 'vertical' (eight-fold 'nature' including 'ego') (van Buitenen). An involvement in the theory of evolution is the notion of multiplicity of inefficient but necessary purushas. The outlook is thoroughly naturalistic and materialistic.

Primordial nature (Prakṛti) is unconscious and dynamic. It is the principle of 'becoming'; changes and creativity are natural to it. But it becomes active only when it comes to be associated with ('impregnated with', Anima Sengupta) the teleological force called the Person (purusha). The important explanatory idea that Sāṁkhya has formulated in this context is that of 'guṇas' ('reals', S.N. Dasgupta), which are fundamental to the fabric of the outer world of objects as well as the inner world of thoughts and feelings [*See* GUṆA]. The three types of 'reals' are sattva, rajas and tamas, which have different connotations such as awareness, activity and inertia; pleasure, pain, and delusion; being, becoming, and resistance; good, bad, and indifferent; wisdom, passion, and dullness. When the three 'reals' are in a state of equilibrium, like three perfect strands of a rope, they are indeterminate, homogeneous and undifferentiated. It is this condition that is called 'prakṛti'. It is the potential source of all energy and change. This is why it is described in classical Sāmkhya as 'productive', 'unmanifest', 'pervasive', 'objective', 'universal', 'unconscious', and 'three-fold real'.

As distinguished from this principle of change, there is the principle which is of the nature of consciousness but altogether unproductive, viz. the purusha, which is beyond the scope of the three 'reals'. It is isolated (kevalin), while the former is necessarily involved. The epic Sāṁkhya brings out the distinction between them by describing them as 'field' (kshetra) and 'knower of the field' (kshetrajña) respectively.

Sāṁkhya is pluralistic inasmuch as it postulates that every 'field' (physico-mental conglomeration) is enlivened by the presence of a particular 'knower of the field' (or purusha). The plurality of purushas is justified on the ground of differences which are congénital, differences in predispositions, abilities and aptitudes, and differences in the 'reals' (GAUḌAPĀDA). The idea of 'field' comprehends the five elements, and as related to them the five sense-organs, mind, individuated awareness (buddhi); viz. the body-mind complex. Sāṁkhya has rejected the Vedānta idea of one ātman, as the absolute principle of pure awareness. While it also rejects the idea of jīva, it concedes the usefulness of this idea by postulating 'a subtle body' (liṅga-śarīra) for each mind-body complex.

There are three Sāṁkhya viewpoints that have been listed in the epic *Mahābhārata* (12, 318): one that postulated 24 principles (which was obviously an earlier version, and which is accepted both by PAÑCHAŚIKHA and by CHARAKA), another that enumerated 25 principles (which is the classical Sāṁkhya, explained by ĪŚVARA-KṚSHṆA), and still another which worked with 26 categories (as represented by Yoga system). The 24 principles are: ten organs of sense (indriyas, five of action and five of cognition), mind (manas), five objects of sense-perception (indriyārtha) and eight-fold prakṛti (the unmanifest, the transactional consciousness, the ego, and five primary forms of matter, earth etc.). The 25th principle accepted in the second viewpoint was purusha as an independent principle. The 26th principle accepted in Yoga is Īśvara.

The system as described by CHARAKA (*CS*, śarīra) is the first of these viewpoints, and it agrees with the viewpoint of PAÑCHAŚIKHA as given in the epic (*Mahābhārata,* 12, 219). It is, as Dasgupta has argued, an early version of Sāṁkhya. But it is certainly not the atheistic and materialistic version that is said to be earliest version. CHARAKA mentions not only purusha but describes him as paramātman. It appears likely that he has adapted PANCHAŚIKHA'S thought to suit the clinical context.

CHARAKA begins his exposition of the system (Śarīra, 1) by defining the human being that is the subject-matter of the science of medicine (according to the commentator). The human being is a conglomeration of six 'elements' (dhātus): five physical elements or primary forms of matter (earth, water, fire, air and akaśa) with 'consciousness' (chetanā) as the sixth. The commentator explains 'consciousness' as "the self associated with mind", which is the ground for consciousness ('chetanādhārah samanaska-ātma'). It is the same person (purusha) that is spoken of as consisting of twenty-four principles; mind, ten sense-organs, sense-objects, and eight-fold prakṛti (the five elements, the transactional consciousness or buddhi, the unmanifest or avyakta and the ego or ahaṁkāra). The commentator explains that the classical Sāṁkhyan principle, purusha, has not been included in this enumeration, as the indifferent (udāsīna) purusha although different from prakṛti, is, like the latter, unmanifest and, therefore, ground under prakṛti; further distinction in this matter, according to the commentator, is of little profit.

CHARAKA further speaks (verse 35) of the person as a conglomeration (rāśi) of the twenty-four factors; and the factor beyond (paraṁ) the twenty-three viz. the 'unmanifest' (avyakta) is spoken of as the supporter of the particular organization (yoga-dhara) of the other factors [*See* PURUSHA]. The conglomeration of factors has been ascribed to the function of rajas; when, however, sattva is in the ascendent, the conglomeration breaks down.

Prakṛti, in CHARAKA'S account, appears to have a two-fold relevance. It is the unmanifest (avyakta), and, in this nature, it is tantamount to the purusha (or the principle of consciousness); and is a series or class of changes brought about by evolution (vikāra). In the latter sense, it is the 'field', while, in the former, it is the 'knower of the field' (verses 60 off). Evolution proceeds, according to CHARAKA, thus: the unmanifest-transactional consciousness-ego-five physical elements and the sense-organs (including mind). CHARAKA speaks of sixteen 'modifications' (vikāras) of the primordial prakṛti: five organs of cognition (seeing, hearing, smelling, tasting and touch), five organs of action (speech, prehension, locomotion, elimination and reproduction), mind, and five physical objects (earth, water, fire, air and ākāśa).

SUŚRUTA also relies on the Sāṁkhya ideology (*SS,* śarīra., 1), but the viewpoint appears to be more in accord with the classical version (admitting twenty-five principles). His description of the unmanifest prakṛti as characterized by the three guṇas (sattva, rajas and tamas), as being eight-fold, and as being the cause of the origination of the world (saṁbhava-hetu) is plain and precise. He not only describes rather tersely the sequential emergence of transactional consciousness (called here mahat) from the unmanifest, and of ego from the former, but gives an account of the three-fold egoity (similar to the account in the classical version vaikārika, taijasa and bhūtādi) and evolutes therefrom: the eleven senses (five of cognition, five of action, and mind which is both, ubhayātmaka), the five 'subtle' elements (tanmātra), and five gross elements (mahābhūta). It is interesting to note that the idea of 'tanmātra' is not to be found in *CS*.

The twenty-four principles that are thus enumerated are described as belonging to the 'unconscious' group (achetana-varga), distinguished from which is the 'purusha', 'the twenty-fifth principle' (so called explicitly by SUŚRUTA), which is yoked to the complex 'effects' (the elements and sense-organs) and 'causes' (the eight-fold prakṛti), and which 'enlivens' the entire complex (chetayitā). SUŚRUTA also credits the purusha-prakṛti conglomeration with a teleological function (for the isolation of the purusha, kaivalyārthaṁ) (śarīra, 1, 8). [*See also* GUNA, INDRIYA, EGO, PURUSHA).

Saṁyoga: The expression signifying 'perfect combination' or 'organization' is defined as yoking several things to constitute a wholesome unity by an unseen force (CHKP. on *CS,* sūtra, 1, 42, 'saṁyag-adṛshṭa-yantrito yogah'); and the context in which the expression has been used is the sustaining organization of the body, sense organs, mind and soul in the individual organism (*CS,* ibid.). Samyoga is also a Vaiśeshika category meaning conjunction, as distinguished from viyoga, disjunction. [*See* VAIŚESHIKA].

Sandhi: [*See* BONE-JOINTS].

Sapta-dhātu: Seven principal constituents of the body, viz. chyle (rasa), blood (rakta), muscle (māmsa), fat-tissue (medas), bone (asthi), bone-marrow (majjā) and semen (śukra). [*See* DHĀTU].

Śarīra: [*See* BODY].

Sātmya: Food, conduct, or medicine that becomes agreeable to one's nature or constitution is regarded as congenial, wholesome or suitable to that individual, for it gets into community with the essence or nature (sātmya, 'sa+ātma'). It becomes natural to the person (*CS,* vimāna, 1, 20, 'yad-ātmani-upaśete'); or, the person becomes habituated to the conditions as a result of long custom. But it is not a negative concept. The significance of wholesome food or conduct does not consist only in not producing any injurious effect on the health but it contributes to positive pleasure and comfort, which are the necessary ingredients of health (*SS,* sūtra, 35, 40-41, 'sukhāyaiva'). Even if the food or conduct is contrary to the natural conditions, and may tell on the health of others, it may not cause any disturbance to the individual whose constitution is thoroughly acclimatized to it. It may in fact result in the well-being of the individual (*CS,* ibid.).

Further, *CS* (vimāna, 8, 118) spells out: sātmya is whatever is wholesome to the individual even when used continuously ('tad yat sātatyenopasevyam upaśeté'). Implied here is adaptability due to habitual use of anything (food, medicine, conduct), not in the sense of development of immunity, but in that of contributing to the welfare of the individual.

This acquired suitability due to habituation may vary depending on several factors, like the nature of the territory one lives in (deśa), the time of the day (kāla), the species one belongs to (jāti, human being, quadruped, bird, etc.), season (rtu, viz, food and conduct prescribed as suitable for the period of the year), the disease one may suffer from (roga), the peculiar kind of physical and mental exertion one has to indulge in for the sake of his livelihood (vyāyāma), the properties of the water one habitually drinks or which is available in the place where he resides (udaka), sleep during daytime (divā-svapna), and the taste that he is used to (rasa) (*SS,* ibid., 35, 40).

Defining the expression as "whatever, when resorted to, conduces to the happiness of the individual" ('yad-yasya sevitam sukhāya sampadyate tat tasya sātmyam'), *SS* (sūtra, 10) distinguishes between two main categories of suitability: (1) conduct (cheshṭā, of three kinds, physical, vocal and mental) and food (āhāra, of six kinds, according to the prevailing taste, rasa).

CS (vimāna, 1, 20), however, classifies suitability into three types: (1) 'superior' (pravara), when all the tastes are habitually indulged in; (2) 'inferior' (avara), when the individual relishes only one taste; and (3) 'middling'(madhya), when the individual habitually relishes two to five tastes jointly. The habit of taking food containing all the six tastes is recommended as best, for each taste has a specific contribution to make towards health. The habit of taking food only of one taste, and the habit of taking food with limited tastes are to be changed to the 'superior' habit of relishing all the six tastes. But the change must be instituted only gradually (kramena eva).

Superiority of the first group (viz. those who have habituated themselves to all the six tastes, sarva-rasa-sātmya) consists in the individuals belonging to this group being endowed with strength, long life, and ability to face difficult situations; while those who are habituated only to one taste (eka-rasa-sātmya) lack these qualities. A combination of these two types (vyāmiśra-sātmya) endows on the individuals moderate strength (cf. *CS,* vimāna, 8, 118).

The expression 'sātmya' acquires a practical significance in the clinical context as a synonym of 'upaśaya', a pathological investigation by homologation (cf. *CS,* vimāna, 1, 20 "sātmyārtho hyupaśayārthah"). The idea of 'asātmya' is involved in one of the three causes of diseases: 'incompatible correlation of senses with their objects' (asātmyendriyārtha-saṁyoga), viz. indulgence in a sensory experience that one is not accustomed to, or beyond ones tolerance threshold. When the disease develops manifest symptoms (rūpa), the investigation of the cause of the disease is undertaken by preliminary administration of drugs on the basis of homologation, so that the cause is traced from the effects (cf. *MN,* 1, 8-9).

Sattva: The word (derived from sat, participle from verb *as,* "to be", 'being', 'real') has many meanings. In the medical context it is used to signify: (1) one of the three guṇas which constitute prakṛti (the other two being rajas and tamas), entering into the human constitution (both physical and mental), and determining by its predominance the personality type and temperament (cf. *SS,* śarīra, 1, 3) [*See* GUṆA, CONSTITUTION, SĀṀKHYA]; (2) a synonym of manas (mind) (*CS,* sūtra, 1, 55, and 56), hence sattvāvajaya [*See* MIND]; (3) dry and powdered sediment left, after the water in which pieces of drugs are macerated and kept for a night is strained and allowed to settle; (4) strength (bala); (5) living being; (6) foetus; and (7) qualities like purity, clarity, generosity, piety, discipline, etc.

Sattva, as a guṇa, is said to be the dominant factor in the ākāśa form of matter and in cognition (prakhyā) (as rajas in activity or pravṛtti, and tamas in conservation or sthiti). Cognition comprehends all awareness of the external objects as well as the experience of the subjective context (or 'I'); and, therefore, sattva is connected with manas as well as buddhi [*See* MIND]. In this context, sattva is the capacity for shining forth (perceptibility) what really exists (sat); it thus has the capacity to relate itself to purusha as pure consciousness. In the sense of the ideal state of being, it is also regarded as 'good' (viz. 'as it should be'), possessed of bodily and mental characteristics which facilitate the individual's advancement towards the *summum bonum.* [*See* SĀṀKHYA, GUṆA].

Sattvāvajaya: The expression 'sattva' has many meanings, but in this context it means mind ('sattva-saṁjñe manasi', *CS,* sūtra, 1, 46). Subjugation of mind (sattvāvajaya) has been prescribed as one of the three types of therapeutic procedures (*CS,* sūtra, 11, 54), the other two being religious and magical techniques (daiva-vyapāśraya) and rational methods (yukti-vyapāśraya). This has the import of psychotherapy and counselling, for it is reduction of mind to restrain itself from unwholesome preoccupation (ahitebhyo 'rthebhyo mano-nigrahah', *CS,* ibid.).

This has relevance to the idea that errors of judgement (pragñāparādha) [*See* PRAJÑĀPARĀDHA] are causes of diseases (*CS,* Sārīra, 1, 102-108). Owing to this reason, the individual's intelligence (dhī), endurance (dhṛti) and memory (smṛti) get vitiated; and this leads to wrong conduct and thereby to ailments and misery. The curative methods prescribed are naturally the control of mind so that the three factors (intelligence, endurance and memory) are not disturbed.

Besides the preventive methods involved in wholesome conduct (sadvṛtta) and 'daily routine' (dina-charyā), Āyurveda also prescribes curative methods of weaking the pathogenic emotions (fear, anger, jealousy, etc) by provoking opposite feelings.

Seasonal conduct: The Indian year is divided into six seasons (rtu) of two months each: winter (hemanta, roughly November-December), cool season (also called winter's close, śiśira, January-February), spring (vasanta, March-April), summer (grīshma, May-June), rainy season (varshā, July-August) and autumn (śarad, September-October). Each season has a characteristic impact upon the human body, and therefore our conduct must be appropriate to the season, so that the impact is not injurious to health. Like daily routine (dina-charyā), seasonal conduct also is a necessary part of hygiene and preventive medicine. [*See* HYGIENE, PREVENTIVE MEDICINE, DAILY ROUTINE]. The conduct prescribed for seasons includes the type of food to be eaten or avoided, drinks that are helpful or harmful, residence, clothing, massage, prophylactic measures, rest, exercise and sex habits that are appropriate to the climatic conditions (*CS*, Sūtra, 6, 1-51, *AHr*, 1, 3, 1-58, *AS*, 1, 4, 3-56).

The six seasons are grouped into two divisions: 'uttarāyaṇa' (cool, spring and summer) and 'dakshināyana' (rains, autumn and winter). The former is the period when strength is taken away (ādāna) gradually, by the northerly course of the sun, which is hot and fierce; and, therefore, the air too is warm and coarse, and the earth dry. In the latter period, when the sun courses in the southward direction, the moon has the upper hand, and the sun becomes weaker, often covered by clouds; the air gets cooler and the earth moist. It is then that the living beings acquire strength (utsarga). The assumption is that during colder months, bodily strength increases, while in the warmer months it diminishes. Winter and the cool seasons are best so far as strength and vigour are concerned; rains and summer are the worst for strength will be at the lowest ebb: autumn and spring are moderate. Dietic and hygienic regulations vary according to these changes in seasons.

(1) Winter: (including winter's close): During the cold months the cool air will drive body-heat into the inner regions; and the heat gathered at the stomachic area increases the keenness of the digestive fire (jātharāgni). More than normal food, therefore, is required to prevent the digestive power from consuming the body ingredients themselves. Food that is fatty, heavy and rich, sour, or saltish in taste, preparations from milk, sweets, dishes prepared in oil, flesh of animals that inhabit water and marshy places are indicated. Use of hot or warm water for bathing and drinking is recommended. Oil-baths, ointments, applications of thick paste prepared from aloés wood (agaru), and massage would keep the body in fine shape. Warm clothes, residence in warm places, and exposure to sun would be appropriate to the season. Sex-activity would not weaken the body in the cold weather. Alcoholic drinks may be used without disadvantage.

Light food which is pungent, bitter or astringent in taste, would contribute to the increase of 'wind' (vāta) in the body; and must, therefore, be avoided. Sleep during day-time would be harmful; and so would be exposure to the cold breeze.

(2) and (3) Spring : During the close of Winter, kapha begins to accumulate, and by the Spring exposure to the sun's rays, it tends to get excited, resulting in many ailments (like chronic cold, pratiśyāya). To counteract this tendency, emetics (vamana) are recommended especially in the month of Chaitra (March-April); daily administration of strong medicated inhalation (nasya) would be helpful. Food taken must be light and easily digested: tastes like pungent, bitter, and astringent are to be preferred. Bathing in cold or lukewarm water and drinking cold or tepid water are advised. Clothing must be warm; sex-activity and some alcoholic drinks are not contra indicated. Physical exercise and massage would be beneficial.

Heavy and oily food is to be avoided, as also sour and sweet tastes. Sleep during the day-time would be harmful.

(4) Summer : This is the season when kapha would decrease, giving place to vāta. Therefore, food taken must be cold, fluid, oily, and tasty; milk, sugar, ghee, and rice are especially commended. Light clothing (preferably cotton garments), sleeping in the open, walking in cool places (river banks, gardens, forests etc), and bathing in cold water would be appropriate to the season. Application of sandal-paste (chandana), fanning oneself, and exposure to moonlight would be measures to cool the system. Sleep during daytime would not be harmful during this period.

But physical exercise, alcoholic drinks, sex-activity, fumigation and food that is saline, sour or pungent are to be avoided.

(5) Rains : The closing days of summer would tend to accumulate vāta, which will be excited during the rainy months. To counteract it, cleansing of the body (śodhana) by oily enemata (nirūhana-basti) is recommended especially in the month of Śrāvaṇa (July-August). The digestive power becomes dull during this season, and, therefore, food taken must be light, and a diet needs to be observed. Use of honey in food and drinks would be beneficial. The use of rainwater for bathing and drinking is regarded as good. Cotton clothes and massage are indicated, and one must reside in a dry place.

Physical exercise, sleep in day-time, alcoholic drinks, fumigation, and sex-activity are to be avoided, as also night-dew and fierce sun.

The Indian rainy season is not a period of continuous rain, and it will be occasionally warm. At times, it seems like winter, and at times like summer. Conduct must vary according to these changes.

(6) Autumn : During the course of the rainy season, pitta tends to accumulate, and in autumn it will get excited under the impact of the sun's rays. This condition is to be counteracted by purgatives (virechana), especially in the month of Agrahāyaṇa (November–December). Food taken must be moderate, cold, and easily digested; bitter and sweet tastes are to be preferred. One should not even eat his fill, let alone overeat. Use of river-water for bathing and drinking, and exposure to moon light are recommended.

Among the details to be avoided during this period are curds, meat of animals that inhabit water and marshy regions, fatty and oily food, application of oil to the body, easterly wind, and sleep by day.

While the above are general principles, they do not apply to all persons uniformly. Conduct should naturally take into consideration the constitutional peculiarities of each individual, the availability of the foods and drinks, and the individual's habits regarding them, the nature of the land in which one resides, and the incidence of ailments that are due to seasonal variation.

Secondary Disease: Secondary disease (upadrava) arises subsequent to, or during, the course of a main disease that is being treated (rogottara-kālaja, CHKP. interprets it as 'roga-madhya-kālaja'), and is dependent upon that disease (viz. the doshas in the background of that disease) for its origination, nature and strength (rogāśraya) (*CS,* 6,21,40; *also SS,* 1,35). It is called 'secondary' in the sense that its onset follows the presence of the 'primary' (or first) disease (*paśchāt jāta iti, CS;* 'purvotpannam vyādhim jaghanyakāla-jāto vyadhir upasṛjati', *SS*).

It is usually caused by the same doshas that had caused the first disease, and therefore the treatment undertaken for the first disease would be adequate to take care of this also. But if the secondary disease becomes troublesome, then it needs to be treated independently, and even prior to the treatment of the first disease (CHKP on *CS*, 6,21,40). For, the first disease would become difficult to cure, if it is attended by secondary diseases.

It is not a rule that all diseases are attended by such complications. They do not, if the treatment is proper and adequate, and if the patient's vital force (ojas) is good. An important detail of treatment, therefore, is to preserve the vitality (bala) of the patient, so that the disease is eliminated, without leading to complications.

Secondary diseases may be caused by improper diet and conduct on the part of the patient, and incorrect diagnosis and wrong medicine on the part of the physician. [*See* DISEASE]

Sense-Organs: Called indriyas (faculties, capacities), they are ten in number: five organs of cognition (jñānendriya, or buddhīndriya: visual, auditory, tactile, olfactory and gustatory. darśna-śravaṇa-sparśana-ghrānana-rasana), and five organs of action (karmendriya: speech, prehension, locomotion, elimination and procreation, vachana-ādāna-viharaṇa-visarga-ānanda). They have corresponding structures (indriya-sthāna) like the eyes, ears, skin, nose and tongue; mouth, hands, feet, organ of elimination and organ of procreation (chakshu-śrotra-tvak-nāsā-jihvā; vāk-pāni-pāda-pāyu-upasthā). It is usual to count mind (manas) as the eleventh organ, partaking of both abilities: cognition and action (*SS*, śarīra, 1,3-4, *CS*, śarīra, 1,17).

The sense-organs are evolved from the sattva-dominated egoity (sāttvika-ahamkāra) with the help of the rajas-dominated egoity (taijasa-ahaṁkāra), which in its turn is evolved from mahat (buddhi) and appropriates the body-apparatus (abhimāna) and represents the principle of separation or individuality (pṛthaktva). The ramification of the phenomenal world starts with egoity; the sense-organs continue this trend and present a still more ramified phenomenal world (*SK*, 25f).

While the sense-organs represent the subjective aspect of evolution from egoity, the objects of sense-perception (vishaya: form, sound, touch, smell and taste, rūpa-śabda-sparśa-gandha-rasa) are evolutes from the tamas-dominated egoity (bhūtādi-ahamkāra). Egoity is included in the eight-fold natural evolutes (prakrti); but the sense-organs as well as the sense-objects are classed under the sixteen modifications thereof (vikāra).

Each of the sense-organs is composed of all the five primary forms of matter (earth, water, fire, air and ākāśa) but one of the forms predominates in each organ: earth in the olfactory organ, water in the gustatory, fire in the visual, air in the tactile and ākāśa in the auditory organs (*CS*, ibid., 24).

The sense-organs require for their function the association of mind (manas) with them. The initial phase of sensory perception is mental, but later the perception is organized in terms of positive and negative valencies (*CS*, ibid., 22). The coordination of mind, sense-organs and the objects is made possible by the unmanifest aspect of prakrti (avyakta) (*CS*, ibid., 35). [*See* SĀMKHYA]

Sindūra: Like bhasmas, sindūras are widely employed in the Siddha system of medicine. They are essentially medicines which contain red sulphide of mercury (rasa-sindūra) processed by several drugs, and which are prepared by a process of sublimation. The sheets or granules of metals initially are ground with mercury to form an amalgam, and then ground with sulphur so as to provide black sulphide of mercury in a black mass (khajjali), which is treated with herbal drugs, infusions or decoctions. The treated mass is dried and powdered, and then subjected to intense heat in a special apparatus [*See* PREPARATIONS] so that the black sulphide of mercury is transformed into granular particles of red sulphide of mercury, sublimated at the top of the flask. The weight of this red sulphide of mercury must be equal to the weight of mercury used. The granular particles are ground into fine powders, which are to be used.

Of the many preparations under this head, the well-known are: siddha-makara-dhvaja (which involves initial grinding of purified gold leaves and purified mercury for six days, and a subsequent grinding for another six days with purified sulphur, a further grinding for six days with the juices of red cotton flowers and aloes mixed, and sublimation after drying the mixture) used in conditions of nervous debility, anemia, emaciation, loss of weight, and loss of sexual vigour; rajata-chandrodaya (involving silver instead of gold) used as an appetiser, haematinic and aphrodisiac; pūrṇa-chandrodaya used in conditions of sexual neurasthenia, neuritis, tuberculosis and wasting diseases; and navagrahi-sindhura used as a stimulant, antitoxic and antisyphilitic. [*See also* BHASMA. PREPARATIONS]

Sirā (Śirā): Meaning 'the tubular vessels which admit the flow of fluids' (saraṇāt), the expression stands for fine capillaries, arteries, veins, or ducts. Sometimes, it is identified with dhamanī [*See* DHAMANĪ], but it is erroneous (cf. *SS,* śarīra, 9, 2). Dhamanīs are twenty-four in number, while the sirās are seven hundred; their functions also differ. The two, however, originate from the same source (viz. umbilicus region, nābhi-deśa), and ramify to cover the entire body. The sirā network represents the vascular system.

The analogy given is that of the trees in a garden being watered by a large number of canals drawn from a central tank (*SS,* śarīra, 7,2). The sirās, principal ones being seven hundred in number (while the secondary and minute ones are almost innumerable), originate from the region of the umbilicus (nābhi) and spread out over the entire body, some ascending, some descending and some coursing across, like the fibres of a leaf emanating from the central vein ('druma-patra sevanīnām iva', *SS,* ibid.). They nourish and support the body from the navel region, which in turn is supported by the vital currents (prāṇa) (*SS*, ibid., 4).

The primary sirās, however, are forty in number: ten of them carry vāta (and are vermillion in colour), ten carry pitta (and are blue in colour, and warm to touch), ten carry kapha (and are white in colour, and cold and hard to touch), and ten carry blood (and are red in colour, and neither too hot nor too cold to touch.) Each group of sirās gets ramified in the appropriate regions into 175 branches. Thus, the total number of sirās in the body is 700.

The arrangement of the 175 sirās that carry vāta, for instance is like this: (a) 34 in the trunk (koshṭha): pelvic region attached to anus and penis, 8; 2 at each side, that is, 4; back, 6; abdominal cavity, 6; chest, 10; (b) 100 in the extremities: each of the legs 25, each of the arms 25; (c) 41 in the region above the clavicles (jatrūrdhva): head, 14; ears, 4; tongue, 9; eyes, 8; nose, 6. Similar is the arrangement for the other groups of sirās, except for the sirās in the eyes (8 of them carrying vāta, but 10 each of the other groups carrying the remaining doshas, including blood) and in the ears (4 carrying vāta, but 2 each carrying the other doshas).

The sirās carrying vāta, when normal, facilitate the normal and specific functions of the body (expansion, contraction, articulation, etc.), clarity of mind, and acuity of sense-organs ('amoham buddhi-karmaṇām'), and, when abnormal, bring about several (actually 80) diseases of vāta. The sirās carrying pitta, when normal, produce a healthy glow of complexion, relish for food and stimulation of the gastric fire, while they produce, when abnormal, diseases (40) of pitta. The sirās carrying kapha, when normal, give unctuousness to the limbs, firmness to the joints, strength and efficiency, and, when abnormal, causes diseases (20) of kapha. The sirās carrying blood normally strengthen the other primary constituents of the body (dhātu), improves complexion, helps the sensation of touch and pain, and contributes to the efficiency of behaviour generally, and, when abnormal, bring about diseases of the blood (*SS*, śarīra, 7,8-14).

It should, however, be borne in mind that the sirās, described as carrying a dosha, do not carry that particular dosha in isolation. In fact, a sirā is a 'carrier of all things' ('sarvavaha') (*SS*, ibid., 15). But the dosha mentioned as specific to the sirā will be the dominant factor in this complex, especially when pathogenic conditions prevail.

As a curative measure, when venesection is resorted to, a distinction is made between the sirās that are fit to be opened and the sirās that should not be opened. Of the 400 sirās located in the extremities, 384 are suitable for venesection; of the 136 sirās located in the trunk, 104 are suitable; and of the 164 sirās in the region above the clavicles, only 114 are suitable. When the sirās that are regarded as unsuitable for venesection are pierced or opened, there is a risk of bodily deformity or even death. (*SS*, ibid., 8). [*See also* BODY and DHAMANĪ]

Sleep: Three conditions (avasthā) of life have since long been recognized: wakefulness (jāgrat), dream (svapna) and deep sleep (sushupti) (cf. *BU*, 2,1,18; 4,3,9; *CHU*, 6,8,1-2; 8,10,1; *KauU*,4, 19); *MāndU*,5, etc.). The explanations in the Upanishadic context are that sleep results from the fatigue brought about during the waking state, that sleep is a state when one does not desire and has no dreams, and that one 'goes into himself' during sleep (*svam-apīti*) (cf. *BU*, 4,3,19-22). It is a state when the sense-organs do not function (viz. they do not prehend their respective objects) and mind ceases to operate (unlike in dream). There is a loss of communication between the individual and his surrounding.

Āyurvedic texts also recognize the three conditions, but explain them as due to the operation of the three guṇas: sattva (wakefulness), rajas (dream) and tamas (sleep) Hārīta (śarīra,1) holds that sleep results when tamas overpowers the individual, and the body rests; and that sleep is a condition of dissolution of the outer self in the inner self in the region between the eyebrows and halfway through the nose (nāsārdhe cha bhruvor madhye līyate chāntar-ātmanā'). *SS* (Śarīra, 4,31), however, explains sleep with reference to the heart, which is 'the seat of consciousness' [*See* HEART]. When the heart (which is produced from the essential and nutrient portions of blood and kapha) folds itself up, it is asleep (nidrā); and when it spreads out, it is wakefulness.

The 'folding up' of the heart is characterized by the choking of the channels that carry consciousness (saṁjñā-vāhanī-srotāmsi), by an excess of tamas in kapha. This sleep is called 'tāmasī-sleep'. It is only this condition that prevails at the time of death or 'dissolution'; only, there is no waking up at that time (anavabodhinī) (*SS*, ibid.).

Tamas is given as the cause of sleep, and sattva of wakefulness. Tamas is deṣcribed as an all-pervasive and illusive energy (vaishṇavī-pāpmā) (*SS*, ibid.). The overpowering of the heart by this is experienced as the insensibility in sleep. The sense-organs do not operate then, and thus the mind is deprived of the objects for its activity. *CS* mentions that when the active self is fatigued in body and mind, he loses touch with his surroundings; and then sleep comes to him.

Seven kinds of sleep are recognized in the texts: (1) sleep that is caused by the excess of tamas in the mind; (2) sleep caused by the vitiation of the kapha; (3) sleep caused by excessive bodily exertion; (4) sleep caused by excessive mental exertion; (5) sleep caused by a complication of disease; (6) sleep that is exotic (indicative of bad prognosis); and (7) sleep caused by the very nature of the night. It is the last one (viz. physiological sleep) that is regarded as proper.

Proper sleep is beneficial to the system: it causes happiness, nourishment, strength, virility and longevity. Lack of sleep or improper sleep causes misery, emaciation, weakness, sterility and early death (*AHṛ*, sūtra, 7). Sleep at the right time makes for the balance of the body constituents (dhātu-sāmya), alertness, good vision, good complexion, and fine digestive power (*SKD*).

Persons who have an excess of tamas in their system tend to sleep heavily; they sleep both during day and night. Those with rajas as the dominant trait, sleep either during daytime or during night; and their sleep is light and disturbed. Persons with sattva as the main trait, sleep peacefully, but never before midnight. Those who suffer from enfeebled kapha, from aggravated vāta, or from physical ailments or mental troubles sleep very little, if at all; and their sleep is usually disturbed (*SS*, śarīra, 4,31).

Insomnia is caused by overwork, diseases (especially of the vāta type), old age, predominance of sattva in the system, suppression of tamas, physical exercise, fasting, uncomfortable bed, smoke nearby, or mental conditions like grief, anxiety and fear. Some therapeutic procedures such as elimination of doshas from the body through purgation, emesis and blood-letting also cause loss of sleep. Among the methods of inducing sleep are massage, (saṁvahana, kneading the body by hand); unction; bath; application of soothing ointment to eyes, head and face; comfortable bed; eating śālī rice with curds; drinking the soup of domestic, marshy and aquatic animals; drinking warm milk; intake of 'fermented drinks' in small measure; and keeping to proper time. Excess of sleep is a disorder and may be corrected by the elimination of doshas from the system through purgation and emesis, physical exercise, blood-letting or methods of suppressing tamas.

Sleep during daytime (divā-svāpa) is said to have bad effects, except in the summer months (*SS*, śarīra, 4): it vitiates kapha and pitta, causes headache, jaundice, timidity, heaviness of the body, loss of digestive power, feeling of kapha overpowering the heart (hṛdayopalepa), oedema, anorexia, nausea, cough, diseases of the throat, obstruction of the circulating channels in the body, impairment of memory and intelligence, and weakness of the sense-organs. It is especially unfavourable for those who are obese, addicted to unctuous food, have an excess of kapha in their system, or who have ingested artificial poison (dūshī-visha).

However, sleep during daytime is recommended for those who have got used to it (sātmī-kṛta), those who are given to heavy manual labour or mental exertion, those who excessively indulge in sex-activity, those who are very old or very young, those who are emaciated and those who suffer from diseases (like phthisis, diarrhoea, colic pain, dyspnoea, hiccough, wasting diseases, abnormal thirst etc.). It is good also for those who are exhausted after a long journey, who are kept awake at night, who are troubled by fear or grief, or who have suffered a physical injury.

SS (śārīra, 4,38) recommends: "Do not keep awake during night, nor sleep during daytime; knowing that those are bad for health, one should sleep in moderation. He will thus be free from diseases, his mind will be in good shape, he will be strong, his complexion will be fine, his body will neither be too fat nor too thin, and he will live long" [*See also* SLEEP DURING DAY, HEART].

Sleep During Day: Night is the time for sleep; and sleep that is induced by the very nature of night and by the diurnal habit of men is regarded as 'nourishing and protective sleep' (bhūta-dhātrī). [*See* SLEEP]. Sleep during day-time (divā-svāpa) is both unnatural and unhealthy. It is in the nature of a weakness or a bad habit (vyasana). It brings about ill-health by interfering with the natural balance of the doshas through tipping the phlegm (kapha); it cuts short longevity, and prevents the fulfilment of the objectives of life. It causes among other diseases jaundice, headache, body pain, heaviness of limbs, accumulation of kapha in the lungs,dropsy, loss of appetite and hunger, hiccough, cough, nasal trouble, itches, boils, dullness of brain, and weakness of the sense-organs.

But it does good during the hot season (grīshma, when the element of phlegm, kapha is at a disadvantage). It is also good for a little time immediately before meals: it would help the digestive process. And those who are used to sleeping for a while after food during day time (that is, for whom day-sleep has become constitutionally accepted, sātmī-krta) should not break the habit; otherwise, the doshas would be excited (*YR*, 355).

Sleep during day-time is beneficial to children, old persons, extremely lean persons, and those who have tired themselves with excess of physical exercise, who have lost sleep during night, who have travelled much, who are fatigued, who are fasting, who are inebriated, or those who suffer from wasting diseases, hiccough, respiratory ailments, colic, excessive thirst, diarrhoea and indigestion. It is positively harmful to those who suffer from haemoptysis, consumption, or from the effect of poison, and to those who habitually drink water at dawn (RJN) [*See* USHAH-PĀNA *also* DAILY ROUTINE, SLEEP]

Śleshma: [*See* KAPHA, DOSHA, TRIDOSHA THEORY]

Snāna: [*See* BATH]

Snāyu: Translated as 'ligament', 'snāyu' (from the root 'snā', or 'snai', snāti śuddhyati dosho anayā, 'the doshas are purified by it' cf. sinew in English) is described as tendonous portions of the muscle (peśī), fibres which pervade the muscle both within and without, and help in 'bearing the load' (bhāra-saha). It is also described as 'vāta-carrying duct' (vāyu-vāhanī-nādī), (SKD), signifying its involvement in biomotor functions. Injury to it, more than injury to the bone, *sirā,* muscle, or joints, may result in serious disturbances in the functioning of the organs of action, paralysis, loss of limbs, or death.

It is a mechanism which securely binds the joints with thread-like structures. There are as many as 900 ligaments in the human body: 600 in the extremities (hands and legs), 250 in the trunk, and 70 in the region above the clavicles (*SS*,śarīra,5,29). Their form is fourfold: (1) ramifying or branching (pratānavatī), as those that are to be found in the four extremities and joints (supar fascia, deep fascia, aponeurosis, etc); (2) circular (vṛtta), or the large ligaments or tendons (kaṇḍara); (3) thick or broad (pṛthu), as the sinews and thick fascias that are found in the chest, back, sides, and head; and (4) hollow or perforated (sushira), as those that are found in the stomach, in the intestines and in the bladder (areolar sheaths etc). "As a boat made of planks and timber fastened together by means of a large number of bindings is enabled to float on water and to carry cargo, so the human frame being bound and fastened at the sandhis or joints by a large number of ligaments is enabled to bear pressure" (*SS*, ibid., 33).

'Snāyu' is functionally divided into three stages: (1) snāyus functioning like secondary body constituents (upa-dhātu), subtle thread-like structures constituted of fat-tissue (medas), and the unctuous and firm qualities of the kapha and appearing as white in most places in the body and as yellow in some places; (2) snāyus functioning like structures (avayava), produced from the former (snāyu as upa-dhātu), and occurring in four forms (mentioned above); and finally (3) snāyus as bindings (bandhana) for the bones and the muscles in joints, and occurring in different forms (twisted, rope-like, round, flat, sheath-like etc.), like capsular ligaments. [*See* BODY]

Srotas: Channels of circulation or tracts within the body are called srotas because of the trickling or oozing (sru, 'to flow') of secretions through them. They are pathways (ayana) for the nutrient products or waste-products of body metabolism to reach their destination (viz. assimilation of nutrient substances by different parts of the body, or elimination of waste products from the body). They carry the dhātus (body-constituents or tissues) that are undergoing transformation (parināma) and that are mobile in character. The body-constituents have their own seats in the system; and during the transformation that occurs at each of these seats, the stable portion which is nourished from the preceding costituent (poshya) is separated from the mobile portion which nourishes the succeeding constituent (poshaka) situated in a different place. But for them, the mobile nourishing portion of one constituent cannot reach the site of the next (viz. nourished) constituent. They are physical structures (mūrti-mantah), definite in their number and specific in their function (*CS*, nidāna, 5,3).

According to an ancient view, cited and rejected by *CS*, (ibid., 4), the human being is nothing more than a bundle of these channels ('Srotasāṁ eva samudāyaṁ'), for they are all-pervasive, all-permissive and carriers of health and disease. *CS* points out that these are only channels of circulation, and as such are different from the substances that are carried through them, from the nourishment that is provided to the different parts of the body through them, and from the destinations towards which they carry the nourishing substances. They constitute a network of open spaces within the body ('khāni chhidrāṇi', *RN*). They are so many in number that some hold that they are innumerable, while others find it possible to enumerate them (*CS*, ibid., 5). And they are distinct from arteries (dhamanī) and ducts (sirā).

The body is composed of several types of these channels, some carrying the basic tissues of one body-constituent to its next (dhātus) some the health-giving or morbid doshas from one part of the body to another, and some the waste products out of the body (mala). *SS* (śarīra, 5,9) speaks of nine openings for the channels that are outward directed: eyes, ears, mouth, nostrils, anus and urethra, and adds three more for women: breasts (for flowing out of milk) and the genetic passage which carries off menstrual blood. There are thirteen kinds of channels (*CS*, vimāna, 5,6; cf. *SS*, śarīra, 9 where only eleven are mentioned), which are gross (sthūla) or clearly distinguishable:

(1) Channels carrying the vital breath from outside to the blood-stream (prāṇa-vaha-srotāṁsi), situated at the heart region and the central cavity (mahā-srotas, viz. alimentary tract).

(2) Channels (two in number) carrying water (viz. serum and lymph) (udaka-vaha-), with their seats in the palate (tālu) and the pancreas (kloman).

(3) Channels carrying food (viz. gastro-intestinal tract) (anna-vaha-), with seats in the stomach (āmāśaya) and the left side (vāma-pārśva).

(4) Channels (two in number) carrying chyle (rasa-vaha-), located in the heart region (hṛdayam) and in the ten vessels (rasa vaha-dhamanī).

(5) Channels (two in number) carrying blood (rakta-vaha-), located in the liver and spleen (yakrt-plīha) and in the capillaries in general (rakta-vaha-dhamanī).

(6) Channels carrying muscle-tissue

(māmsa-vaha-), located in the ligaments (snāyu), and skin (tvāk̄).

(7) Channels (two in number) carrying fat-tissue (medo-vaha- located in two kidneys (vrkkau) and ormentum (kati-pradeśa, vapa-vahanam).

(8) Channels carrying bone-tissue (asthi-vaha-) (not mentioned is *SS*), located in the adipose-tissue (medas) and the buttocks (jaghanam).

(9) Channels carrying bone-marrow (majjā-vaha-) (not in *SS*), located in the bones (asthīni) and joints (sandhayah);

(10) Channels (two in number) carrying semen (sperm) (śukra-vaha-), located in the two testicles (vrshanam) and pudendum (śepha).

(11) Channels (two in number) carrying urine (mūtra-vaha-), located in the bladder (basti, urethra) and the two kidneys (vamkshṇau) located in the anus (guda) and large intestines (pakvāśaya); and

(12) Channels (two in number) carrying faeces (purishavaha).

(13) Channels carrying sweat (svedo-vaha-) (not in *SS*) located in the adipose tissue (medas) and in the follicles of hair (loma-kūpa).

All the channels, however, are utilized by the three doshas for their circulation. Health of the system is maintained by the proper (viz. normal, prakrti-bhūtatvāt) functioning of these channels (*CS*, vimāna, 5, 6). And the circulation along the channels is kept normal by taking adequate food, eliminating the waste-products from the system, attending to the natural urges of the body, and taking physical exercise.

If, however, the circulation along the channels is impeded or arrested, owing to some cause, internal or external, the substances in that particular channel accumulate, and thereby the tissue-metabolism is affected. The process of digestion (dhātu-pāka) at that particular seat becomes improper; there will then be 'uncooked' or 'improperly cooked' products (āma) available for circulation. They do not flow smoothly, and remain as lumps along that channel or get into other channels which are functioning properly, and cause disturbances there. This is how diseases are caused.

There are characteristic ways in which the normal functions of the channels are disturbed, and there are also specific treatments prescribed to correct the disorders:

(1) Channels carrying the vital breath (prāṇa-) are disturbed by suppression of natural urges, indulgence in ununctuous things, taking exercise when hungry etc. The disorder is manifested by prolonged, scanty, aggravated, shallow or quick respirations, accompanied by sounds or pain. The treatment for this disorder is the same as that for respiratory disorders.

(2) Channels carrying water (udaka-) are disturbed by exposure to heat, indigestion, intake of alcohol or excessively dry food, or not drinking sufficient water. The disorder is manifested by dryness of the tongue, palate, lips, throat and pancreas (kloman), and excessive thirst. Treatment is the same as that for abnormal thirst.

(3) Channels carrying food (anna) are disturbed by improper and untimely food and by poor digestive power. The symptoms are distaste for food, indigestion, vomiting, colic pain, abnormal thirst, loss of eye-sight, and so on. Treatment is the same as that for digestive troubles.

(4) Channels carrying chyle (rasa) are disturbed by an over- indulgence in food which is heavy, cold and oily, and also by worry and fear. Symptoms are swelling, consumption, troubles in breathing etc. Treatment is by fasting.

(5) Channels carrying blood (rakta) are disturbed by over-indulgence, by unctuous and hot food and drinks, and by exposure to sun and fire. Symptoms are pallor of the face, blushing, fever, burning sensations, haemorrhage, redness of the eyes. Treatment is

blood-letting.

(6) Channels carrying muscle-tissue (māṁsa) are disturbed by eating heavy and coarse food and by sleeping soon after eating. Symptoms are swelling, atrophy of muscles, varicose veins etc. Treatment is by surgery, use of alkalis and cauterization.

(7) Channels carrying fat-tissue (meda) are disturbed by lack of exercise, sleep during daytime, eating fatty food, and intake of alcoholic drinks. Symptoms are excessive sweating, oily skin, parched palate, swelling of body, abnormal thirst etc. Treatment is emaciation therapy.

(8) Channels carrying bone-tissue (asthi) are disturbed by excess of physical exercise, manual labour where bones are rubbed and pressure is applied on them, and by eating food which promotes vāta. Symptoms are pain in teeth and bones and pathological conditions of hair and nails. Treatment is by pañcha-karma (five eliminations), and enema of milk and ghee boiled with bitter drugs.

(9) Channels carrying bone-marrow (majja) are disturbed by crushing, excessive liquification, injury and compression of marrow as also by eating food-stuffs that are mutually antagonistic. Symptoms are pain in the finger-joints, giddiness, fainting spells and deep-seated abscesses of finger-joints. Treatment is by the diet of sweet and bitter taste, indulgence in sexual activity and timely elimination of the doshas.

(10) Channels carrying semen (śukra) are disturbed by untimely sexual intercourse, suppression of natural urges, undergoing surgical operations, application of alkalis, cauterization etc. Symptoms are impotency, delayed emission, blood-stained emission etc. Treatment is the diet of sweet and bitter taste and timely elimination of doshas.

(11) Channels carrying urine (mūtra) are disturbed by eating food, drinking water or having sexual intercourse while there is the urge for micturition and for suppression of natural urges, especially by persons prone to wasting diseases. Symptoms are excessive urination, retention of urine, impairment in the composition of urine, discharge of thick urine, pain while urinating, numbness of genitals, or constipation. Treatment includes the remedies prescribed for difficulty in urination.

(12) Channels carrying faeces (purīsha) are disturbed by suppression of urges, eating food excessively, and eating when the food previously eaten has not been digested, especially by people with weak digestion. Symptoms are retention of stools in bowels, distention of the abdomen, foul smell, watery stool, and painful evacuation. Treatment is the same as for diarrhoea.

(13) Channels carrying sweat (sveda) are disturbed by excessive physical exercise, exposure to heat, indulgence in cold and hot things, intake of unbalanced food, worry, grief and fear. Symptoms are absence of sweat, excessive perspiration, coarseness of body, burning sensation, horripilation, etc. Treatment is the same as for fever.

Generally, the vitiation of any channel is manifested by exaggeration or inhibition of normal functions, tumours and shifting of the course of substances (dosha, dhātu and mala) to channels not proper to them.

Strength: Known as 'bala', it is regarded as three-fold: (1) 'natural', innate or congenital (sahaja), dependent upon ones own physical constitution and mental make-up, and not upon any extraneous aids; (2) 'due to temporal factors' (kālaja), dependent upon the seasonal variations and upon ones own age; and (3) 'rational' or acquired (yuktija), dependent upon the food one takes or the conduct one adopts (*CS*, sūtra, 11,36).

Śukra: Counted as the last of the seven body constituents (dhātu), this is the generative fluid, derived from the bone-marrow (majjā) during the course of its 'cooking' in its own 'fire' (majjāgni). Although the Sanskrit expression refers to the reproductive substance or impregnating fluid in the male animals (semen, sperm), it is said to be present in females also, being secreted during the orgasm. It contributes to strength, complexion and nourishment in both men and women.

This generative substance (śukra) is cool, white and viscous fluid that has the property of strengthening the body; it is described as the 'essence of the body system' ('vapuh-sāra') and as the best support for life ('jīvasyāśraya-uttamah'). It is present all over the body, even as butter in milk or jaggery-juice in sugarcane (*SS*, śarīra, 4, 20). But its chief region is below the urinary bladder (vasti). "It passes through the ducts situated about two fingers breadth on either side (vas deferens) and just below the neck of the bladder and finally flows out through the canal" (ibid., 22).

Its chief function is to reproduce (impregnate); it also strengthens and invigorates the body, and produces fondness for the opposite sex. It is ejected out during sexual congress, through the urinary outlet.

Although composed of all the five primary forms of matter, it is principally 'water' (as semen). It is the last of the constituents, and therefore, during its being 'cooked' in its own 'fire' (śukrāgni), it does not generate any other constituent. Derived from it, however, is vitality (ojas) as the secondary constituent (up-dhātu). [*See* VITALITY]

Among the diseases pertaining to this fluid are sterility, impotence, begetting diseased and deformed offsprings. Semen, vitiated by deranged doshas becomes coloured (reddish black in vāta, yellowish or bluish in pitta and dirty white in kapha), causes pain in its flow, has foul smell and acquires clotted character. Likewise, catamenial fluid (ārtava) in women can also be vitiated (*SS*, śarīra, 2,3-4). [*See also* DHĀTU GARBHA, DEVELOPMENT].

Suppression of Urges: Suppression of natural bodily tendencies or impulses or physiological urges (vega-dhāraṇā) (delay in answering calls of nature) forms an important subject in Indian medicine, especially in preventive medicine ('rogānutpādanīya'); for such suppression produces ailments of various kinds, many of them serious [*See* PREVENTIVE MEDICINE]. Allowing freedom for the discharge of these impulses is, therefore, regarded as essential to health. "The wise person will not suppress the urges when they have arisen" (*CS*, sūtra, 7,3).

The rationale of this hygienic principle is given as follows: the formation of urges within the body is the function of vāta, especially the 'downward-breath' (apāna), located principally near the lower abdomen [*See* DOSHA]. In order to discharge this function, the vāta will become excited. If the discharge of impulses are suppressed (viz. are not allowed to be discharged), the excited vāta would be obliged to continue in the excited condition. This would bring about diseases.

Thirteen bodily tendencies (urges) are enumerated as natural, the discharge of which would help maintain health: the wind that goes out of the anus (vāta or adho-vāta), faeces (purīsha, vit), urine (mūtra), sneeze (kshavathu), thirst (pipāsā or tṛṭ), hunger (kshut), sleep (nidrā), cough (kāsa), heaving due to exertion (nihśvāsa or śrama-śvāsa), yawning (jṛmbhaṇā), tears (aśru), vomiting (chhardi), and semen virile (śukra, retas); sometimes, belching (udgāra) is also included in the list of impulses.

Texts describe the diseases caused by the suppression of each of these impulses, and also suggest remedial measures in each case (*CS*, sūtra, 7,5-25; *AS*, 1,5,4-25; *AHr*, 1,4,4-24): Suppression of (1) downward wind: phantom tumours, flatulence, colic, fatigue, pressure on the heart; (2) faeces: cold, headache, eructation, swellings; (3) urine: bodily pain, calculus, pain in the urinary tract etc.; (4) sneezing: headache, weakness of sense-organs, torticolis or stiffness of neck facial paralysis etc. ; (5) thirst: dryness of mouth, weakness of body, distraction of mind, deafness, fainting, heart-diseases; (6) hunger: body pain, loss of appetite, faintness, weakness, colic, giddiness; (7) sleep: heaviness of eyes and head, sloth, yawning, stiffness, weakness, fainting, indigestion, giddiness; (8) cough: increase of cough, dyspnoea, loss of appetite, diseases of heart, hiccough; (9) heaving due to exertion: difficulty in breathing, phantom tumours, diseases of the heart, syncope or fainting; (10) yawning: same as in sneezing; (11) tears (due to pleasure or sorrow): chronic rhinitis, cold, diseases of eye, headache, diseases of heart, torticolis, phantom tumours, loss of appetite, giddiness; (12) vomiting: erysipelas, skin diseases, diseases of the eye, itching, anaemia, fever, cough, dyspnoea, swelling; (13) semen-virile: discharge of semen with urine, pain in the penis, vagina, and anus, burning in heart, body-pain, suppression of urination, impotency.

While non-suppression of bodily urges is a hygienic measure, suppression is prescribed for mental impulses such as greed, fear, anger, sorrow, and arrogance (*CS* sūtra 7,23-29). "One who is eager to maintain his health and accomplish his welfare must always restrain the impulses such as avarice, jealousy, hatred, envy, and anger" (*AHr.* 1,4,24). One must also refrain bodily from undertaking exertion beyond his capacity (sāhasa), and from activities of the body, mind and speech that are unworthy (aśasta) (*CS*, ibid., 26). Even when tendencies such as these exist naturally (for example, desire to physically hurt, steal, insult, and condemn, and illegal sex-gratification), there is merit in suppressing them (ibid., 28 and 29). Suppression of these unbecoming tendencies of the mind will not lead to any diseases; on the other hand, non-suppression of them may eventually result in distress and disease.

This is an aspect of Indian medicine which brings out the importance of morality in maintaining health. The assumption is that there are within the individual constitution, tendencies which will disturb the physiological balance and tendencies which will ruin the functional integrity of the individual. The former are to be discharged, so that the balance is restored; and the latter suppressed, so that the individual's integrity is maintained. [*See also* HEALTH, HYGIENE, DAILY ROUTINE].

Sutures: Known as sevanī, they are tendinous bands looking like sutures, from which the muscles on either side arise (*SS*, śarīra, 5, 14, cf. *Bhishagratna*, vol II, p.162, fn.). They are seven in number, five in the head, one in the root of the tongue, and one under the genital. Incision made in any of these sutures spells danger to the person., (*SS*, ibid.). [*See* BODY (HUMAN)].

Svabhāva-Bala-Pravrtta: A variety of diseases, brought about by natural causes such as hunger, thirst, sleep, old age etc. Two varieties in this are recognized: (1) due to time, or normal ageing, diseases which occur periodically despite all care that is taken (such as good food, wholesome drinks, nourishing drugs etc.) and (2) not due to time or normal ageing diseases which occur owing to lack of sufficient care or absence of proper medication. These are also called 'ādhidaivika' (*SS*, sūtra, 24). [*See* DISEASES]

Svapna: [*See* DREAMS]

Svarasa: [*See* EXPRESSED JUICE]

T

Taila: Although, literally *taila* means only sesamum oil (from *tila*), it is generally employed for all oil preparations in which decoctions and pastes of drugs are involved, and which acquire the colour, odour, and taste of the drugs used although their consistency is that of the oil. Most of the preparations are for external application and for a bath; but some are meant for internal use (with warm water or milk; some are prescribed as post-prandial drink). [*See* MEDICATED OILS]

Tamas: One of the three gunas constituting prakrti [*See* GUṆA, PRAKṚTI], it stands for mass, inertia, resistance to activity, or conservation (sthiti) (distinguished from sattva, which is perceptibility and brightness, and from rajas, which is activity), obscuration, darkness, gloom. It is characterized by heaviness, ignorance, blindness, delusion, gloom, error, sloth, dullness and also emotions like sorrow, despair, fear, despondency, anxiety etc. Its colour is black (as sattva's colour is white, and rajas' red). Its involvement in the human constitution is also recognized [*See* SĀMKHYA, GUNA, CONSTITUTION]

Tāmbūla: Chewing betel leaves (*Piper betle*) with areca nuts (tāmbūla-charvana) after a meal is highly commended in Āyurvedic texts (even in *CS* and *SS*), and is a practice even now much in vogue all over the country. The usual (and minimum) ingredients are fresh betel leaves (nāgavallī), areca nuts (pūga), lime (chūrna) and catechu (khadira). Also added are coriandrum sativum (dhānya), Myristica fragrans (jāti), scented seeds of Hibiscus abelmoschus (katuka), Elettaria cardamomum (sūkshmaila), flower stalk of Syzygium aromaticum (lavaṅga), and extract of Cinnamomum camphora (karpūra). Sometimes tobacco also is added. There are several varieties of tāmbūla, some with nine ingredients and some with thirteen. Royalty and nobility in medieval India encouraged the inclusion of gold leaves, bādām, kuṁkuṁ-keśarī, sandal, dālchini, etc.

Chewing is said to pacify all the three doshas, and cause cheerfulness (saumanasya); it cleanses the mouth, removing all foetid odours; it makes the mouth fragrant. More importantly, it causes an extra-secretion of saliva, which will aid the digestive process.

Chewing betel leaves is recommended after a night's sleep, after a bath, after the meals, and after sexual activity in the night.It is also useful after vomiting, or when some organic poison has entered the stomach. It adds to convivality in assemblies of like-minded people.

It is advisable, however, to chew in moderation (viz. not more than three or four times a day), for excessive chewing impairs the physique, diminishes strength, injures eyesight, dulls the complexion of the skin, loosens teeth and roots of hair, and causes deafness; it aggravates both vāta and pitta, and makes blood tend towards haemoptysis (rakta-pitta). While chewing in moderation helps digestion, excessive chewing weakens the digestive power. Chewing must never be resorted to when one is hungry, or when a purgative has been taken; nor when one is having diarrhoea. Persons with weak teeth, troubled eyesight, ulceration in the mouth, persons infected with poison, or suffering from hysteria, diabetes, epilepsy, asthma, consumption, heart-troubles,haemoptysis or reaction to excessive drinking of alcoholic beverages (madātyaya) must avoid chewing.

While chewing, care must be taken to spit out the first and second parts of the juice, for the first part (viz. the mouthful juice of first chewing) aggravates pitta and is toxic(visha) and the second is heavy (causing indigestion) and purgative. From the third part, the juice is like ambrosia, preventing disease and senile decay.

Chewing betel leaves and so on is an ancient practice in India (dating back to the second century B.C.) and probably the Tāntrik cults encouraged it and made it widespread. It has remained obligatory on festive occasions; and large numbers of Indians are addicts to it even today. The practice is also prevalent in other tropical countries like Thailand, Vietnam, Malaya, New-Guinea, Indonesia, South China, Madagascar and Philippines; it is also popular in Burma and Sri-Lanka.

There are a few works dealing especially with the practice of chewing betel leaves. Instances are *Tāṁbūla-mañjarī (JOI,* M. S. University of Baroda) and *Tāṁbūla-kalpa-saṁgraha* of Narasiṁha-bhatta (noticed by P. K. Gode). Mythological accounts of the origin of the practice are to be found in some of the purānas (for example, *Skanda-purāṇa,* 6, 210), (cf. medieval compilation in Sanskrit of useful information about the practice, *Tāṁbūla-mañjarī,* ed. by J.S. Pade, Poona Oriental Research Institute) [*See also* FOOD].

Taste : The Sanskrit word for taste, rasa, has many meanings, of which four are relevant to Indian medicine (1) 'taste', one of the seven body constituents (dhātu), (called chyle), (2) mercury, and (3) pharmacological preparation. [*See* RASA, DHĀTU, MERCURY and PHARMACY). We are concerned here with the first of the meanings. It is defined as the object of the gustatory organ, viz. the tongue (*CS,* 1, 1, 'rasanārtho rasah'), as a quality that is perceived by its contact with the mucous membranes of the mouth. Its relevance to pharmacology is in the context of the direct action of a drug on the nerve-endings in the mouth, especially the tongue.

Like the drug (dravya), of which the taste is a property, and to which it is related as a dependent detail, taste is composed of all the five primary forms of matter (pāñcha-bhautika). It is principally a property of 'water', in which, however, taste is unmanifest (avyakta). It becomes manifest only when 'water' is combined with the 'earth' element. Therefore 'water' is said to be the main generative source (yoni) of taste (also *SS,* sūtra, 42), while 'earth' is the auxiliary or cooperative cause. The other three elements (fire, air and ākāśa) enter into this initial combination, and become responsible for numerous tastes.

Although tastes are theoretically innumerable, only a few of them are manifest (viz. apprehended by the tongue). And the expression 'rasa' is confined to such clearly manifest (vyakta) tastes. There are tastes which are altogether unmanifest (avyakta), or only slightly manifest (īshad-vyakta), or manifest only at the end (ante-vyakta). These are known as 'secondary tastes' (anu-rasa) (*AS,* 1, 17 and Hemādri on *AHr*). The distinction between the two is made on the following counts: (1) the rasas reside in the substance and are easily and fully recognized by the organ of taste, for example, pungent taste in pippalī (*Piper longum*) and astringent taste in harītakī (*Terminalia chebula*), whereas the anurasas cannot be so easily apprehended, and can be recognized only by its action on the constitution (for example, the sweet taste in harītakī); (2) the rasas are present in the substance in their fresh state as well as in the dry state (for example, the sweet taste in grapes), while the anurasas may be present in the fresh state of the substance but disappear in its dry state (like in the sweet taste of pippalī); and (3) the rasas are apprehended as soon as they come into contact with the tongue (like the sour taste of butter-milk), while the anurasas are recognised only later, neither as soon as tasted or in the middle but at the end (like the bitter taste in buttermilk). The prefix 'anu' in the latter case signifies 'little': ('alpo rasah', HEMĀDRI on *AHṛ*). Even when recognized at the end, it is but slightly. Altogether, sixty-three varieties of tastes are enumerated, of which only six are 'rasas' proper.

The apprehension of tastes is dependent upon several factors like attention (pravṛtti) to the object being tasted, the healthy condition (svastha) of the gustatory organ, the adequate quantity (matrā) of the thing tasted, and dissolution of the subtle properties of the thing with taste in the bodhaka-kapha. The last factor is considered especially important, for when the tongue is perfectly dry there can be no perception of the distinction between tastes.

The relation between a substance and its taste is one of reciprocal dependence; the substance is the ground while the taste is a figure thereon; they stand in the same relation as body and soul (*SS*, 1). The constitutional peculiarity of the substance determines the particular taste that is characteristic of that substance. The six tastes that are now generally accepted in Indian thought are: sweet (madhura), acid or sour (amla), saline (lavana), pungent (kaṭu, or kaṭuka,), bitter (tikta), and astringent (kashāya) (*CS*, 1, 1, 65).

CS, contains an interesting account of different views regarding the number of rasas. BHADRA-KĀPYA held that taste was really one, the object of the organ of gustation (viz. tongue), and not distinct from water. Taste, according to him, is a positive experience emerging at the tongue, although the tongue is capable of apprehending the absence of taste also. The Brahmin ŚAKUNTEYA argued that tastes are two-fold: emaciating (chhedaniya) and nourishing (upaśamanīya). But these are, in fact, actions of tastes, and not themselves tastes. PŪRṆĀKSHA-MAUDGALYA added a third variety of taste to the aforesaid, namely having in common both of them (sādhāraṇa). It may mean, sometimes nourishing and sometimes emaciating. Oil is given as an example of substances which emaciate the fat, and nourish the lean. HIRANYAKSHA-KAUŚIKA held that tastes were of five kinds: palatable (to the tongue, svādu) and wholesome, (hita, good for the body), palatable but unwholesome, unpalatable but wholesome, and unpalatable and unwholesome. While palatable or otherwise could be regarded as tastes, wholesome and unwholesome are effects rather than tastes. KUMĀRA-ŚIRĀ-BHĀRADVĀJA regarded tastes as five in number in accordance with the five primary forms of matter: earth, water, fire, air and ākāśa. These are actually distinctions among substances, and although tastes have substances as their ground, they may not be influenced by the distinctions among them. According to the royal sage VĀYOVIDA, tastes are six-fold: heavy, light, cold, hot, unctuous and dry, which are actually properties of substances rather than varieties of taste. The prince of Videha, NIMI, thought that tastes are seven in number, adding 'alkaline' (kshāra) to the standard list of six. But 'alkaline' is more a substance than a taste. BAḌIŚA DHĀRMĀRGAVA held that one more taste, viz. 'Unmanifest' or imperceptible (avyakta) must be added to the list of seven. But perceptibility or otherwise is a condition of tastes; it cannot itself be a taste. And finally, KANKĀYANA, the physician of the Bāhlīka region, argued that tastes are in fact innumerable on account of the wide variety of substances, properties, actions and their combinations.

The discussion is concluded by the statement of the view of ĀTREYA-PUNARVASU that tastes are only six in number ('shaḍeva rasāh', *CS*, 1, 26, 9, cf. also *AS*, 1, 18 and INDU on it, 'neither more nor less'). The six tastes are in the direct experience of people ('āsvādāt', *RVS*, 3, 5), and there is no seventh. Other categories of gustatory experience simulating tastes are to be classified 'secondary tastes' (anurasas), which are unmanifest in actual experience.

However, taste is not the fixed property of a substance: one taste can change into another, owing to several factors like the passage of time (kāla), the nature of the container (pātra), association with other substances (saṁyoga), the impact of sunlight (ātapa), cooking on fire (pāka), pharmaceutical processes (bhāvanā), climatic peculiarities of the place (deśa), natural transformation (pariṇāma), infection by worms etc (upasarga), and unnatural transformations (vikriyā) (cf. *RVS* and comm.).

Taste, being a property of substances, cannot itself have properties. But each taste, having a characteristic physical constitution, acts in a specific manner on the body (on the body constituents, on the doshas and on the waste products). The physical constitution of each taste is dominated by two of the five primary forms of matter, (although all tastes have all the five forms), and this must be inferred from the action of the tastes which can be observed. And the testimony of the wise ancients, who had the power intuitively to apprehend this matter, must also guide us in ascertaining the physical constitution of the tastes ('āgama-vedanīyah'). This ascertainment is important because the correction of disorders would otherwise be impossible: the drug selected must be able to correct the errant dosha and help maintain balance. An attempt has also been made to correlate the twenty properties of substances that *CS* enumerates ('gurv-ādi') with the six tastes.

The inferred physical constitution of tastes, their emergent properties, the various seasons in which tastes are on the ascendent and the drug-action dependent upon the different tastes are given below (*SS,* 1, 42; *CS,* 1, 26; *AS,* 1, 18):

(1) Sweet (madhura): predominantly composed of 'earth' (therefore, heavy) and 'water' (therefore, unctuous and cold); the season that favours the action of this taste is early winter (hemanta); pacifies vāta and pitta but vitiates kapha; responsible for the increase of chyle, blood, muscle, bone, bone-marrow and vitality; good for the eyes, hair and complexion; good for body strength; clears blood and chyle; removes thirst, burning sensation, fainting spells; causes worms in the stomach; facilitates oleation and satiation; causes pleasure; softens; heals wounds; promotes secretion of milk.

(2) Sour or acid (amla): predominantly 'earth' (according to *CS;* but 'water' according to *SS,* therefore, unctuous) and 'fire' (therefore, warm and light); the favouring season is the rains (varshā); pacifies vāta, but vitiates pitta and kapha; makes teeth sensitive; facilitates discharge; causes perspiration; clears mouth; affords flavour; causes burning sensation in mouth and neck; good for the heart; makes hair stand erect; helps digestion; gives appetite; causes burning sensation in the inner cavities.

(3) Saline or saltish (lavaṇa): predominantly 'earth' (therefore, heavy according to *SS,* or 'water' and therefore, unctuous according to *CS,* and *RSV*) and 'fire' (therefore, warm and sharp); the favouring season is autumn (śarad); pacifies vāta, but vitiates both pitta and kapha; quickly dissolving; moistening; softening; flavouring; causing burning sensation in the mouth, cheeks and throat; internally purifying; helping digestion; causing slackness; counteracting all other tastes; clearing the bodily channels; softening all the organs of the body.

(4) Pungent (kaṭu): predominantly 'air' (therefore, rough and light) and 'fire' (therefore, warm and sharp); summer is its favourable season; pacifies kapha, but vitiates vāta and pitta; irritates the tongue as soon as it comes into contact with it; appetiser; digestive; flavouring; purifying; oppressing; reduces bulkiness, sloth and phlegm; counteracts poison and intestinal worms; removes itching sensation; loosens the joints; detrimental to semen, adipose tissue and secre-

tion of milk; gives a burning sensation in the mouth, nose and eyes, causing also watering in these regions; brings on headache;

(5) Bitter (tikta): predominantly composed of 'air' (therefore, rough and cold) and ākāśa (therefore, light); the season that favours is late winter (śiśira); pacifies pitta and kapha, but vitiates vāta; removes all other tastes as soon as it is perceived by the tongue; although by itself it is undesirable, it enhances relish (flavouring); clears the throat and cleanses the mouth; cooling; expectorant; appetiser; removes fainting spells, fever, and itchiness of the skin; galacto-depurent; dries up urine, excreta, adipose tissue (medas) and fat (vasā);

(6) Astringent (kashāya); predominantly 'air' (therefore, rough and cold) and 'earth' (therefore, heavy); the season that favours is spring (vasanta); pacifies pitta and kapha, but vitiates vāta; clears the tongue; benumbing, and favours inactivity; causes obstructions in the throat and dryness of the mouth; produces pain in the heart; brings about heaviness; heals wounds, etc; emaciates the tissues.

The six tastes, in the above order (which is according to *CS*, but 'pungent' coming after 'bitter' according to *AHṛ*) are decreasingly potent; 'sweet' is the most potent (prakarsheṇa balāvaha) and 'astringent', the least. Pungent, sour and saline are tastes that have potencies (vīrya) which are progressively higher degrees of 'heat' (ushṇa); and likewise bitter, astringent and sweet are tastes that are progressively 'cold' (śīta) in their potency. Tastes are also grouped in six triads according to the predominant properties of the physical substances that enter into the composition of the tastes: (1) sticky or viscid (snigdha): sweet, sour and saline; (2) dry and parched up (rūksha): astringent, pungent and bitter; (3) cold (śita): astringent, sweet and bitter; (4) hot (ushṇa): saline, sour and pungent; (5) heavy (guru): sweet, astringent and saline; and (6) light (laghu): bitter and sour.

Tastes are again classified according to their impact on the doshas (1) tastes that pacify (śāmaka-rasa): (a) sweet, sour and saline for vāta, (b) astringent, bitter and sweet for pitta, and (c) pungent, bitter and astringent for kapha; (2) tastes that vitiate (kopaka-rasa) : (a) pungent, bitter and astringent for vāta, (b) pungent, sour and saline for pitta, and (c) sweet, sour and saline for kapha (*CS*, vimāna, 3, and *AS*, 1, 1). There are, however, some exceptions. Sweet generally vitiates kapha, but honey (which is sweet) does not. Sour vitiates pitta, but āmalaka (emblica), although sour, does not. Salt also vitiates pitta, but rock-salt (saindhava-lavaṇa) does not. Pungent taste generally vitiates vāta, but śunṭhi (*Zinziber officinale)* and pippalī (*Piper longum*) which are pungent in taste do not vitiate vāta. Bitter taste also vitiates vāta, generally; but guḍūchi (*Tinospora cordifolia*), which has this taste, does not vitiate vāta. Astringent taste is usually cold and paralysing; but harītaki (*Terminalia chebula*), although astringent in taste, is warm and activating (cf. *DGV*).

SS (1, 42) suggests a dichotomous classification of tastes on the premise that the entire world is constituted by two principles 'sun' (or fire) and 'moon' ('agnī-shomīyatvād jagatah'): tastes belonging to the Sun group (āgneyāh viz. pungent, sour and saline) and tastes belonging to the Moon group (saumyāh, viz. sweet, bitter and astringent). The former are warm and produce burning sensations (vidāhi); they vitiate pitta, bring about faintness. The latter are cold and pacify the burning sensation (śāmaka); they pacify pitta. (cf. also *RVS*, commentary).

It is difficult, however, to identify substances which have only the taste indicated in therapy. In fact, most of the substances that are available will be found to have more than one taste. A list has been available of sixty-three varieties of substances possessing more than one taste (cf *CS,* 1, 26, 15-17 and *SS,* 1, 42, 23). There are only six things, in which only one of each of the tastes dominates, like sweet in raisins, saline in rock-salt, and pungent in pippalī (*Piper longum*). Fifteen in the list possess two predominant tastes; twenty have three tastes; fifteen have four tastes; six of them have five tastes. One of them has all the six tastes. While the thing with all the six tastes manifest has not been named, all the tastes in the unmanifest state are said to be present in poison. HĀRĪTA mentions that meat of the black antelope has all the six tastes in manifest condition.

While treating diseases, the physician is expected to ascertain the condition of the doshas, and select drugs having suitable tastes. During the course of treatment, he must select the tastes at the commencement, at a later stage, and at the end, so as to counteract the errant dosha. In diseases that are caused by vāta, treatment is commenced with drugs saline in taste, followed by drugs sour in taste, and completed by drugs sweet in taste. The order of drugs would facilitate progressive pacification of the errant dosha. Likewise, in diseases caused by disturbances of pitta, treatment begins with drugs bitter in taste, proceeds later with drugs sweet in taste, and is concluded with drugs of astringent taste. In diseases due to the disturbances of kapha, treatment begins with 'pungent', followed by 'bitter', and ends with 'astringent'. Even while eating food, the person who is interested in maintaining health is advised to begin with eatables that are sweet in taste, later eat sour and saline things, and then articles with other tastes (*SS,* 46, 15).

During digestion of food, three phases are recognized: in the first phase, the food is undigested (āma), and then, due to the preponderance of sweet taste, kapha (gastric-mucous) emerges as the by-product; in the second phase, the food is digested in the stomach primarily and duodenum only partly (pachyamāna), where, owing to the preponderance of the sour taste, pitta (digestive fire) emerges as the by-product; and in the third phase, the food is digested in the intestines fully (pakva) due to the preponderance of pungent taste, vāyu, emerges as the by-product. All the tastes in the food that is eaten are thus transformed into three main tastes (first sweet, then sour, and finally pungent) in three distinct and progressive stages (called avasthā-pāka). If, during the first stage, the food that is eaten has an excess of sweet, the kapha produced then would be more; if on the other hand, if pungent taste predominates in the food that we eat, the production of kapha would be less. Similarly with the other stages. *CS* considers vipāka as a special transformation of tastes incidental to digestive metabolism, and as having the same physiological effect as the tastes. Vipāka thus is said to be three-fold; sweet (madhura), sour (amla) and pungent (kaṭu). [*See* DIGESTION, VIPĀKA].

The tastes of drugs (or eatables) which are sweet, sour and pungent do not undergo any change in taste when they are digested. But the saline taste of the things eaten change into sweet taste when digested; bitter taste, likewise, is transformed into pungent, as a result of digestive and metabolic changes (vipāka); astringent taste is also converted into pungent as a result of these changes. Digestion is described as a process where the tastes are 'cooked' by the body heat. The distinction made between food and drugs is in terms of taste in the former and potency (vīrya) in the latter. Tastes build up the body constituents..

When tastes are excessively ingested, each of the tastes may give rise to abnormal conditions, and may bring about diseases. Due to an excess of things sweet in taste being eaten, the individual may become obese and inactive, lose appetite, develop cold, cough and hiccough, and fall victim to diseases born out of kapha disturbances; he may be stricken by scrofula, elephantiasis, urinary disorders, ulcers, intestinal obstructions, and worms. Excess of sour taste may lead to disorders of blood, swelling, sensitivity of teeth, burning sensations in muscle, heart-burn, skin irritations, anemia, troubles with eyes, delusions, haemorrhage, and disorders of pitta. Excess of saline taste exposes one to impotence, premature grey hairs, baldness, haemorrhage, loosening of teeth, loss of sensory activity, dyspepsia, psoriasis, and disorders of blood and pitta.

Excess of pungent taste leads to impotence, fainting spells, delusions, burning sensations in the skin, weakness, depression, morbid thirst, emaciation, tremor, body pains, and other disorders of vāta and pitta. Excess of bitter tastes would dry up the body constituents (dhātu), roughen channels within the body, cause weakness, emaciation, vertigo, depression, and other disorders of vāta. Excess of astringent taste brings about dryness of mouth, pain in the heart region, blocking of the internal channels, suppression of the secretion of urine and the development of excreta, abnormal thirst, paralysis, hoarseness of voice, vertigo, tympanitis, facial paralysis, and disturbances of vāta. [*See also* GUṆA, VĪRYA, FOOD, DIGESTION, VIPĀKA].

Temperament: That individuals differ on account of the dominance of one or the other doshas (vāta, pitta, and kapha) at the moment of conception, and that individuals in whom the doshas are not in a state of balance at the moment of conception are prone to diseases, are accepted in Indian medicine (*CS,* sūtra, 7, 39-40). The individual's equipment from this earliest phase of his life is known as 'bodily constitution' (deha-prakrti), which is intimately associated with the temperament derived from the three doshas (tri-dosha-prakrti).

Apart from physical and physiological differences that the body obtains amongst the three bodily constitutions (with regard to, general body-build, body formation, bodily strength, complexion, warmth, articulations or joints, digestion, aggravation of dosha, bowel habits, sensory functions, speech etc),there are psychological differences which may be described as temperamental. Differences also obtained as regards sleep, dreams and conduct. In all these differences, mental symptoms are characteristic.

The main differences as regards mental traits are three-fold : vātala or śuddha (where vāta or sattva dominates), pittala or rājasa (where pitta or rajas predominates) and śleshmala or tāmasa (where kapha or tamas predominates) (*CS,* śarīra, 4, 36). Each of these divisions is again classified into several temperamental types (called 'kāya' in *SS*): śuddha into seven, rājasa into six, and tāmasa into three (*CS,* śarīra, 4, 36-39).

The types under śuddha are: (1) brāhma (honest, restrained, righteous, wise, creative, courageous, equitable, clear-headed, tolerant, and endowed with verbal skill); (2) ārsha (pious, ritualistic, generous, calm, humble, detached, equitable, eloquent, artistic, and with good memory); (3) aindra (given to a high standard of living, compelling attention and obedience, pious, energetic, indefatigable, virtuous, opulent, pleasure-loving, and with farsight); (4) yāmya (virtuous, dependable, firm, impressive, energetic, free from envy, hate and confusion, and detached); (5) vāruna (brave, firm, clean, fussy, orderly, fond of water-sports, hard-working and prompt); (6) kaubera (opulent, money-minded, luxury-loving, full of self-respect, virtuous, fond of company, sensual, clean, open in anger or generosity); and (7) gāndharva (interested in stories, music, dancing and poetry, loving flowers, anointments, fine clothes and sense-pleasures, fond of the company of women, tolerant, and free from envy or jealousy).

The temperamental types under rājasa are: (1) āsura (courageous, arrogant, self-willed, authoritative, violent in temper, envious and jealous, self-centered, devoid of compassion, and fond of flattery); (2) rākshasa (intolerant, unforgiving, irritable, violent, hard-hearted, gluttonous, indolent but also hard-working, occasionally envious, given to excessive sleep, and fond of meat); (3) paiśācha (indolent, unclean, slovenly, irregular and abnormal in food habits, fond of company of women, coward but given to frightening others, annoying in habits and conduct); (4) praita (gluttonous, annoying in habits and conduct, envious, critical of others, greedy, indiscriminate, and averse to work); (5) sārpa (coward normally but brave when excited, painstaking, fond of food and sport, prompted frequently by fear); and (6) śākuna (fond of food, sports and sex, frivolous, intolerant, devoid of possessiveness, unstable and unreliable).

The types under tāmasa are: (1) pāśava (forbidding and frightening, lecherous, dull-witted, of poor memory, and outlandish in food habits); (2) mātsya (coward, dull-witted, greedy and gluttonous, unsteady, irritable, given to wanderlust, easily frightened, and fond of water); (3) vānaspatya (indolent, impassive, gluttonous, indifferent to higher aspects of life).

Actually the temperamental types are infinite in number (aparisaṅkhyeya-bheda), but the major types that are frequently met with are enumerated under three heads: śuddha, rājasa and tāmasa, which are fundamental and universal divisions (*CS*, ibid., 40.). [*See also* CONSTITUTION].

Three-fold Therapy: When the bodily doshas are vitiated, and health is thereby disturbed, there are three possible methods that can be applied to cure the bodily ailments: (1) 'internal cleansing' (antah-parimārjana), especially for curing diseases caused by wrong food etc., for example, medicines for internal administration, methods like purgation, enemata, errhines, sweating, and so on; (2) 'external cleansing' (bahih-parimārjana), for example, applications, fomentation, affusion, unction, massage etc; and (3) 'surgical treatment' (śastra-praṇidhāna), like incision, excision, puncturing, scraping, probing, suturing, application of alkalies and use of leeches for blood-letting. (*CS*, sūtra, 11, 55).

While they are mainly meant for curing bodily ailments, they may also be used in mental diseases which have bodily involvements (like epilepsy and insanity) (CHKP. on above).

Toxicology: The importance of toxicology (visha-vaidya, agada-tantra) in ancient times was in the context of power politics and romances in royal households. Administration of poison through food and drink to eliminate an unwanted person was a common practice. The skill of the court physician was required both to administer poison and to antidote it. Thus, the theoretical and practical aspects of toxicology constituted the necessary equipment of medical practice. Also, the prevalence of poisonous reptiles, rodents, wild animals and poisonous vegetation in the country necessitated the knowledge of plant and animal poisons as also the expertise in handling them. Organic and inorganic poisons had their medicinal value in curing intractable diseases. [*See* POISON]

Toxicology was thus classed as one of the eight classical disciplines of Āyurveda (ashṭāṅga), and was practised extensively in the country, especially by the rural and tribal physicians (jāngali-vaidya). Bites of poisonous snakes, scorpions, spiders and insects were frequent occurrences, and had to be treated. Enemies who attacked a territory would leave behind poisoned water, earth, air, roads and vegetation. An investigation of the nature and extent of poison was necessary before antidoting the poison. Medical texts contain detailed descriptions of poisoned water etc., and also measures for the elimination of poison from them.

The curious institution of 'poison-girls' (visha-kanyā-yoga) (cf. *SS*, Kalpa, 1) appears to have been prevalent in some parts of the country. Infant girls were got used to poison by the daily administration of minute doses, and when they grew up their body would be saturated with poison. They would altogether be unharmed by the poison made natural inside their bodies; but whoever came into intimate contact with them, would promptly be affected. Such girls would be reared, and sent to seduce princes and other noblemen, only to kill them. They would gain entry into the seraglios of enemy camps, and spread death fast. Girls who were born on Tuesdays, Saturdays or Sundays, and on the second, the seventh or the twelfth days of the lunar month, and in the constellations of kṛttikā Śata-tāraka, or āśleshā were selected for this dangerous game. (For details regarding guarding against poison cf. *SS*, ibid., 5-32)

Selection of vegetable poisons, and the preparation of powerful potions from minerals and animal products were also employed for therapeutic purposes. 'If taken in a small and proper measure (mātrā), even the poison would function like the life-giving nectar; and if taken all of a sudden (sahasā), or in excess (ati-mātra), or in an improper manner, even nectar would lead to all sorts of troubles, and finally death'. When poisons are used as drugs, the patient is required to follow numerous precautionary measures in food and habits. And there are well-defined pharmaceutical techniques to purify or refine poison, when it is used as a drug or as a corrective. Besides these details, toxicology also deals with the purification of substances (food, water, air) afflicted by poison. Characteristic symptoms of the presence of poisons, assessment of the extent of toxicity, and the management of the patient in different stages of toxic effect are also dealt with in manuals of toxicology. [*See* POISON)

Treatment: Treatment (chikitsā, bheshaja) is broadly grouped into three types (1) involving supernatural influences (daiva-vyapāśraya); (2) involving human reason and rational methods (yukti-vyapāśraya); and (3) involving control of mind (sattvā-vajaya) (*CS*, sūtra, 11, 54).

The first type may be called magico-religious. It recommends incantations (mantra), herbs (aushadha), precious stones (maṇi), auspicious rituals (maṅgala), sacrifices (bali), oblations (upahāra), expiatory rites (prāyaśchitta), ceremonial fasting (upavāsa), propitiatory rituals (svastyayana), worship (praṇipāta), and pilgrimages (gamana). This therapeutic system is inherited from the Atharva-veda background, and relies heavily on invoking supernatural aid to counteract the influences of 'unseen forces' (adrshṭa) that manifest themselves as diseases.

The second type is the rational therapeutic system or the treatment proper, which employs almost exclusively the natural substances (diet and drugs), prepared as medicine, by the wisdom and skill of the physician ('āhāra-dravyāṇām yojanā'). This is the system of medicine that CHARAKA, SUŚRUTA and others have sought to crystallize, codify, and organize on a scientific basis. [*See* RATIONAL MEDICINE].

The third type of treatment recognizes the great role that mind plays in causing diseases as well as curing them, and recommends its control or withdrawal from unwholesome impact from the external world. Self-restraint, discipline, yogic exercises, and methods of calming the mind are recommended here.

Indian medicine recognizes that treatment comprehends curing the diseased condition of the patient (ārtasya roga-nut) as well as enhancing the efficiency of the healthy person (svasthasya ūrjaskaram). The former aspect aims not only at removing the diseases by using vegetable drugs, mineral recipes and medicines from animal source, but at preventing the recurrence of the disease. The latter aims at giving strength (vrshya) by the employment of elixirs (rasāyana) and aphrodisiacs (vājīkarana) (*AS*, 1, 1, 12).

The guiding principle of treatment in Āyurveda involves that preventing the disease (prāgeva) is better than curing it, and that treating the disease in its early stages (taruṇeshu) is better than tackling it in its advanced condition. The physician should be able to foresee the nature of the disease by judging the first symptoms (vikārānām pūrva-rūpam), and act immediately so that the disease will not develop. Besides the prophylactic emphasis, SUŚRUTA urges that treatment should neither be too early (ap rāpte kriyā-kāle), nor too late (prāpte), too little (hīna,) nor over-much (atirikta); otherwise, even the readily manageable conditions grow out of control (sādhyeshv api na siddhyati). Further, lack of skill consists in planning major treatment (mahat-karma) for minor ailments (vikāre alpe), or inadequate treatment (kriyā laghvī) for serious diseases (mahāgade).

Treatment is said to be of three kinds: 'diabolical' (rākshasī), involving violent methods like surgery and cauterization; 'human' (mānushī), involving milder methods like the use of herbal drugs, fastings, purgatives and tonics; and 'divine' (daīvī), involving alchemical preparations. The first is considered as 'lowest', and is recommended only when the other two fail. Alchemical treatment also is fraught with danger, and requires the guidance of an extremely competent physician; it is indicated only in rare and normally intractable conditions. Herbal medicine is, therefore, the most suitable for most ailments, and least violent and risky.

Treatment is again classified into three varieties, depending on the action of the drug or treatment on the body. The first variety of treatment cleanses the interior (antah-parimārjana), as when drugs are ingested, or dietary regulations observed. This mostly relates to the diseases caused by food. The second variety purifies externally (bahih-parīmārjana), as when sweating, oleation, poultice, and ointments are employed. The third variety is the use of surgical instruments (śastra-pranidhāna): excision, incision, scarification, puncturing, probing, drainage, cauterization, suturing, extraction of foreign bodies, cupping and blood-letting.

Treatment is preceded by the ascertainment of causes of diseases symptoms and pathology (hetu-liṅga-jñāna), and the determination of the method of treatment (aushadha). Diseases are caused by the imbalance of the doshas, and the disturbances in the bodily constituents and the elimination of waste products [*See* DOSHA, DHĀTU, MALA, DISEASE, HEALTH, PATHOLOGY]. Whatever methods restore the imbalance and correct the disturbances are collectively termed 'treatment' (chikitsā), or the 'job of the physician' (bhishajām karma). The body has its natural mechanism to restore the imbalance and correct the disturbances and the physician only helps it (svabhāvasya sāhāyyaṁ)

His assistance is mainly two-fold: (1) 'cleansing' (samśodhana) the body of morbific diathesis internally with the help of emetics (vamana), enemata (basti), blood-letting (asra-vimochana) etc., or externally by surgical operations, cauterization, use of alkaline preparations etc., and (2) 'pacification' (samśamana) or restoration of the disturbed doshas with the help of drugs, stimulants (dīpana), fasting (kshut), restriction of water (trt), exercise (vyāyāma), fomentation (ātapa) etc. Diet regimen and wholesome conduct are factors that greatly assist the treatment undertaken.

Disease (vyādhi) is essentially a symptom or a group of symptoms caused by a number of factors. Treatment does not aim at the elimination of the symptoms, for temporary alleviation will only lead to the re-appearance of symptoms, later or elsewhere. Symptomatic cure is not rational (viśuddha) that is, it is not based on correct principles of medicine. Real treatment should remove the cause first, and the symptoms will of their own accord disappear, never to appear again (*AHr,* 1, 13). Therefore, the mode of therapeutic action should be 'counteracting' the cause of disease (hetu-viparīta). In many cases, however, symptoms also need to be handled independently, when the mode of therapeutic action is described as 'counteracting the symptoms' (vyādhi-viparīta). A combination of the two is the third mode of therapeutic action recommended in Indian medicine. The essential concept underlying treatment is, in the words of SUŚRUTA, "briefly, therapeutic action (kriyā-yoga) is the elimination of the causes of diseases (nidāna-parivarjanaṁ)"

Numerous treatment procedures are in vogue among the practitioners, and have been described elaborately in medical texts. Five of them are classical and major, and are collectively called pañcha-karma: emetics (vamana), purgatives (virechana), enemata (basti), oily enemata (snehana), and nasal therapy (nasya) [*See* PAÑCHA-KARMA]. Other methods include the employment of tonics (bṛmhaṇa), astringents (staṁbhana), respiratory, cardiac, gastro-intestinal and nervine stimulants (dīpana), diuretics and purgatives (śodhana), local application of smoke through pipe (dhūpana), eye-instilling (āśchyotana), eye-ointments (añjana), suppository (varti), ointments (lepa), poultice (pradeha), and elixirs (rasāyana).

Treatment also includes the wise utilization of water, air, sunlight, fasting, and exercise (especially for 'cleansing', saṁśodhana). Drugs extracted from natural substances are mainly vegetable (from fruit-bearing trees, from flower-and-fruit bearing trees, from plants that live for a year, and from creepers and bushes), although medicines from animal sources (like, honey, milk, fat, marrow, flesh, urine, bones etc.) and from mineral sources (like gold; the group of five metals: silver, copper, lead, zinc, and iron; sand, lime, realgar, salt, red ochre, etc.) were also prescribed [*See* PLANTS, MEDICINE]. Ayurvedic treatment was heavily herbal, and all parts of a plant were used for medicinal purposes (roots, bark, solid interior, stalk, fruits, flowers, leaves, pods, thorns, shoots etc.), as also gum, ash, oils, milk, potash and juice from plants [*See* AUSHADHI].

Treatment in the system known as 'Siddha-āyurveda' consists of herbal medicine (aushadhi), yoga, alchemical preparations (rasa-vaidya) and incantations (mantra). It has a branch devoted to elaborate pharmacological preparations (kalpa), and another devoted to astrological considerations (jyotisha).

Tridosha theory: The theory of the three doshas (vāta, pitta, kapha) [*See* DOSHA] is fundamental to Indian medicine (both Āyurveda and Siddha systems). Corresponding ideas may be found in Greek and Arabian systems of medicine also (and hence in the Yunāni system). [*See* ARABIAN MEDICINE, GREEK MEDICINE, YUNĀNI SYSTEM]. Attempts have been made to draw parallels, and identify the three doshas with the humours wind, bile, and phlegm (hawā, khūn and balgâm), and with the nervine force, metabolism, and survival.

The Indian theory, however, goes back to the Vedic period (*RV,* 1, 34 and 6, *AV,* 1, 12, 3), and is greatly influenced by the Sāṁkhya doctrine of the three guṇas [*See* SĀMKHYA] rajas, sattva and tamas, which are universal principles at work and generative of the five primary forms of matter. Earth is essentially tamas; water is a combination of sattva and tamas; fire is a combination of sattva and rajas; air is rajas; and ākāśa is sattva. Air and ākāśa combine to produce vāta; fire produces pitta; and water and earth combine to produce kapha (or śleshman). (cf. *SS,* uttara, 2,

1-8; 3, 1-20 and *AS*, 1, 20). While it is usual to identify vāta with rajas, pitta with sattva and kapha with tamas, *RN* (sec. 21) identifies kapha with sattva, pitta with rajas, and vāta with tamas.

In the human body, whatever is gross, dense, compact, hard, heavy, and stable is the earth principle; whatever is moist, unctuous, cold, slow unifying, liquid and soft is the 'water' principle; whatever is hot, burning (cooking, digestion,) acute, light, dry, radiant, lustrous and clear is the 'fire' principle; what is cold, dry, pain-giving, rough, mobile, clear and light is the 'air' principle; and whatever is soft, porous, light and subtle is the ākāśa principle. The bodily forms of matter are produced from the three doshas, which are present in the body: in the lower parts (vāta), middle parts (pitta) and upper parts (śleshma) ('vāta-pitta-sleshmānah eva deha-sambhava-hetavah;.... tair eva...... adho-madhyo-rdhva-samnivishtaih śarīram dhāryate, *SS*, sūtra, 21). They preserve the bodily structure and functions, like three pillars ('sthunābhih tisrbhih') of a house. They cause grave disturbances and even death, in pathological conditions (*SS*, ibid., cf. also *CS*, sūtra, 1, *AHr*, sūtra, 10).

The dosha, known as vāta, sustains the body, regulates breathing, contributes energy, creates enthusiasm and all bodily movement, and is responsible for mental processes. Pitta, the second dosha, takes care of digestion, generates body-heat, helps vision, and stimulates intelligence, understanding and courage. Kapha causes steadiness and softness, and makes the joints efficient (*AHr*, 1, 11, 1-5). The three doshas together maintain the integrity of the psychophysiological system.

The three doshas are chiefly located in the region of the heart (vāta), the umbilicus region (pitta), and the chest and stomach (kapha). But they are pervasive all over the body; their function differs according to different locations (sthāna). And each of the three doshas has again been grouped into five kinds, in accordance with their specific location and function [*See* DOSHA].

According to *SS*, these doshas are concomitant causes working in cooperation with blood (rakta) and semen (śukra) (*NiS*, on *SS*, sūtra, 21, 3). Blood is regarded in this tradition as the fourth dosha; its importance consists in the fact that the other doshas are never aggravated independently of blood viz. their aggravation and disturbed condition of the blood go together), and in fact, the doshas are transported to the various body constituents only through this liquid medium. [*See* DOSHA, VĀTA, PITTA, KAPHA, PAÑCHABHŪTA THEORY, RAKTA].

U

Upa-dhātu: Secondary or emergent body-constituents [*See* DHĀTU], which are produced as a result of the action of 'fire' in each of the seven body-constituents (dhātvagni). The digestive process in each of the body-constituents (dhātu-pāka) involves the generation of supporting and nourishing material which is utilized by the body (poshaka-dhātu), and the separation of this from the waste products which are eliminated from the body (kitta). The nutrient material is then circulated all over the body through an appropriate channel [*See* SROTAS].

This nutrient material which occurs as a byproduct in the body metabolism is also responsible for the formation of secondary body-constituents (upa-dhātu) (*CS*, chikitsā, 8, 39 and 15, 17; cf. also CHKP. on the latter). They are secondary in the sense of supplementing the sustaining work of the main constituents while the nutrient material (poshaka-dhātu) and the secondary constituents are like products of the digestive action The former are subjected to changes that transform them, while the latter are final products, not subject to such transforming changes.

Among secondary body-constituents, the following are listed: breast-milk (stanya) from chyle, catamenial discharge (rajas) from blood, muscle-fat (vasā) from muscle, sweat (sveda) from fat-tissue, teeth (danta) from bone, hair (keśa) from bone-marrow and vitality (ojas) from sperm or semen (cf. *BP, SaS,* 1, 5). Other details of the body that are included under the head of secondary body-constituents are tendons (kandara), blood-vessels (sirā), the layers of the skin (6 of them, shadtvacha) and ligaments (snāyu).

The expression also denotes seven 'minor' metals: sulphate of copper (tuttha), mica (abhra), red arsenic (manah-śilā), antimony (nīlāñjana), yellow orpiment (haritāla), vitriol of copper (rasāñjana) and makshikā (?) [*See* DHĀTU].

Urges: [*See* VEGA]

Ushah-pāna (Drinking water at dawn): Drinking water, or inhaling water through the nostrils, soon after one gets up early in the morning viz. immediately before sunrise [*See* DAILY ROUTINE] is regarded as hygienic and prophylactic. There is a saying that meals must be ended by drinking butter-milk, the day by drinking milk, and the night by drinking water.

Water for such drinking must not be hot, or ice-cold. It is best if it is drawn from the well directly. Well-water is reputed to be warm in the cold season, and cold in the hot season. This warmth or coolness is, therefore, natural. If well-water is not available, water kept in a copper vessel all through the night is to be preferred. The quantity of water to be drunk is suggested to be about eight 'handfuls' (prasrti, hollowed palm, equivalent to the measure of two palas), or 64 tolas (viz. about 32 ounces).

If inhaled through the nostrils, the quantity suggested is 48 tolas (24 ounces). Eyes will become strong and eye-sight keen; intelligence will be sharpened; there will be no signs of old age; and the individual will live long, free from diseases. Such inhalation of water through the nostrils is not indicated for persons who are wounded, who have boils, or who suffer from distension of stomach, flatulence, constipation, hiccough, and diseases due to kapha and vāta.

Water drunk at dawn is said to clear the system of many ailments: diseases of the eyes, of the head, of the neck, of the ear, colic pains, enlarged liver and spleen, chronic diarrhoea, piles, haemorrhagic diseases, obstructed micturition, obesity and dropsy. It is recommended that the water is to be drunk (or inhaled through the nostrils) even before one has cleared his bowels (anujjhita-mūtra-vit). This would not only cleanse the internal organs, but decrease the element of kapha inside the body, and thus prevent cataract of the eyes (which is ascribed to excess of kapha). It will also help move the bowels properly and regularly.

Those who habitually drink water at dawn should also take care to bathe everyday (twice during hot weather) and use buttermilk, vegetables (other than leafy ones), and rice (boiled in water). They should avoid meat, milk, oil-fried food, excess of physical exercise, fasting, exposure to sun's rays, warm food, fomentation for the body, and sleep during daytime.

V

Vaidya: The word is derived from vidyā (knowledge), and hence means 'knowledgeable', 'learned'. But the meaning has narrowed down to 'well-versed in the art and science of healing', viz. a physician, used as a synonym of bhishak [*See* BHISHAK].

Four kinds of physicians are recognized (*Mahābhārata,* 'Rāja-dharma'): (1) one who cures diseases (rogahara, viz. a general physician); (2) one who removes poison (visha-hara); (3) one who extracts foreign substances from the body (śalya-hara, viz. a surgeon); and (4) one who counteracts black magic (krtya-hara). Whatever the particular calling, he is expected to be very clever (pratyutpanna-mati), brilliant (dhīmān), hard-working (vyavasāyī), soft-spoken (priyam-vada), devoted to truth and virtue (satya-dharma-para) (*SKD*). 'The physician who is ill-dressed, harsh in speech, arrogant, vulgar, or who visits uninvited is to be avoided, even if he is as brilliant as Dhanvantari himself' (ibid).

There are three types of physicians according to *CS,* (sūtra, 11, 50-53): (1) 'pseudo-physicians' (bhishak-cchadma-dharā), flaunting the customary paraphernalia of physicians (medicine-box, books, etc.) while being entirely ignorant of the medical art or science, and posing as very able while not knowing how to diagnose a disease or treat; (2) 'feigned physicians' (siddha-sadhitāh), who consort with the wealthy and celebrated folk and pass off for competent physicians, while not at all being so; and (3) physicians who save lives of people (jīvitābhisarāh), who are knowledgeable, trained, experienced, insightful and intent on the welfare of the patient. [*See also* PHYSICIAN].

Vaiśeshika: An ancient system of thought that sought to take a rational view of things, and to construct a philosophy based on perception and reason. According to S. N. Dasgupta, it represents an old school of Mīmāmsā (*HIP,* vol.I, pp. 280-285). It has also been suggested that the Vaiśeshika system was redacted earlier than BĀDARĀYANA'S Vedānta-sūtra, and was ready, therefore, much before the formulation of the Nyāya system. While it is unlikely that CHARAKA had before him the Nyāya-sūtra that we know of today, it is certain that he was acquainted with the Vaiśeshika-sūtra (from which he is found to quote, *CS,* sūtra, 1, 35-38). We also find that the Vaiśeshika system is silent on the yoga methods, which are advocated in the Nyāya-sūtra (4, 2, 38-42). Scripture (śabda) is not regarded as a valid means of correct knowledge (pramāna) in the Vaiśeshika system, while it is accepted by the Nyāya and Yoga schools; and Vaiśeshika-sūtra does not even refer to analogical reasoning (upamāna) as one of the means, as the *Nyāya-sūtra* and *CS* do. The Vaiśeshika-sūtra altogether ignores the concept of god (īśvara), which the Nyāya system seeks to affirm and justify, and which is tacitly assumed in the Yoga system as well as in the medical schools. Thus the Vaiśeshika system appears to be of great antiquity.

Although the Vaiśeshika thought was systematized by PRAŚASTA-PĀDA (fifth century A.D.), the author of the commentary (bhāshya) on Vaiśeshika-sūtra, the thought-complex itself reaches back to a distant past. The supposed founder of the school, KANĀDA (–Aulūkya), may have lived before the rise of the Buddhist schools, and before BĀDARĀYANA compiled his Vedanta-sūtra. We find references to the contents of the Vaiśeshika-sūtra in the Vedānta-sūtra and in *CS*.

PRAŚASTA-PĀḌA'S commentary on KAṆĀDA'S aphorisms is known as *Padārtha-dharma-saṁgraha*. However, this work, which discusses the six Vaiśeshika categories in order (substance, quality, activity, generality, particularity and inherence), can hardly be called a commentary, for it is an independent and elaborate treatise, preceded by brief explanations of the original aphorisms. Glosses and annotations on this Bhāshya helped further the systematization of the Vaiśeshika outlook. Of them, the most important are ŚRĪDHARA'S *Nyāya-Kandalī* (about A.D. 991), UDAYANA'S *Kiraṇāvalī* (about A.D. 948), SRVATSA'S *Nyāya-līlāvatī*, JAGADIŚA'S *Bhāshya-sūkti* and ŚAṀKARA-MIŚRA'S *Upaskāra* (about A.D. 1425). Among the later works that projected effectively the Vaiśeshika viewpoint, VIŚVANĀTHA'S *Bhāshā-paricheda* (1634) and JAGADĪŚA'S *Tarkāmrta* (1635) may be mentioned.

The Vaiśeshika approach was incorporated into the Nyāya-system in manuals like VARADA-RĀJA'S *Tārkika-rakshā* (A.D. 1150) and KEŚAVA-MIŚRA'S *Tarka-bhāshā* (A.D.1275). And the Nyāya approach was accommodated within the Vaiśeshika framework in works like VALLABHA'S *Nyāya-līlāvatī* (twelfth century and ANNAṀ-BHATTA'S *Tarka-Saṁgraha* (1623). The two viewpoints fused, thus occasioning an integrated approach. [*See* NYĀYA-VAIŚESHIKA].

The Vaiśeshika system is a critical study of the six categories comprehending reality: substance (dravya), quality (guṇa), activity (karma), specificity or individuality (viśesha), generality or commonness (sāmānya), and the relation of inherence (samavāya). A seventh category was later added to these positive categories: non-existence (abhāva). The purpose of the system was to describe the independently existent, sensorily cognizable, linguistically expressible category (padārtha). And category was defined as whatever could be denoted by verbal symbols, i.e. words (abhidheyāh padārthāh), and thus become objects of knowledge (prameya). This knowledge was considered as essential to the practice of dharma (for which Veda is the authority), which would lead to the correct knowledge of reality (tattva-jñāna), which in turn would generate salvation (nihśreyāsa). Salvation in the Vaiśeshika system was the ultimate and irrevocable dissociation of the soul from the body-complex. Later, under the influence of the Nyāya thought, this dissociation of the soul from the body as interpreted was elimination of all misery.

The substance, is defined as the ground (āśraya) on which the other categories like quality and action are founded (āśrita), and as independently existing. It cannot be reduced to anything else. Substances are nine in number: the four primary physical elements (earth, water, fire and air); ākāśa which is all-pervasive, eternal, and functions as the vehicle of sound; time (kāla), which is unitary, objective, and independent of human involvement (in contradistinction with the Sāṁkhya view that time has only a psychological reality); space (dik) which is relative and unitary; the soul (ātman), which is all-pervading but distinct for each individual; and mind (manas) which is atomic in nature and locus for memory.

Of special interest in the Vaiśeshika thought is the idea of adrshṭa (unseen influence), which is regarded as the source of all action and all motivation. The movement of the needles towards the magnet, the combining movements of the atoms, the upward movement of fire, and sideward movement of air, movement of water inside the plant-body, circulation of blood in the animal body, transformation of the food that is eaten into blood and flesh, inclinations of the mind, passing of the soul from the body into other bodies, the fruition of action done in this or other lives and so on are all ascribed to the influence of adrshta. It is distinguished from all other categories that are 'seen' (dṛshṭa); this is something for which no explanation can be given, and which can in no way be observed directly. It explains the cosmological processes as well as the individual nature and behaviour of plants and animals (including human beings).

The concept of adṛshta has an ethical aspect also, inasmuch as it is regarded as being occasioned by rituals like bath, fasting, observance of restraint, study, charity, performance of sacrifices, purity in food and so on. The purpose of religion is to gradually eliminate the accumulated influences of adṛshta and thereby to prevent the necessity for being born again (viz. the obtainment of salvation).

The soul is a substance that is eternal, omnipresent and pluralistic. Souls are many, different in different bodies, but capable of being perceived by all individuals internally as possessing qualities evident in psychological processes like cognition and happiness. There are two kinds of souls: individualized and pluralistic (jīvātmā), and universal, creative and unitary (īśvara). [*See* ĀTMAN].

Mind is inferred from the fact of non-sensory internal perceptions. While the sense-functions are structure-specific, we do experience many sensations simultaneously; and this is due to the mind. Further, the external sensations are incapable of monitoring and organizing themselves; mind not only organizes the activities of the sense-organs, but also enables the soul to attend to them.

Āyurveda relies heavily on the Vaiśeshika theories of matter and organization of the world. It accepts the Vaiśeshika argument of creation (ārambha-vāda), the atomic theory, the rôle of physical and chemical changes, and the notion of mind. The doctrine of five primary elements (pañcha-bhūta) that is basic to Āyurveda is drawn directly from Vaiśeshika sources. But the borrowal from Vaiśeshika in Āyurveda is tempered to a considerable extent by the influences of the Nyāya and the Sāṁkhya approaches. [*See also* NYĀYA, NYĀYA-VAIŚESHIKA, PRAMĀṆA, ĀTMAN *and* PAÑCHA-BHŪTA].

Vājīkaraṇa: Classed as the eighth branch of Indian medicine, it is a system which deals with the methods and drugs for increasing sexual potency (vājī-karaṇa actually means 'making a horse out of a man', horses being known for their heightened sexual vigour). This branch of medicine is intended to invigorate and increase the sexual potency (vīrya) which has become (due to ill-health, old age or over-indulgence) insufficient (alpa), diseased (dushṭa), 'dried up (viśushka) or degenerated (kshīṇa); and to maximize pleasure during sexual congress (praharsha-janana) (*SS*, sūtra, 1, 1).

For the emaciated and for those with insufficient potency, it provides an increase in vitality and enhancement of strength; and for those whose body-constituents are normal and balanced, it provides satisfaction (*Vaidyaka-saṁgraha*, 2). It is widely resorted to among those afflicted with sexual debility, sexual inadequacy or poor quality of semen.

But one who desires to take this line of treatment must always be self-controlled (nityam-ātmavān), for on it depends virtue, wealth, love of people and fame, and due to it the offsprings would possess desirable qualities (*CS*, chikitsā, 2).

Vanaspati: [*See* PLANTS].

Vāta: Derived from the root 'vā' ('to move'), the word stands for one of the three doshas in the body which are responsible alike for health and diseases. [*See* DOSHA]. Composed predominantly of two primary forms of matter, ākāśa (representing sattva) and air (representing rajas), it is essentially 'air' (vāyu) with rajas as the main guṇa (although it has all three guṇas). It is the most important among the doshas as it is the principal support for the structure and function of the human system (tantra-yantra-dhara) (*CS*, sūtra, 12; *SS*, nidāna, 1, 5-8; *AHṛ*, śarīra, 3, 8-9; and *AS*, 1, 16).

Among its physical properties are: dry, non-sticky, cold in action, coarse, light, expanding, mobile, minute, and penetrating. It has no taste or colour. In the body, it is responsible for all actions (like breathing, sensations, sensory cognitions, bodily responses, internal circulations, systemic transactions, evacuations, regulation of the body constituents and mental processes), for the organization of all the parts of the body, for a proper appetite and for general energy and enthusiasm. It is described as the very life (prāna) of the individual, as it sustains the body and directly governs all functions of the body, speech and mind. The other two doshas (pitta and kapha) and all the body constituents (dhātu) are regarded as 'lame' (pangu), and they become active only when inspired by vāta, even as the clouds move only when, and wherever, the wind carries them (*SaS*, 1, 5).

The regions in the body where vāta prevails are principally the large intestine, the waist, thighs, ears, bones and the skin (*AHr*, sūtra, 12).

However, when vāta is disturbed, general disorganization of the body takes place; limbs may slacken, movements may become spasmodic and uncoordinated, tearing or throbbing pains may be felt in different parts of the body, some organs may become inactive and lose their sensation, the excretory process may be suspended, muscles may contract, abnormal thirst may be experienced, tremors may occur, bones may get dry and develop cavities, body movements may get arrested, colour of the skin may darken, limbs may grow cold, and the body may emaciate.

The normal vāta is aggravated by anything in excess: manual labour, physical exercise, food, mental exertion, travel, sexual indulgence, loud talking, wasting of the body constituents, keeping awake during night, carrying heavy loads, fasting for a long time, and eating at irregular times, fear or grief, suppression of natural urges. Blocking of the internal channels of circulation may also result in the aggravation of vāta. Season, time of the day, and the developmental stage too have their impact on the dosha. Vāta is aggravated in the cold and rainy seasons, especially when the weather is cloudy and stormy. It is aggravated during evenings and late in the night (when the digestive process is nearing its completion). It is also aggravated in old age, and in wasting diseases.

The treatment of the disorders of this dosha involves prescription of diet and drugs which are unctuous, hot, stable, saline, sour, sweet, strength-giving, use of oils, exposure to the sun, bathing, massage, enema, inhalation therapy, application of warm ointments, rest, sleep etc. There are as many as eighty disorders which are listed under the vāta-disorders.

Vāta (or vāyu) is five-fold in its function: 'moving out' (praspanda), 'carrying upward' (udvahana), 'filling' (pūrana), 'separating' (viveka), and 'supporting' (dhāranā) (*SS*, sūtra, 15 and also nidāna, 1 etc.); and as these functions are discharged it is called prāna, udāna, vyāna, samāna and apāna respectively (*SaS*, 1, 5, 27).

(1) Prāṇa-vāyu: This air, moving about the nostrils and mouth, is chiefly located in the interior of the heart (hrdayāntara), although its field of activity covers the thoracic region, face, ears, nose, tongue and the brain. It is mainly concerned with respiration and maintenance of the action of the heart, mind, sense-organs, arteries, veins and nerves. It helps ingestion of food and the transportation of food to the stomach by way of esophagus, spitting out, sneezing and eructation. Disorders of this aspect of the dosha manifest themselves as sneezing, cold, cough, bronchitis, asthma and hoarseness of voice.

(2) Udāna-vāyu: This air which tends to move upward, has its seat mainly in the umbilicus (nābhi-deśa), lungs in the thoracical region and larynx in the throat. As it moves up, it produces and regulates sounds by causing appropriate vibrations of the vocal chords. It is mainly concerned with vocalizations (speech and music), actions, and efforts to preserve body strength. Its disorders include diseases of the eyes, ears, nose and throat.

(3) Vyāna-vāyu: The air that moves about all over the body has its special seat in the heart, and its movement is characterized by speed. It concerns itself mainly with the transportation of chyle (rasa-saṁvahana) and blood to all parts of the body. It is also responsible for five kinds of action, viz. contraction, expansion, upward movement, downward movement, and other general movements. It helps perspiration. The opening and closing of eyes, yawning, and the movement of spermatozoon inside the vaginal cavity are also ascribed to this aspect of vāta. The diseases of this aspect include impairment of circulation, diseases like fever and diarrhoea, and ailments all over the body.

(4) Samāna-vāyu: This air which is an ally of 'fire' is situated near the seat of the 'stomachic fire' ('agni-samīpasthah', viz. digestive tract, gastro-duodenal region), and moves about the abdominal region (koshtha). It is mainly concerned with admitting food into the stomach, and with helping in its digestion by inflaming the 'digestive fire' (pāchakāgni). It controls and sustains the secretion and flow of juices within the body. It also separates the nutrient portions of the digested food (sāra-bhāga) from the waste-products (kitta), and assists in the elimination of the latter. Disorders of this aspect of vāta include indigestion, diarrhoea and defective assimilation.

(5) Apāna-vāyu: The air that tends to move downward, pushing in due course by-products (urine, faeces, semen, menstrual blood) towards their exits. It is located in the lower part of the digestive tract (pakvāśaya, large intestine), and functions in the region covered by gluteal, vesical, genito-urinary organs and thighs (śroṇi-basti-medhro-rugocharah, *AHr,* sūtra, 12). Its main function is to retain and regulate the discharge of urine through the urethra faeces through the rectum, semen through the urethra, and menstrual fluid through the vagina. It also holds the foetus in the womb until the moment of discharge, and helps in the delivery. Its disorders include diseases of the urinary tract, colon, bladder, anus and testicles, obstinate urinary diseases. constipation, and flatulence.

Besides these, five other and minor varieties of vāta are mentioned (*BP*): 'nāga' (which is responsible for articulation), 'kūrma' (responsible for opening the eyes), 'krkala' (responsible for hunger), 'devadatta' (responsible for yawning) and 'dhanañjaya' (spread all over the body).

These are aspects of the same vāta, differing in their names, locations and functions. But all them are together responsible for balancing inside the body the doshas, the body constituents (dhātus), and the digestive fires (agni), for transacting with the outside world (vishayeshu samprāpti), and for maintaining the life of the individual (cf *SS,* nidāna, 1). [*See also* DOSHA, PRĀNA, APĀNA, UDĀNA, VYĀNA *and* SAMĀNA].

Vatī: Derived from vat ('to encompass', 'to connect'), vatī is a preparation in the form of pills or tablets, where a drug or several drugs are dried, finely powdered and ground into soft pastes before they are rolled into pills by the fingers (to which they must not stick) and dried in the sun or in shade (according to prescription). Minerals are also used as ingredients, but after they are reduced to ashes (bhasma or sindūra); where mercury is used, it will be in the form of the kajjali *Aethiops* *mineralis*) thereof. [*See* PILLS].

Vayah: [*See* AGE, DEVELOPMENTAL STAGES].

Vega: Derived from vij ('to agitate', 'to move quickly'), the word means in the medical context, natural urge (for elimination), reflex, excitement, and effect of poison on the human body. Usually, however, it is taken in the sense of natural urges of the body (urination, expulsion of faeces, flatulence, vomiting, yawning, sneezing, shedding tears, hunger, thirst, sleep), which call for urgent satisfaction. By restraining these urges (postponing their satisfaction), one becomes prey to bodily disturbances and diseases. (*See* SUPPRESSION OF URGES].

Vega-dhāranā: [*See* SUPPRESSION OF URGES, VEGA].

Vikāra: [*See* DISEASE].

Vipāka: Literally, 'ripening', 'change of state', 'cooking', the expression refers to the changes that occur in the food as a result of digestion (pariṇāma-lakshaṇa. *RVS*). "Cooking (pāka) means a change of form (svarūpa) and taste (rasa) of substances; it is the transformation of taste as a result of transformation of form. Vipāka is so called because the transformation occurs specially (vi) when the digestive processes are completed (jāraṇa-nishṭhā-kāla)". It is this activity in the body that builds up the body constituents of the food that we eat, increase or decrease the morbid factors, and help assimilate food or drug.

Digestion of food is said to occur in two distinct stages: (1) the preliminary stage (pra-pāka), occurring in three phases (or avasthās, hence called avasthā-pāka) of gastro-intestinal digestion: (a) 'undigested' (āma) phase, commencing soon after the food is ingested through the mouth, and before it gets into the stomach and duodenum; the prevailing taste-mode in this phase is 'sweet' (madhura); and the emergence of kapha as a by-product (mala) is the distinguishing detail of this phase; (b) 'partly digested' (vidagdha or pachyamāna) phase, in the region of stomach and duodenum, where the emergent taste-mode would be 'sour' or 'acid' (amla), and the dosha as byproduct would be pitta; and finally (c) 'fully digested' (pakva) phase in the large intestine, where the taste-mode is transformed into the 'pungent' or 'acrid' (kaṭu), and the emergent dosha is vāta; and (2) the culminating stage (nishṭhā-pāka, also called vipāka) which follows the completion of digestion of food in the above three phases and the beginning of the separation of the chyle (rasa) from faecal matter (mala) (*CS*, 6, 15, 9-11). [*See* DIGESTION, MALA].

The expression vi-pāka is explained as meaning 'the completion of the act of digestion' (*CS*, 1, 26, 66 'vipākah karma-nishṭhayā' commentator; nishṭhā= 'nishpattih, kriyā-samāptih'), or the end-result of the digestive process which is the combined effect of the three phases of the pra-pāka (avasthā-pāka) mentioned above. The prefix 'vi' to the main word referring to digestive transformation signifies the sense of 'special' or 'subsequent'. The transformation here is special in the sense that it is not regional (as the avasthās imply), but systemic. Whatever the taste of the food that we eat, they are all changed into sweet, sour and pungent in order, during the three phases of gastro-intestinal digestion. The tastes undergo a final change in this 'subsequent' stage (nishṭhā-pāka) and enter into the general stream of chyle (rasa as one of the seven body constituents), and thus conveyed to all parts of the body. [*See* RASA].

The concept of vipāka as current in present-day Āyurveda was crystallized by *AHṛ* (1, 9, 20), although all the implications of the concept were adequately spelt out in *CS* and *SS*. This work refers to the association of the 'digestive fire' (jātharāgni, especially referring to the heat that is responsible for intestinal digestion) with the finally transformed tastes (rasānāṁ pariṇāmānte, ibid., the expression 'rasānāṁ, however, is taken by HEMĀDRI to mean 'substances having tastes', 'rasavatāṁ dravyānām'). The transformation of tastes also involves in the subsequent stages the activity of 'elemental fire' (bhūtāgni) and 'body constituent fire' (dhātvagni), so that the transformed tastes are involved in the general rasa as a body constituent, and in the other six body constituents (dhātu) [*See* AGNI].

In the final transformation of tastes under the impact of intestinal digestion (jātharāgni) in vipāka, if the emphasis is on the changes in tastes as properties of substances we have three possible kinds of vipāka: sweet, sour and pungent (*CS, AHṛ,* and *AS*). If, however, the emphasis is on the changes in the substances themselves, we would have two varieties: 'heavy cooking' (guru-pāka) and 'light-cooking' (laghu-pāka) (*SS,* and *RVS*). The former is said to be the view of Ātreya-Punarvasu, while the latter is ascribed to DHANVANTARI. Attempts have been made to reconcile the two views. What in the former view is called 'sweet' (madhura) is the same as that called 'heavy cooking' in the latter view; the other two vipākas in the former view are combined in the 'light-cooking' of the latter view.

According to the view held by ĀTREYA-PUNARVASU and the followers of that tradition, sweet and saline tastes are converted to sweet taste during the post-digestive transformation (vipāka), sour into sour, and the other three (pungent, bitter and astringent), generally (prāyaśah) into pungent (*CS,* 1, 26). This view rests on the doctrine of the three doshas. The view advocated by the DHANVANTARI tradition (and held by *SS* and *RVS*) on the other hand, relied upon the doctrine that all things are constituted by five primary forms of matter (pāñcha-bhautika theory). The properties of these five forms are an important consideration in the classifying of the vipāka categories. If, during the post-digestive transformation the property of heaviness (guru) which is the property of two forms of matter, 'earth' and 'water', predominates, then the vipāka is styled as 'guru-vipāka'. The two forms of matter themselves undergo changes: they become cold, unctuous, heavy and rough. The resultant taste is sweet. If, on the other hand, the property of lightness (laghu), which is the property of the other three forms of matter (viz. fire, air and ākāśa), the transformation involves the properties of lightness, coarseness, smoothness and sharpness. The resultant taste is pungent. The properties of substances are responsible for the vipāka ('guṇāh vipākayoh kāraṇaṁ', *RVS,* 1, 123). This view is therefore known as 'guṇa-vipāka-vāda' or as 'bhūta-vipāka-vāda'. The transformation, according to this view, is slow when the property of heaviness prevails (chira-pāki), whereas it is quick when the property of lightness prevails (achira-pāki).

Prior to the wide acceptance of these two views, there were other views such as the one that held that there were six vipākas in accordance with the six tastes (yathā-rasa-vipāka-vāda), and the one that argued that it was difficult to ascertain which taste would become powerful, and that the powerful taste suppresses the weak taste (aniyata-vipāka-vāda).

The post-digestive transformations are significant inasmuch as they act upon the doshas, body constituents (dhātus), and the production and elimination of waste matter in the body (mala): The sweet-vipāka, unctuous and heavy in property, induces the dominance of kapha, and increases the production of semen; it helps in the elimination of urine and faeces. The sour-vipāka, unctuous and light in property, induces the dominance of pitta, but hinders the production of semen; it too helps in the elimination of urine and faeces. The pungent-vipāka, coarse and light in property, induces the dominance of vāta, and hinders the production of semen ; it facilitates the discharge of urine and faeces (dysuria and constipation).

Tastes are different from their final (post-digestive) transformations, for the former are immediately (āśu) apprehended as gustatory experience (āsvāda) while the latter are delayed (vilaṁbita) and progressive changes (pariṇāma). The former are regional in action and effect (sthānika), while the latter are systemic (sārvadehika). The former are available for direct observation (pratyaksha), whereas the latter can only be inferred (anumāna). [*See also* PRAPĀKA, ANIYATA-PĀKA-VĀDA, GUNA-PĀKA, DIGESTION, TASTE].

Vīrya: [*See* POTENCY].

Visha: [*See* POISON].

Vishamāgni: Meaning 'irregular fire', it refers to the condition of the 'digestive fire' (jātharāgni) being erratic under the influence of excess of vāta. Sometimes food is easily and quickly digested, and at other times with difficulty and slowly. The digestive condition is associated with distention of the abdomen, colicky pain, diarrhoea, ascitis, heaviness of the limbs, dysentery and a gurgling sound in the intestines. [*See* AGNI, ATYAGNI, JĀTHARĀGNI, DIGESTION, SAMĀGNI, VĀTA].

Vitality (Ojas): An important concept in Indian medicine, ojas is variously translated as vitality, bodily strength, vigour, energy, force, and power. The words bala and tejas are used as synonyms (for example, *SS,* 1,15, 30 and 31). The word also means virility, water, and metallic lustre. In medical literature in India it is used in different contexts to mean 'vital fluid' (rasa), 'the life-giving blood' (jīva-śoṇita), 'bodily warmth' (dehoshmā), and 'phlegm' (kapha). The expression in Sanskrit means 'lustre', 'support', 'strength', 'light'. Its use is as old as the Vedic corpus, as the possession of Indra and Vrtra, the valiant heroes of many battles. It is meant here only as bodily vigour and force. It is suggested that the concept in Indian medicine is only a theoretical concretization of the Vedic concept (J.Filliozat).

Attempts have been made to equate the concept of ojas with those of albumin, glycogen, vitamin, internal secretion of the ovary, prostatic secretion, protein, endosperm, calorific radiation of activity and so on. But the correspondences are both incomplete and uncertain; and suggestions of conceptual identity are far-fetched. The biochemistry of ojas is as yet obscure.

It is a physical substance which is essential to active life; it contributes strength and vigour to the body, and makes all the functions in the body go on smoothly. All living beings are sustained by it; they are alive, because it is there, and its absence is death. (*CS,* 1,30,8). It begins its course as the very essence of the embryo (sāram ādau garbhasya), continues uninterrupted throughout life. There is another view that it is formed during the eighth month in the life of the embryo.

There are several time-honoured theories regarding the nature, status and function of this substance even in the field of Indian medicine (cf. CHKP on *CS,* 1, 30, 7; *NS* ed. p. 185). The general view, however, is that it is fluid in form, having the quality of flowing (saraṇa), white in colour (with tinges of red and yellow), unctuous (snigdha), slimy (picchila), cold (śītala), soft (mrdu), pure (śuddha), sweet in taste (madhura), endowing stability and firmness to the body parts (sthira), unique in its structure (vivikta), and the principal seat of life (prānāyatanam uttamam) (*SS,* 1,15,25). It is associated with the moon (soma), and is therefore cooling (*SS,* ibid), although the commentator interprets this detail as meaning agreeable, gentle and placid (saumya, *NiS*). Another view associates it with moon and fire (agni-somātmaka).

There is a discussion about its nature, whether it is or not a dhātu (body constituent, dimension of the physiological framework). It is usual to enumerate seven of them, viz. chyle (rasa) as the primary product of digested food, blood, flesh, muscles and tendons, fat, bone, bone-marrow, and vital fluid [*See* DHĀTU]. Some authorities are inclined to regard ojas as the eighth dhātu, on the assumption that it is a product of the seventh, viz. vital fluid. Some consider it as a secondary constituent (upa-dhātu).

The prevailing idea, however, is that even as the bee makes honey collecting nectars from different flowers, ojas is formed from the essences of the seven dhātus (cited in CHKP on *CS,* 1,30,7). Therefore, ojas being essentially indistinguishable from the dhātus, cannot be regarded as a separate dhātu, or as an upadhātu. Besides, the seven dhātus support the body (dhāraṇā) as well as nourish the body (poshaṇa), while ojas discharges only the former function.

In any case, ojas is generally described as a special product of the essential factors inherent in all the seven dhātus, and as located principally in the heart (hṛt), which is the seat of consciousness ('hrdayam chetanāsthānam ojaś chāśrayam', *SaS,* 1,5), although it pervades the entirety of the physical constitution, accompanying the seven dhātus in their course. Its main function is to support the body and provide the necessary force or energy for all functions, bodily and mental. It also enables the organism to endure the pain resulting from disease, and sets into motion the processes within the body to counteract the disturbances caused by diseases. If there is a weakening of ojas, these are impeded, and the body begins to disintegrate.

Two kinds of ojas are recognized in *CS* (1,30,7; and also *AHr*): 'higher' (paraṁ) and 'lower' (aparaṁ). The former abides in heart, and is of the form of 'eight drops' (ashta-bindu), that is, slight in quantity (alpa-pramāna). The heart is where consciousness and life are concentrated (chaitanya saṁgraha), and ojas as the core of both these is located here; 'it is therefore that the physicians regard the heart as the most important' (*CS*, ibid. cf. also CHKP on it). When this ojas is alright, the individual will be healthy, and will have the feeling of well-being. When, on the other hand, it weakens, death results, even if all the other dhātus are alright.

The other kind of ojas (viz. the 'lower') abides principally in the 'veins' (dhamanī) of the heart, and is 'half-a-handful' (ardhāñjali, or two palas) in quantity. It is this that pervades the entire body by its flow. Deficiency in this is not fatal, although it leads to serious ailments. In diabetes, for instance, it is this ojas that flows out in urine.

There are authorities who reject the validity of this two-fold division of ojas (for example HĀRĀNA-CHANDRA and GANGĀDHAR-KAVIRĀJA, the author of *Jalpa-kalpa-taru* on *CS*). In actuality, the two 'kinds' of ojas are only two levels of its operation. There is no difference in the nature, role or functions in ojas, despite the 'higher' and 'lower' levels of operation. The 'heart', where the 'higher' ojas abides, is the core of the being, the very focal point of the organism's life. Thus, the 'higher' ojas is merely the vital power of the organism. The 'veins of the heart' (where the 'lower' ojas is said to abide) is the physical heart, viz. the organ. Depending upon its health is the vitality that is involved in activities. Ojas is transformed into physical strength which radiates from the heart.

There are three ways in which ojas can be weakened or lost: injuries (abhighāta, persisting wasting disease, kshaya), and causes such as anger, sorrow, worry, fatigue, and hunger. (*SS,* 1,15,26-27). It is thus that the ojas gets lost through the very pathways that carry the body constituents and principles (dhātus). The patient then becomes incapable of carrying on his normal activities.

Symptoms of vitiated ojas are: (1) dislodgement from its proper place in the body (viśramsa), leading to loosening of the bone-joints, numbness of limbs, wasting of flesh, dislodgement of the doshas from their natural centres, and disinclination to engage in normal activities of body, mind and speech; (2) change in normalcy (vyāpat), as a result of contact of the dhātus with deranged doshas (dosha-dūshya-samparka), leading to heaviness of limbs, numbness, rigidity, excitation of vāta which results in dropsy, change in complexion, drowsiness and somnolence; (3) wasting (kshaya), leading to fits of fainting, loss of flesh, stupor, delirium, incoherent speech, and finally death.

Vyādhi: Ailment or illness in general. It is more usual to employ the expression to mean physical distress, in contradistinction to mental pain, agony, or anxiety (ādhi). But there is also an interpretation that emphasizes the rôle of the mind in fighting against the disease: "Vyādhi is where the mind resolves to counteract the disturbances in the body" ('viśesheṇa ādhīyate abhiniveśyate pratīkārāya manah iti vyādhih', *SSM*). [*See* DISEASE].

Vyāna: One of the five kinds of vāta, it is the wind that spreads all over the body, and is responsible for the circulatory system and for the bodily movements. [*See* VĀTA].

Vyāyāma: Derived from vi+ā+yam, (to extend', 'to pull asunder') the word signifies exercise, effort, struggle, or any exertion, involving bodily fatigue (āyāsa), gymnastics, sports, playing with heavy clubs, drawing a bow with chain, etc. [*See* EXERCISE]

W

Walking: Walking (chaṅkramana) is regarded as a very good physical exercise, but it should not fatigue the body. When the body is taxed, it is unhealthy; it cuts short life, and harms vision (*SS*, chikitsā, 24). Otherwise, it gives strength, increases longevity, stimulates the 'gastric fire', and sharpens the sense organs; it reduces obesity and counteracts the accumulation of kapha (*RN*, 2). [*See* EXERCISE]

Y

Yakshmā: Originally pulmonary disease, consumption. But the term came to stand for disease in general. It is more usually employed to signify the co-existence of two or more diseases, or the presence of a large number of symptoms. [*See* DISEASE]

Yathā-Rasa-Vipāka-Vāda: The view that during digestion and assimilation of food, all the six tastes (sweet, sour, saline, pungent, bitter and astringent) are severally involved in the resultant (post-digestive) transformation. Each taste brings about its own vipāka (prati-rasam pākah). The view is also called 'rasa-sadrśa-vipāka-vāda' (cf. *SS* and *RVS*). [*See* VIPĀKA, DIGESTION]

Yātudhāna: Literally, 'a travelling spirit', but

frequently a term for any evil spirit or demon that causes diseases. The term is also employed to mean a sorcerer.

Yoga: Yoga is the general name for diverse bodily and mental practices, currently in vogue in the country and coming from very ancient times. These practices achieve certain physical and supernormal powers, and obtain the ultimate liberation from the miseries of life. There are evidences that such ascetic practices were in vogue, even during the Indus civilization; and we have copious references to them in the Vedic literature. It is also suggested that practices which were of numerous kinds came to have different philosophical outlooks justifying particular practices. Thus Yoga represents a motley collection of practices and ideologies.

However, PATAÑJALI, whose *Yoga-sūtra* is the most influential treatise on Yoga, attempted to construct a system which was at once theoretical and pragmatic. He affiliated this system to the Sāṁkhya complex of thought. Subsequently, Sāṁkhya and Yoga have come to be regarded as twin-systems. References to the two systems together are to be found even in the Upanishads (for example *Katha* and *Švetāśvatara*). *Mahābhāratha*, for instance, refers to them as the 'enduring two' ('sanātane dve'): they are complementary to each other as theory and practice, as gnosis and askesis, as philosophy and religion, as wisdom and power (*Śānti-parvan*, Moksha-dharma, 316-2). Sāṁkhya held that the necessary precondition for liberation was the discriminatory wisdom (viveka-jñāna); and Yoga sought to teach the method to attain it. It is usual to describe Yoga as 'the Sāṁkhya system which postulates a godhead' (seśvara-sāṁkhya).

Sāṁkhya was but one of the affiliations of Yoga. It appears that the expression 'Yoga' originally signified the Nyāya-Vaiśeshika thought-complex. KAUṬILYA, who refers to Sāṁkhya, Yoga and Lokāyata as constituting the 'rational method' (anvīkshikī) meant by Yoga only the Nyāya-Vaiśeshika system and not the Yoga of PATAÑJALI. VĀTSYĀYANA, the celebrated Nyāya commentator, differentiates Yoga from Sāṁkhya on the ground that the former subscribes to the view that the effect is unprecedented in the cause, and therefore something totally novel (i.e. ārambha-vāda, which is exactly the view of Nyāya-Vaiśeshika, and which is peculiar to this system), while the latter subscribes to the theory of preëxistence of effect in the cause (i.e. sat-kārya-vāda) (*Nyāya-bhāshya,* 1,1,29). It is obvious that Yoga here does not refer to Patañjali's Yoga, which follows closely the Sāṁkhya thought.

The employment of the expression 'Yoga' in *RV* includes different shades of meaning such as 'yoking', 'harnessing', 'connecting' or 'linking', 'achievement that is positive and productive', and 'magical power'. PĀṆINI crystallizes the meaning by deriving the word from yuj (samādhau, 'to focus or concentrate'), and alternately from yujir (yoge, 'to yoke or connect'). *Bhagavad-gītā* employs the word in both senses; but PATAÑJALI's work refers only to the methods for focussing or concentrating, and the idea of 'yoking' (uniting, harnessing) has little relevance in the framework of his thought. The Vaiśeshika school was referred to as 'yoga', because it believed that the 'combination' (yoga or samyoga) of atoms was responsible for the world. Yoga also meant 'rational method' (yukti), in which sense it was applied to Nyāya.

The most celebrated and the earliest classic on Yoga is the masterly aphoristic manual ascribed to PATAÑJALI (about second century): *Yoga-sūtra* in four books dealing with the definition, the psychophysical constitution of man, the methods of bringing mind under control, acquisition of supernatural powers, and doctrines peculiar to this system. Although it is usually assumed that PATAÑJALI was the founder of the Yoga system, the work itself claims that he was only an editor or redactor of the Yoga ideology and discipline. The systematization and crystallization of ideas and practices that generally went under the name of Yoga may be ascribed to him. In fact, his work is regarded as a part of the Sāṁkhya teachings (*Sāṁkhya-pravachana*).

The Yoga, as crystallized by PATAÑJALI, adopts the methodology, which is significantly medical in approach: understanding the disease which needs to be eliminated (heya or symptom), understanding the causes and the course of the disease (heya-hetu or diagnosis), understanding the condition that would prevail when the disease is eliminated (hāna or health), and understanding the method by which the elimination of disease is effected (hānopāya or treatment). Yoga had intimate association with the medical sciences from very early times. The origin of Yoga is actually ascribed to the ancient 'medicine-men', magician-priests of tribal relevance. Even the classical Yoga recommends medicine (aushadha) for attaining perfection (*Yoga-sūtra* 4, 1); and Indian medicine has special value for Yogic exercises, charms and spells. Among the curative methods common to Yoga and Indian medicine may be cited fasting, regulated breathing, sweating, abstinence from indulgence, postural perfection, relaxation, exercises, and employment of spells.

CHARAKA is influenced by the Sāṁkhya-Yoga complex. [*See* SĀṀKHYA]. But he does not treat them together. Even as his Sāṁkhya corresponds to the older version of Pañchaśikha, anterior to the classical Sāṁkhya of Īśvara-Kṛshna, his Yoga also appears to be older than the *Yoga-sūtra* of PATAÑJALI. True to the spirit of Sāṁkhya, CHARAKA relies on reason and analysis; although influenced by Yoga, he postulates the presence of godhead whose grace is curative. It is important, however, to note that in his system it is the rational approach to treatment (yukti-vyapāśraya) that figures prominently and not treatment by appealing to divine intervention (daiva-vyapāśraya), although he does mention this. It may be recalled that in PATAÑJALI'S system too the mention of 'a personal god' (īśvara) is both casual and paradoxical.

While the classical Yoga follows the Sāṁkhya ideology closely, there are some considerations that are especially dealt with in Yoga. Of them, important is the classification of spontaneous activities of the mind-stuff (observation, pratyaksha; erroneous notions, viparyaya; fantasy, vikalpa; sleep, nidrā; and memory, smṛti). The account of the major dimensions of personality stresses (kleśa) grouped under nescience (avidyā), egoity (asmitā), approach tendencies (rāga), aversions (dvesha) and survival impulses (abhiniveśa, 'clinging to life') is another significant contribution of Yoga. The description of the vital force (prāṇa) as responsible for normal life and stresses therein, as also for the reintegration of life, involves the theory of differential gunas [*See* GUṆA] and the doctrine of transcendence of the guṇas by askesis. In this, the Yoga system goes beyond the Sāṁkhya framework.

Yoga seeks to provide a constructive account of the totality of human possibilities, intellectual and emotional, taking into consideration the spontaneity of human nature, compounded of the three guṇas. The purpose of Yoga praxis is to enhance the sattva component, so that it dominates over the other two gunas. This is the rationale for the Āyurvedic prescription of 'right and healthful living' (sad-vrtta and svastha-vrtta).

There is a brief disquisition concerning moksha and yoga in *CS* (śarīra, 2, 137-156). Moksha, the summum bonum of human endeavour and life, is defined here as the complete annihilation of all phenomenal involvement (*CS*, ibid, 137, 'moksho nivṛttir-nihśeshā', cf. CHKP on it: 'absolute annihilation of body,' 'ātyantika-śarīrādyucchedah').

Yoga is the means towards this end (ibid., 'yogo moksha-pravartakah'; CHKP. takes the expression 'pravartaka' in the sense of 'kāraṇa', 'cause'). In both yoga and moksha, there is a non-recurrence of all sensations ('vedanānām avartanam'), sensations which provide the dimensions of phenomenal involvement. Sensations being the products of contact between the soul, organs of sense-knowledge, mind and the objects of the sensory organs, yoga and moksha are characterized by the absence of such contact. The absence is temporary and limited in yoga, while it is permanent and absolute in moksha (CHKP).

CS (ibid. 138-139) further explains that such contact (between the soul, sense-organs, mind, and sense-objects) éngenders the experiences of happiness and misery, and when mind is settled firmly in the soul ('ātma-sthe manasi sthire'), these experiences are at once eliminated. It is mind that prompts the sense-organs to apprehend the sense-objects [*See* MIND], and when the mind is withdrawn from its association with the sense-organs it can be settled in the soul (viz. "absorbed in the awareness of the soul" CHKP) without distractions. The mind is no longer under the influence of sensations (nor is thereby involved in the phenomenal world), its positioning in the soul endows on it certain supernatural powers (vaśitva). They are the eightfold magical powers: (1) entrance intc another body at will (āveśa); (2) reading the thoughts of others (chetaso jñānaṁ); (3) accomplishing all things at will (arthānāṁ chandatah kriyā); (4) extraordinary vision (drshti); (5) extraordinary audition (śrotram); (6) remarkable powers of recall (smrti); (7) extraordinary brilliance (kānti); and (8) the capacity to become invisible when desired (adarśana) (*CS,* ibid., 140-141). These attainments are due to the utter purity of mind, viz. the mind that is completely free from the influence of passion (rajas) and dullness (tamas).

Yoga, being the accomplishment of mind's purity, along with the annulment of the past actions [*See* KARMA], leads to moksha, which indeed is complete and final dissociation (viyoga) from all phenomenal contacts, and therefore a state which precludes renewal of contacts or rebirth (*CS,* ibid., 142).

Yogavāhī: Any substance which, when used along with a drug, helps to enhance the effective properties of the drug, without forsaking its own properties, is called a yoga-vāhī (like honey, an alkali, mercury) or that 'which carries the properties of the drug added to it' (*CS,* sūtra, 27, 249). It is a medium for mixing medicines.

Yukti: Yukti has many meanings: union, connection, reasoning, device, artifice, expedient, stratagem, and application. In the medical context, however, the word is used in the sense of application of reason to diagnose and treat diseases, for 'success of medical practice is founded in rational application; and one who is adept in reason is superior to one who is merely acquainted with drugs' (*CS,* sūtra, 2, 16). Rational application takes into consideration mainly two factors: dosage (mātrā) and time (kāla). Even poison, if used judiciously and with reason, can be made to function like a restorative (*CS,* sūtra, 24, 60). [*See* PRAMĀNA, YUKTI-VYAPĀŚRAYA, MEDICINE, TREATMENT].

Yukti-vyapāśraya: Treatment of diseases by the employment of reason, viz. clinical examination (parīkshā), diagnosis (nidāna), and employment of drugs, prescription of diet, etc. This forms the theme of the Indian medical texts (*CS, SS, AHṛ, AS, MN, SaS,* etc.). It is distinguished from two other types of treatment, daiva-vyapāśraya (treatment by harnessing divine and occult influences) and sattvāvajaya (restraining the mind from unwholesome objects, psychotherapy) (*CS,* sūtra, 11, 54)

It broadly includes three varieties of treatment: (1) internal cleansing (antah-parimārjana, viz. drugs that enter inside the body and become effective in curing disease mainly caused by food); (2) external cleansing (bahih-parimārjana, viz. drugs and treatment that cure only by coming into contact with the body from outside, like fomentation, massage, unction etc); and (3) use of surgery (śastra-praṇidhāna, viz. using instruments, alkalies and leeches). (*CS*, sūtra, 11, 55). [*See* RATIONAL MEDICINE, TREATMENT].

Appendix

Conceptual Framework of Indian Medicine

For CHARAKA, Āyurveda was just a "science of life": it "instructs us about life".[1] SUŚRUTA, on the other hand, suggests that Āyurveda is that "by which life is obtained or examined".[2] Life in both definitions stands for health, or 'diseaselessness' (*ārogya*). And the basic postulate is that man is a conglomeration of elements, a pattern of factors: and when these elements or factors are properly balanced (*sāmyagyoga*) it is beneficial (*hita*) and pleasant (*sukha*). The balance involves the sense-functions (*kala*), sense-objects (artha) and the three-fold behaviour (*karma*-bodily, vocal and mental). Treatment (*chikitsā*) becomes necessary when the effective balance gets weakened (*hīna*) or distorted (*mithyā-yoga*). While Āyurveda in theory concedes the curative value of Ātharvanic practices (*daiva-vyapāśraya*), it attaches importance to rational methods like proper medicine, beneficial diet, and favourable habits.

Among the Indian systems of thought it is Āyurveda that openly recognizes reasoning as an independent and important instrument of knowledge (*pramāṇa*). This naturaly marks a point of departure from the primitive mentality of reliance on magic, and signifies the dawn of what may be called the 'scientific' spirit. The methods of Āyurveda are interesting: observation (*pratyaksha*), examination (*parīksha*), inference based on reason (*anumāna* or *yukti*), discussion with colleagues (*sambhāsha*), formulation of hypotheses (*pratijñā*), and diagnosis (*nidāna*). There is a special value assigned to advice from competent authority (*āptopadeśa*).[3]

Āyurveda accepts another treatment procedure based on Yoga ideology, 'mastering the mind' (*sattvāvajaya*). This consists in restraining oneself from excess, from unwholesome sense-functions, and controlling one's own mental status. CHARAKA argues that most of our troubles are due to folly or errors of judgement (*prajñāparādha*): and to avoid or eliminate the troubles, one must 'live correctly' (*sadvṛtta*). Correct living, according to Āyurveda, does not involve supernatural sanction or Vedic authority. It is wholesome, integrated living which adequately satisfies the three fundamental motivations: urge for self-preservation, the desire for material provisions which make life comfortable, and a longing for better states of existence, here and hereafter. Ethics is thus judiciously subordinated to pragmatic considerations.

Although Āyurveda is by its Tāntric background committed to the body-principle (*dehatattva*) and to the idea of making the body efficient (*kayasādhanā*), there is in it an acceptance of what may be called the 'psyche' (*atman*), a spiritual principle different from, and independent of the body. The person (*purusha*) who is regarded in this system as the frame of reference for all medical speculation and object of treatment is a configuration (*samavāya*) of the body (including the sense-organs), mind, and the psyche, organised into a single system in the manner of a tripod.[4] The body is grossly material, made up of the five physical elements (*pañchabhūtas*): space (or ether), air, fire, water and earth. Senses are sensitive sockets in the body made up of the same elements. Mind too is likewise physical, but subtly so. It transcends the senses and is therefore termed meta-sensory (*atīndriya);* the senses are activated by it, guided by it, and in that capacity it is described as 'supporting' or 'providing the ground' (*adhishthāyaka*). The 'psyche' upholds, bears up and preserves these factors; and, therefore, it is 'the upholder' (*dhārin*). In so doing, it actively binds the factors into a single system; in other words, it is a designer (*anubandha*). Life (*jīvita*) is thus an organisation, a phenomenological unity (*samyoga*).

The individual person is thus essentially dynamic and is a product of transaction which is known in Āyurvedic literature by two expressions: *karma-purusha* (CHARAKA) and *samyogi-purusha* (SUSRUTA): The former word emphasises the activity aspect of the individual, while the latter, the integrational aspect. Both words bring out the phenomenological, transactional, and dynamic characters of the individual. The person may be viewed as the field of activity, providing motivation for all action, and organising the physical factors that go to make up the body.[5] In this sense it is described as 'one with a body' (*śarīrin*). The psyche is involved in this field as a factor, no doubt as an important factor,but as one of the factors nevertheless.

Āyurveda explains the function of this factor which 'upholds' the other factors (known collectively as the body-mind complex). The psyche, when active, excites the mind (*manas*) into action, for the psyche is invariably associated with the mind (which incidentally is a doctrine peculiar to Āyurveda).[6] The cognition occasioned by mind may not necessarily be of the external world, for, as explained by CHARAKA'S commentator CHAKRAPĀṆI, there can be no cognition of the external world without the participation of sense-organs. In the absence of sense participation, cognition of the psyche as is occasioned by the mind alone persists. This is not transactional cognition, but introverted cognition (*ātmajñāna*), independent of objects (*nirvishaya*), indeterminate, unstructured and devoid of form.

But this introverted cognition is not to be construed in terms of ātmajñāna of the Vedānta. Here it is purely a psycho-physical process, only unstructured and indeterminate. And CHARAKA specifically subscribes to the notion of psychophysical parallelism.[7] His doctrine of invariant association of mind with the psyche would adequately explain also the formulation of the phenomenological person (*samyogi-purusha*).

Āyurveda's indebtedness to the Sāmkhya school of thought has expressed itself in the concept of the 'subtle-body' (*sūkshma-śarīra* or *lingadeha*).[8] Constituted by consciousness, ego, eleven senses, and five subtle elements, this body is said to survive the physical body and transmigrate; "like a little thing no bigger than a thumb, yet pervading the entire body even as a small lamp lights the whole room".[9] This body is called 'linga' because it merges thoroughly with the constitution.

In Āyurveda, this body is composed of air, fire, water, earth and mind: it is exceedingly subtle and is carried over (*ātivāhika*). This is sometimes referred to as 'elemental consciousness' (*bhūtātmā*), a mass of fine particulars integrated and directed by the psyche (*jīva*). The individuals as determined by this subtle mass of directions within is the *karma-purusha*, whose disorders medicine seeks to correct.[10] The subtle body is a substrate, a foundation, a ground for the psychophysical constitution to take shape and function. The foetus is said to be formed as a result of the father's sperm (*śukra* or *sattva*) and the mother's blood (*śoṇita* or *rajas*) coming together, but not until the subtle body has migrated into this union.[11]

This subtle body, mind, heat-power (*agni*), watery contents (*soma*), breath (*vāyu*), and the five senses (cognitive functions) are together described as the vital currents (*prāṇāh*), which are located in one hundred and seven vital centres (*marmas*), of which head, heart and pelvis (*vasti*) are considered most important.[12] Sensory and mental functions are associated with the head, while consciousness (*chitta*) is located in the heart. It is interesting that CHARAKA calls heart by the characteristically Sāmkhyan word for elemental consciousness, 'mahat'. It is in the heart that all modes of consciousness are gathered, and all vital currents are centred.[13]

Human constitution, according to SUŚRUTA, is distinguished by the functions; physiological functions (like breathing), reflex actions (like winking), sensory functions (*vishayopalbdhi*), intellectual functions (like decision, *niśchaya*, inquiry, vicarana, scrutiny and apperception, *vijñāna*, memory, *smṛti*) and energetic application (*adhyavasāya*). These functions are organized on the basis of a network of elemental modifications that work together to 'uphold' the body (*dhātu*).

There is a normal pattern that may be described as 'health'. When in this normal pattern all processes are properly balanced in an equilibrium the flow is unitary and at an even pace (*samayogavāhi*); the factors that 'uphold' the body, viz., *dhātus*, are in their proper natural proportions (*prākṛta-māna*) so that the balance (*sāmyāvasthā)* is maintained. When, however, these factors are deficient or in excess, the balance is disturbed, and disease results.

Disease thus is essentially in the nature of departure from normalcy or disturbance (*vikāra*). There are forces within the body that make the body foul (*mala*) and disturb its processes. It is important to note that there are also forces within the body which strive to keep the body clean and its processes even (*prasāda*). The aim of Āyurveda as a curative discipline is to strengthen the prasāda forces against the mala forces. The struggle between them is normal and natural, and health is a necessary concomitant of this struggle. The job of a physician is merely to aid nature in its normal struggle,[14] so that the proper balance of the basic design in the body (*dhātu-sāmya*) is secured.

Important in Ayurveda is the notion of equivalence of macrocosm (*bramāṇḍa*) and microcosm (*piṇḍāṇḍa*), inherited from the Tāntric tradition. The structure of the individual organism is essentially similar to the structure of the universe.[15] This refers to the five primary elements (*pañchabhūtas*) that enter into composition; earth (density, solidity), water (cohesion, liquidity), air (expansion, movement), force (heat, light) and ether (space, extension). The body is as material and physical as the world around it; its growth, maturation, decay and disappearance follow the same natural laws.

The primary elements combine and modify to produce and maintain the inorganic as well as organic world. In the organic world however their modifications assume a particular pattern, best illustrated in the human body. But the Āyurvedic theory applies equally to human beings as to the lower animals or even plants. There are not only branches of Āyurveda to treat elephants (*Hastyāyurveda*), cows (*Gavāyurveda*) and horses (*Aśvavaidyaka*), but there is a discipline which specializes in maintaining the health and curing diseases of plants (*vrkshayurveda*). There are treatises written on these branches, and there in no doubt that these specialities were once actually practised.

SUŚRUTA quotes an ancient opinion : "The constitution (*prakṛti*) of human beings is physical : it is made up of air, fire and water."[16] Of the five classical elements (the *Pañchabhūtas*) these three were held in high regard even by the vedic poets who personified them as wind-gods (*maruts* or *vāyu*), fire-god (*agni*) and water-god (*varuṇa*). The wind-god is the most powerful; it is indeed the soul fo all gods, essence of the very worlds, first-born of the natural order, king of the cosmos.[17] The fire-god was the living divinity in a sacrificial society. And waters were "the causes of creation", rich in *rasas* and containing the 'liquor of immortality'.[18] Perhaps this recognition follows the earlier thought-complex. In any case, the five primary elements in the cosmos were supposed to be represented by these three in man. In the Tantra-Samkhya speculation, each of the elements is characterised by one or more of the three modes of being *(guṇa)* : *sattva, rajas,* and *tamas.* The earth element is characterized by *tamas,* air by *rajas.* In the human body the air factor is composed of the elements ether and air; the fire factor by the element fire, and water factor by the elements earth and water.

These factors are named in Āyurveda *vāta* (or *vāyu*), *pitta,* and *kapha* (or *śleshman*), characterized by the three modes *rajas, sattva* and *tamas* respectively. It is usual to translate these factors as wind, bile (gall) and phlegm (mucus), following the humoral doctrine of the Greeks. While the Indian factors theory and the Greek humoral theory are not identical, we may take these expressions as meaning more or less what the Sanskrit term connotes.

These factors are the component parts of the functional system that we call an organism; and in their normalcy they support the body-mind complex, and therefore they are called 'dhātus'. But when they are thrown out of balance, or are excited, they can be troublesome. They become, in that condition, pathogenic and are called '*doshas*'. In Āyurveda, the expression 'dhātu' (elements or component parts) is confined to the seven structural aspects; plasma-tissues or chyle (*rasa*), blood (*rakta*), flesh (*māmsa*), fat (*medas*), bone (*asthi*), marrow (*majjā*) and sperm (*śukra*). And, therefore, the three factors that were mentioned earlier are generally, though incorrectly, called *doshas* (pathogenic factors).[19]

It is essential to distinguish *dhātus* from *doshas*; the former are structural while the latter are entirely functional. *Dhātus* are body-constituents while *doshas* are behavioural processes. It should, however, be noted that some authorities have taken even *dhātus* as not so much structural as functional aspects; an even proportion of the *dhātus* (*dhātu-sāmya*), for instance, is interpreted in terms of satisfaction in sense-function (*prīṇana*), a quality of chyle; a contribution to vitality (*jīvana*), a characteristic of blood; production of oiliness (*sneha*) representing fat; support of the burden (dhāraṇā), namely bones; filling up of cavities (*pūraṇa*), the work of marrow; and reproduction (*garbhotpāda*) by means of the sperm.

Even then, the *dhatus* are essentially specific in their function, and are actually bound with physical organs. The *doshas,* on the other hand, are rather abstractions. When *vāta* is referred to as wind, *pitta* as bile and *kapha* as phlegm, they are not to be taken in their actual specific connotations; it would probably be nearer the Āyurvedic intentions if we regard them as the windy aspect, the fiery mechanism and the watery network in the organism respectively. But they are not merely philosophical expressions without actual parallels in the body; their areas of function have been specified, their ascendance periods have been noted, their excitation, deficiency and distortion have been described.

The *dosha* concept is really very old, as old as *Ṛgveda* I,34,6 and I, 12,3) and probably older. We have references to wind and bile in *Ṛgveda* itself, and phlegm in *Śatapathabrāhmaṇa.* The Vinaya texts (370-360 B.C) contain the idea of *dosha* and *dhātu.* We find the three-*dhātu* theory in the *Mahābhārata* (12,343,83-85).

We read in the *Atharvaveda* about bile being the liquid fire (*agne pittam apām asi,* 18,3,5). KĀTYĀYANA'S *Vārttika* on PĀṆINI (5,1,38), prepared about 300 B.C., mentions the appeasement (*śamana*) and excitation (*kopana*) of the three *doshas.* And there may have been different schools of thought with regard to the nature and function of the *doshas.* There was a line of thought which regarded the *doshas* as merely discrepancies, as the expression really means, and counted the three factors mentioned above under *dhātus* (constituents). SUSRUTA, for instance, held the three as responsible for the formation of the body, with the active co-operation of blood (and sperm according to his commentator DALHAṆA[20] CHARAKA on the other hand, was inclined to emphasise that these three factors were indeed agents of discrepancies and causes of all morbidity, quite distinct from the dhatus.[21]

By the time, however, when Āyurvedic thought became crystallized *dhātus* and *doshas* were regarded as as structural constituents and functional factors respectively of the human body, viewed as both basic to health and as sources of disturbance. The notion of 'mala' as the group of waste products (faeces, urine, and sweat) that render the body foul unless they are promptly eliminated, highlighted the constituent elements that contribute to health (*prasāda-dhātu*) and those that cause disturbance and disorder (*mala-dhātu*). The *doshas* in balance (*svamāna*) are bound up with the former, while being out of balance they relate to the latter. The *dhātu* by itself is regarded as neutral, preserved and destroyed by *dosha* and *mala.* This explains the paradoxical interpretation in Ayurveda of 'discrepancy' (*dosha*) as a constituent factor. The '*tridosha*' theory is as valid in understanding normal health as in pathology.

The factors (*doshas*) are said to depend upon *dhātu* and *mala,* and when they themselves become errant they disturb and pollute the latter two. They are essentially emergent and functional, although each of them is associated with different bodily areas and physiological functions. Each factor is in actuality a complex of processes working in a common direction and resulting in a common benefit or disturbance. A *dosha* has its emergent aspect (*chaya* arousal in its own specific areas) excitational aspect (*prakopa,* overflowing from their own areas into other regions), and the normalization or tranquillization aspect (*prasamana,* returning to their own areas of action). Normal health involves necessary and sufficient arousal of the *doshas;* disease is a result of excitation and treatment consists of the normalization of the *doshas.*

The three constitutional factors are intimately interconnected in a complex network of behaviour patterns. In the life-span of an individual, early years are dominated by kapha, middle age by pitta and old age by vata. During the first four hours of the day (morning) and of the night kapha will be in ascendance; the hours between 10 and 2 during night is the period of the ascendance of vāta. Ascendance of a factor is a natural phenomenon all through an individual's life, and in all his activities. Even when he eats his food, for instance, in the beginning kapha will predominate, but when food starts getting digested pitta will become important; and then vāta will take over. The involvement of human constitution in the natural order is emphasized by the periodical ascendance of the three doshas in the several seasons of the year. In winter (hemanta, November-December), rains (varsha, July-August) and the cool season (śiśira, January-February) vāta is said to be the king; in summer (grīshṃa, May-June) pitta rules; and in spring (vasanta, March-April) kapha dominates. The occurrence of diseases as well as their treatment procedures take into consideration the individual constitution with reference to the ascendance of the factor and the time of the year. Health is considered to be result of a proper balancing of the factors (samadosha), for disease is symptomatic of an imbalance in them (doshavaishamya).

In the body, the area of arousal of vāta is below the navel (between the pelvic region and the rectum); the area of pitta is the region between the heart and the navel (midstomachic region and the small intestines); and the area of kapha is the region above the heart (chest and throat). While vāta fills all the interspaces in the body (like bladder, intestines, ear, skin and so on), pitta is active in liver, blood, spleen, heart, eyes, and skin; and kapha in the upper parts of the stomach (āmāśaya). Vāta is related to the element air and ether; pitta to the fire element, and kapha to earth and water. To repeat what was said earlier, the three principles in the body are comparable to the three principal elements air, fire and water in the cosmos. And they represent the rajas, sattva and tamas modes of being, respectively. Of these, vāta is the most important factor; it is the prime mover. It is because of this factor that the other two become active. But the pitta factor (fire in the body) is principally associated with digestion, and there is a school of Āyurvedic thought that regards all ailments as fundamentally due to indigestion. But even this 'fire' is fanned by vāta or wind.

Due to the excessively unstable nature of the vāta, the factors get frequently thrown out of balance and so disturbances of the factors are thus inherent in nature. Causes of health, they can be causes of trouble also. What is important in health, or in disease, is the particular pattern of the factors, for the three factors always function together although they occur in varying proportions and intensities. It is interesting that Āyurveda emphasizes that the factors combine : For instance, when kapha is in ascendance (already dominated by tamas), vāta flares up and gets combined with the general tamas of the body, sleep, (*nidrā*) results. The pitta (dominated by sattva) flares up and combines with the general rajas to produce delusions (*bhranti*); an excited wind (rajas) also enters into it. The same bile combining with tamas results in the fainting spells (*mūrchhā*). The phlegm (dominated by tamas) and wind (rajas) together combine with the general tamas and bring about drowsiness.

The combinations and the ascendance of the factors in the constitutions are responsible for personality types (*prakṛtis*). Āyurveda speaks of the pure wind-type (śuddha-vāta-prakṛti), the pure bile-type (śuddha-pitta- prakṛti) and the pure phlegm-type (śuddha-kapha-prakṛti). These are types in which the mentioned factor is obviously assertive, the other two being subordinate to it. But pure types are rare; more frequent are the mixed types. Although this classification was originally with reference to the pathogenic factors only, it assumed a general significance in course of time. When two of the factors combine in equal proportion to determine a type, it is called 'pair-determined' (*dvandvaja*). And when all three factors are involved more or less significantly but not equally, the constitution is miscellaneously assorted (*samnipāta*).[23] When, however, the three factors combine in equal quantity and strength, the type is perfectly balanced (*sama*). The ascendance-tendency of the factors commences even at the foetal stage of development, and becomes settled in late childhood. Influencing factors include heredity (*kula*), vocational affiliation (*jāti*), climate and country (*deśa*), age (*vayas*), and 'the inclinations of the subtle body' [24]

The wind as a factor sustains the whole bodily system, the physical machinery as well as the physiological functions (including psychological processes) : efficiency of the sense-organs and alertness of mind are both dependent upon it. Being associated with rajas, it is described as red in colour, productive of energy, and highly unstable (or constantly in motion). Dryness, lightness, instability, cold; roughness and solidity are given as its characteristics. In function it is five-fold : (1) 'forward breath' (prāṇa, breath that governs respiration and prevails in the whole body from toe to nostrils, especially located in the head and moving in chest and throat, contributing to mental alertness and sense efficiency), (2) 'downward breath' (apāṇa, prevailing in the lower regions but moving in navel, intestinal canals, sex-organs and legs, contributing to the production of sperm, and responsible for expelling faeces and urine), (3) 'pervading breath' (vyāna, prevailing in the heart but pervading all over the body, characterized by great speed in circulation helping sensory-motor functions, blood circulation, reflexes like winking, all sensory perceptions, and distribution of the vital sap to all parts of the body), (4) 'ascending breath' (udāna, prevailing in the chest but moving in throat, nostrils, palate, skull and navel, responsible for speech, intentions, energy, strength, memory and complexion), and (5) 'equalising breath' (samāna, prevailing in close proximity to the 'stomach fire' and moving in the digestive organs, heart, navel and the joints, helping digestion and assimilation).

The concept of multiple breaths, as was mentioned earlier, is an old one, perhaps per-vedic. In vedic literature, especially in the early Upanishads, we find that breaths three to ten in number are mentioned.[25] Āyurveda has defined its functions as well as its anomalies. When wind as a factor is excited, sense function is weakened, insensibility for touch sets in, pain in body is felt, constipation occurs, one feels thirsty and restive, palpitation and trembling are noticed, and one gets weak and emaciated

The constitution that is dominated by this factor, known as 'vāta prakrti' is identified by several physical and psychological traits. Scanty hair, lean and fragile figure, high body-temperature, dry skin, dark complexion and low voice suggest this type. The person belonging to this type has a weak constitution and has frequent trouble with his digestion; his resistance is low and immunity poor, with the result that he is often sick. His ailments are mostly of the nervous system. His intelligence, however, is above average, and receptivity high; he is imaginative. But he is likely to be nervous, timid, suspicious, jealous, quick in his likes and dislikes, fickle-minded, and rather talkative. He is a light sleeper and when he dreams, he soars in the sky.

The second factor pitta is described as 'bodily fire' (*dehāgni, kāyāgni*). According to SUŚRUTA this is the only fire in the body. It digests all that we eat and is responsible for warmth, digestion and metabolic changes. The concept of bodily fire is a collective one: it includes 'digestive heat' (*pachakagni*), the five elemental fires (*bhūtāgnis*), and the fires of the seven constituents (*dhātvagnis*); covering enzymes and hormones of metabolism.[26] It is described as hot, yellow liquid exuding an unpleasant odour; it is a 'fiery liquid'. The five-fold aspects of this factor are: (1) 'cooking or digestion' (*pāchaka,* prevailing in the midregion between the upper and lower parts of the stomach, composed of the five elements, responsible for assimilation and digestion, and contributing to the other pittas in the body), (2) colouring (*rañjaka,* prevailing in the upper parts of the stomach, where undigested food is received, liver, and spleen, responsible for the conversion of chyle into blood);[27] (3) 'realizing' (*sādhaka,* prevailing in the heart, and responsible for intellection, memory and self-regarding), (4) 'perceiving' (*lochaka* or *ālochaka,* shining in the eyes and responsible for visual perceptions), and (5) 'irradiating' (*bhrājaka,* lustre-giving and illumining, occurring as a quality of the skin as complexion). When this factor is excited one is dejected, feels thirsty, sweats much, and may even faint; there appear on the face pimples and there is excessive heat within the body.

The constitutional type determined by this factor is charactered by good appetite and good digestion, unsteady muscles, loose joints, glowing complexion, and premature greying, His body tends to be soft and odorous. He frequently has burning sensations in parts of his body, and his urine is often high in colour; his eyes too have a yellowish tinge. His sleep is easily disturbed. He is intelligent and inclines to be imaginative. He is irritable, impatient and rather boastful. He is proud, sometimes haughty; he is prone to anger and can be cruel. His perseverance, however, is poor, and his moods change quickly. His dream-contents reveal association with heavenly bodies (sun, moon, and stars). He has greater stamina than the previous group, but is susceptible to ailments of the digestive system.

The third factor, kapha or śleshman is related to the earth and water elements and to the *tamas* mode of being. Therefore, it inclines its possessor to heaviness, dullness and indolence. Its main function appears to be to neutralize the heat that is produced by pitta, which would otherwise burn the system down; it also unites the joints (and that is why it is called śleshman, from the root *ślish,* "to connect") and eliminates friction. It is this factor that gives firmness and strength to the body, and also the capacity to resist disturbances within the organism.

Its five-fold functions are: (1) permeation of the entire body with watery essence (*klédaka*, moistening, with stomach as its principal centre and enhancing the activity of the other phlegm centres), (2) supporting the action of the heart (*avalambaka,* located in the chest, imparting energy and strength), (3) salivation. (*bodhaka,* chief centres being throat and tongue, ensuring gustation), (4) co-operation (*śleshmaka*, located in the joints, uniting them firmly and lubricating), and (5) cooling the sense-organs (*tarpaka*, located in the head and favouring all sensory activities). When this factor is excited, the body becomes dense and hard, with a tendency towards cold and numbness of limbs; digestion is disturbed and sleep becomes excessive; there is an inclination to be drowsy, and the skin pales.

The constitution dominated by kapha, is distinguished by a well-integrated body mechanism. Persons belonging to this type are endowed with a robust physique, are well-proportioned, and are rather heavily built. They are inclined to obesity; they are vigorous in sex-activity, courageous, and free from envy and greed. They are the healthiest of the three groups; their powers of endurance are great. They do not sweat much; their gait is firm, and the steps even. Their digestion, however, is rather weak. Their sleep is heavy and not easily disturbed. When they dream, it is usually about watery stretches like lakes and rivers. When they do fall ill, the ailments are usually of the respiratory and lymphatic systems. Dominated by *tamas,* their temperament tends to be indolent and indulgent.

An interesting consideration in Āyurveda is what is called literally 'the stomachic fire' (*jāṭharāgni*) or 'the bodily fire' (*kāyāgni,* according to Bhela). That there is a fire within man that keeps him alive and active is indeed a very ancient notion, by no means peculiar to Indian people. That the organism is enlivened by a mysterious fire that glows within, concealed in the dark recesses of the heart, is a belief that is almost universal. Vedic literature contains this notion : "This pan-human fire (*agnire-vaiśvānarah*) inside man, by means of which the food that we eat is cooked....."[28] The association between fire and water is likewise an old belief. The Veda considers fire as the descendant of water(*āpām napāt*); there is mention of 'the fire of the clouds'. Āyurveda developed this ancient idea into a semi-scientific concept.

Within the stomach, at a distance of about two inches from the navel, to the left in man and to the right in women, is supposed to be the seat of this 'fire'. Although small like a grain of paddy or of barley, it lights up the whole being, and its heat pervades the entire body. In obese persons it is said to be of the size of a barley-grain, while in slim persons it is atomic in size. It is present in all living beings. In minute organisms like flies and insects, it is 'like mere air'. Another view locates this fire in the mystic space within the heart-lotus (*dahara-puṇḍarīka*), extremely subtle and yellowish, flaming like a light. A third view regards it as a spring of sour water located in the visceral cavity. Bhela records Ātreya-Punarvasu's view : the 'bodily fire' which is of the nature of heat (*ushmā*) and light (*tejas*) digests the food we eat. Even as the sun quickly dries up the puddle and small water holes by his rays, the 'fire' in the stomach digests all food that enters.[29] This is the principal agent not only in cooking (*pāka*) but in 'specially cooking' (*vipāka*) so that the food is absorbed into body-tissues. It is responsible for the transformation of what we eat into organic juices (*rasas*), which are the primordial substances of the organism, and the essence of which is water. CHARAKA cites the opinion of the ancient Vāryo-vidas : "Organisms are born of rasa, and so also are the various diseases, because waters are rich in these juices, and they are the causes of creation".[30] Bhela makes the position more explicit : "The heat, residing in the organic juices in the body, continues gathering up life; man is after all born of these juices, and therefore it is the juices that go by the name of life".[31] One is reminded of the vedic description of fire as the descendant of water (*ápām napāt*). That the stomachic fire is intimately connected with the 'fiery liquid' (pitta) is also to be considered in this context. Bhela speaks of the five-fold functions of this 'fire', but his explanations are more intriguing and psychologically significant.

'Perceiving' (*ālochaka*) as a function of stomachic fire is two-fold, according to Bhela; one specialized in the visual apparatus, and the other covering general consciousness. The former generates knowledge by the contact of the sense-organs with ego and mind, while the latter, located in between the eyebrows on a mound (or at 'the road-cross'), is responsible for the subtle 'thoughts' which are not only prehended, but retained, remembered, recalled, and projected as occasion demands. 'Irradiating (*bhrājaka*), in Bhela's opinion, refers to the specific characteristics and functionings of the various organs in the body. 'Colouring' (*rañjaka*) is appropriating the external sense-objects as one's own, because of the ego, and inclining towards them with an emotional set. 'Performing' or 'relating' (*sādhaka*) is achieving of the proximate and distant objective, with regard to object thus appropriated. Cooking (*pāchaka*) is digesting the various kinds of food eaten, a physiological function but with a mental involvement.[32]

Bhela's analysis opens up an interesting mass of psychological speculations (to be dealt with by the present author in a separate publication), but it is sufficient here to note that Bhela preserves an old tradition of the association of the stomachic fire with waters within the viscera. He likens it to a lamp that is placed in the hollow of a bitter-gourd (*iksvāku-kośa*) and set floating. When the water is undisturbed, the lamp burns steadily; but when it is disturbed, the lamp is no longer steady and constant.[33] All the three essential factors (vāta, pitta, and kapha) are involved in it; they determine its nature, although it is a fire that burns by its own fuel.[34] The excitation or disturbance in the factors bring about changes in the 'fire.' An excitation of the wind will produce ' irregular fire' (*vishamāgni*); an excess of pitta will intensify the fire (*tīksṇāgni*); and when the kapha is excited, we have the 'sluggish fire' (*mandāgni*). The changes in the 'fire' have their direct impact on the digestive process. When, however, the three factors are evenly distributed in the body, the fire will be steady and even (*samāgni*) which makes for sound health. Man's life rests on this 'fire.' His strength, vitality, health, pleasures and sorrows are all rooted in this. The warmth (*ushmā*) that makes man alive indicates the presence of this 'fire'; when it cools, he dies.

The Āyurvedic concept of 'stomachic fire' is an important aid in reconstructing the early phase of *ātmāvāda*, which matured in the Upanishads. The *śaktivāda* of the tantras is undoubtedly related to it. The five fundamental elements (*pañchābhūta*), the three constitutional factors (*tridosha*), the seven essential substances that emerge from the organic juice (*rasādi-saptadhātu*), the three modes of being (*guṇa*), the intra-organic energetics and psychological integration are all involved here. The notion of 'the fire within the visceral waters' appears to hold the key for understanding the transitional stage between the old tantra culture and the classical vedic tradition. Being a practical discipline, Āyurveda was interested in understanding the causes of disturbances of the fire as well as in the methods of restoring its normalcy. The Ayurvedic regimen and treatment procedures are meant to calm the waters within (and this signifies the purification of the constitution, *sattvāśuddhi*) so that the fire in it retains (or resumes) its natural glow (and this is the prototype of the vedāntic and yogic 'getting back to the original nature', *svarūpāvasthānam*). The importance attached to nature (*sva-bhāva*, being in one's own natural mode) in Āyurveda is to be considered in this context. Health is significantly termed 'abiding in oneself' (*sva-stha*), 'composure', 'being at ease', 'in comfort'. This refers to the even and steady 'fire' in the still waters deep within the constitution. The early Sāmkhyan concept of 'purushāvastham-avyaktam', has probably relevance here. The state of equilibrium (*sāmyāvastha*) of the Sāmkhya school of thought and the process of perfect settling down (*samādhi*) of yoga are no doubt intimately related to the 'even fire' (*samāgni*) of Āyurveda.

NOTES

1. *CS*.1,30,20: आयुर्वेदयतीति आयुर्वेदः।
2. *SS*,1,1,14 आयुरस्मिन् विद्यतेऽनेन वाऽऽयुर्विन्दतीत्यायुर्वेदः।
3. आप्तो नामाऽनुभावेन वस्तुतत्त्वस्य कात्स्र्येन निश्चयत्वात्
रागादिवशादपि नान्यथावादी यः स इति चरके पतञ्जलिः।
quoted in Nāgeśa-bhaṭṭa's *Laghumañjūsha* as the opinion of Patañjali in his commentary on *Charakasaṁhitā*.
4. *CS*.1,1,45 सत्त्वमात्मा शरीरंच त्रयमेतत् त्रिदण्डवत्।
लोकस्तिष्ठति संयोगात्तत्र सर्व प्रतिष्ठितम्॥
5. *SS*.1,1,21: पञ्चमहाभूतशारीरिसमवायः पुरुष हत्युच्यते, तस्मिन्
क्रिया सोऽधिष्ठानम्।
6. *CS*.4,3,26: न ह्यसत्वः कदाचिदात्मा सत्वविशेषाच्योपलक्षते
ज्ञानविशेषः॥
The psyche cannot at any time be without 'mind', so that there is always some sort of knowledge or other. Chakrapāni, the commentator, explains: यत्रु केवलमनोजन्यं आत्मज्ञानं तभ्दवत्येक सर्वदा।
Cf. also इदमेव चात्मन्श्चेतनत्त्वं यदिन्द्रियसंयोगे सति
ज्ञानशालित्वं न निकष्टस्यात्मनश्चेतम्.....।
7. *CS*. शरीरमपि सत्त्वमनुविधीयते सत्त्वं च शरीरम्।
8. Cf. Isvarakrsna's, ***Sāmkhya-kārikā*,40**
9. Cf. ***Sāmkhyapravachana-bhāshya*,5,103:**
यथा दीपस्य सर्वग्रहव्यापित्वेऽपि अङ्गुष्ठपरिमाणत्वम्
10. *SS*.3,1,16 स एष कर्मपुरुषः चिकित्साधिकृतः
11. *CS*.4,2,3,: cf. *Chakrapani*.
यद्यपि शुक्ररजसी कारणे तथापि यदैवातिवाहिकं सूक्ष्मभूतरूप्रशरीरं प्राप्रवतः तदैव ते शरीरं जनयतः नान्यथा॥
Also cf. *SS*.3,1,16.
12. *Chakrapāni* on *CS*.8,9,16: हृदि मूर्न्धि च वस्तौं च नृणां प्राणाः प्रतिष्ठिताः।
Elsewhere (4,7,9) head, heart, throat, navel, rectum, bladder, vital fluid, sperm, blood and flesh are given as the seats of *prāna*
13. *CS*: हृदयं चेतनाधिष्ठानमेकम् The entire body is said to **be founded *(samśṛita)* on the heart (1,30,5).....**
तत्र चैतन्यसंग्रह... प्राणवाहानां श्रोतसां मूलम्.... अन्तरात्मनः श्रेष्ठमायतनम्॥
14. योगक्षेमौ शरीरस्य स्वभावपरिकल्पितौ। स्वभावस्य तु साहाय्यं कर्तव्यंभिषगुत्तमैः।
15. ब्रह्माण्डकलितं सर्वं पिण्डाण्डेऽपि च वर्तति। सारुप्येणोभयं ज्ञेय उभयत्र गुणाधिकम्॥

16. *SS*.3,4,80: प्रकृतिमिह नाराणां भौतिकीं केचिदाहुः। पवनदहनतोयः कीर्तितास्तासु तिस्त्रः॥
17. *Rgveda*, **10,168,3-4.**
18. *Ibid*.10,129,1 and 3: 1,23,19.
19. Thus *Ashtānga-sūtra* 1,13, and 1,6: रसासृङ्मांसमेदोऽस्थिमज्जशुक्लानि धातवः।... वायुः पित्तं कफश्चेति त्रयो दोषास्स्मासतः।
20. *SS*, *sūtra*, 1,5,12 देहसम्भवहेतवः। Dalhana comments शुक्रार्तवादि सहकारितया देहजनका अभिप्रेताः।
21. Vāgbhata, for instance, looks upon the factors as polluting agents (*doshas*) while the *dhātus* are the polluted (*dūshya*). The body, according to him, is an organisation of *doshas*, *dhātus*, and *malas*. (शरीरं च दोषधातुमलसमुदायः)
22. as illustrated in *Ayurveda-sūtram* (edited with Yogānanda-nātha's commentary, by R. Shama Sastry, Oriental Library Publications, University of Mysore, 1922).
23. Bhela speaks of the mixed types as **Samsrstā-prakrti'. According to him, 'pure' types are the best; 'pair-determined are of middling qual-** ity; and the 'miscellaneous' the worst. संसृष्टप्रकृति विद्यात् संसृष्टैश्चापि लक्षणैः। निवृत्त (एकात्म) प्रकृतिर्धन्या द्वन्द्वा भवति मध्यमा। सन्निपातात्मिका या तु जघन्या सा प्रकीर्तिता॥ ***(Bhelasamhita*. vimāna 4,26-27).**
24. Cf. S. Venkataraghavan, "The Scope and Importance of the Doshas", *Chakra* (New Delhi), Vol III, 1971, pp. 124-127.
25. For instance, three *prānas* mentioned in *Br.-up*.,3,1,10, and *Ch-up*., 1,3,3, four in *Br. up*., 4,4,1, six in *Br. up*., 1,5,4, seven in *Br.-up*., 2,2,3 and ten in *Br.-up*., 3,9,4. In *Maitri* 2,6, five are described: *prāna* that goes up (य ऊर्ध्वं उत्क्रामति), *apāna* that goes down (योऽयं अवांग् संक्रामति), *vyāna* that favours other breaths (येन वा एता अनुगृहीता), ***samāna* that sends the thickest part of nourish-**ment into *apāna* and brings the minutest in each member (योऽयं स्थविष्ठो धातुरन्नस्यापाने प्रापयति)
26. *udāna* which disgorges and swallows what is drunk and eaten. (योऽयं पिताशितं उद्गिरति निगरति) cf. S. Venkataraghavan, *op. cit*.
27. Chyle is the subtle essence of fiery nature which results from well-digested food (आहार्यस्य सम्यक्परिपाकस्य यस्तेजोभूतः सारः परमसूक्ष्मः स रस इत्युच्यते *SS*, sūtra, 14,1.). Dalhaṇa explains it as the 'heated thing' (*ghrta*), a fluid which softens, nourishes and vitalizes the body. Located in the heart, it proceeds through twenty-four arteries(*dhamanīs*) to all parts of the body, keeping them alive. When it reaches liver and spleen, it acquires the red colour and becomes blood (स खल्वाप्यो रस यकृत्प्लीहानौ प्राप्य रागमुपैति *SS*, *ibid*).
28. *Br.-up*, 5,8,1: अयं अग्निर्वैश्वानरो योऽयं सन्तःपुरुषे येनेदमन्नं पच्यते यदिदमद्येत॥
29. *Bhelasamhitā*, śarira, 4, pp.85-86 (Girijādayālu Śukla's ed.).
30. *Ibid*., 4,13-14 देहिनां भोजनं भुक्तं नानाव्यञ्जनसंस्कृतं। सूर्यो दिवि यथा तिष्ठन् तजोयुक्तो गभस्तिमिः विशोषयति सर्वाणि पल्वलानि पयांसि च। तदूच्छरीरिणां भुक्तं जाठरो नाभिसंस्थितः॥ **Cf. the typical Ayurvedic view of *jātharāgni*:** नाभेरूर्ध्वं द्रव्यङ्ग्लै वागभागे नृणामग्निर्जाष्ठरे। योषितां तु भात्येत्वाम दक्षिणे व्रीहितुल्यस्तरयैवोष्मा न्युपृतः सर्वदेहे। स जीर्णकारी वदन्ती केचिद्वैश्वानरीं दीपशिखामथान्ये। नीवार शूकप्रतिमां च पीतां कुक्ष्युद्भवोह्याम्लरसोऽयमग्निः।
31. *CS*, *sūtra*, 25, 13: रसजानि तु भूतानि व्याधयश्च पृथग्विधाः, आपो हि रसस्यस्ताः स्मृताः निर्वृत्तिहेतवः॥
32. *Bhela-samhitā*, sarīra, 4,35: ऊष्मा रसस्थो देहेऽस्मिन् जीवं संग्रह्य तिष्ठति। रसोद्भवः पुमान तस्माद्रसो जीवनमुच्यते॥
33. *Ibid*., śarīra, 4, adhyāya, pp.86-87 (Miśra's ed.)
34. *Ibid*., verses 22,23 (pp.89): जाठरो जलसंभुतः पाचकः पवनैस्सह। प्रदीप्यते नृणां कोष्ठे सति स्वेन्धनपूरिते॥ इष्वाकुकोशमास्थाय यथा दीपः स्थिरेऽम्भासि तिष्ठति स्तिमिते सक्तो न यथा जलितेऽम्भासि॥
35. *Ibid*., स्वेन्धनपूरिते..........